Cystic Fibrosis
A Guide for Patient and Family

Third Edition

Cystic Fibrosis
A Guide for Patient and Family

Third Edition

David M. Orenstein, M.D.

Antonio J. and Janet Palumbo Professor of Cystic Fibrosis
Director, Antonio J. and Janet Palumbo Cystic Fibrosis Center
Children's Hospital of Pittsburgh;
Professor of Pediatrics
School of Medicine
University of Pittsburgh;
Professor of Health, Physical and Recreation
Education (Exercise Physiology)
School of Education
University of Pittsburgh
Pittsburgh, Pennsylvania

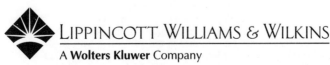

LIPPINCOTT WILLIAMS & WILKINS
A **Wolters Kluwer** Company
Philadelphia · Baltimore · New York · London
Buenos Aires · Hong Kong · Sydney · Tokyo

Acquisitions Editor: Danette Somers
Developmental Editor: Maureen Iannuzzi
Production Editor: Melanie Bennitt
Manufacturing Manager: Colin J. Warnock
Cover Designer: Christine Jenny
Compositor: Lippincott Williams & Wilkins Desktop Division
Printer: Maple Press

© 2004 by LIPPINCOTT WILLIAMS & WILKINS
530 Walnut Street
Philadelphia, PA 19106 USA
LWW.com

Printed in the USA

Library of Congress Cataloging-in-Publication Data

Orenstein, David M., 1945–
   Cystic fibrosis : a guide for patient and family /David M. Orenstein.—3rd ed.
     p. cm.
   Includes bibliographical references and index.
   ISBN 0-7817-4152-1
   1. Cystic fibrosis in children–Popular works. 2. Cystic fibrosis–Popular works. 3.
  Patient education. I. Title.

RJ456.C9074 2003
616.3'7—dc22   2003056496

10 9 8 7 6 5 4 3 2 1

To all those patients and families who have so enriched my life,
and have taught me so well,
"it's not just what you're given,
but what you do with what you've got."
Si Kahn

Contents

Contributing Authors

Louise T. Bauer, R.N.   *Nurse Coordinator, Antonio J. and Janet Palumbo Cystic Fibrosis Center and Pediatric Pulmonology Department, Children's Hospital of Pittsburgh, Pittsburgh, Pennsylvania*

Robert J. Beall, Ph.D.   *President and Chief Executive Officer, Cystic Fibrosis Foundation, Bethesda, Maryland*

Preston W. Campbell, III, M.D.   *Executive Vice President for Medical Affairs, Cystic Fibrosis Foundation, Bethesda, Maryland*

Maria I. Clavell, M.D.   *Department of Gastroenterology, Children's Hospital of Pittsburgh, Pittsburgh, Pennsylvania*

Garry R. Cutting, M.D.   *Department of Pediatrics, Johns Hopkins University School of Medicine, East Baltimore Campus, Baltimore, Maryland*

Raymond A. Frizzell, Ph.D.   *Department of Cell Biology and Physiology, University of Pittsburgh, Pittsburgh, Pennsylvania*

Judith A. Fulton, R.D.   *Nutritionist, Antonio J. and Janet Palumbo Cystic Fibrosis Center, Children's Hospital of Pittsburgh, Pittsburgh, Pennsylvania*

Michael R. Knowles, M.D.   *Professor of Medicine, University of North Carolina School of Medicine; Director, Adult Cystic Fibrosis Center, Chapel Hill, North Carolina*

Geoffrey Kurland, M.D.   *Medical Director, Lung Transplant Program, Children's Hospital of Pittsburgh, Pittsburgh, Pennsylvania*

David M. Orenstein, M.D.   *Antonio J. and Janet Palumbo Professor of Cystic Fibrosis, Director, Antonio J. and Janet Palumbo Cystic Fibrosis Center, Children's Hospital of Pittsburgh; Professor of Pediatrics, School of Medicine, University of Pittsburgh; Professor of Health, Physical and Recreation Education (Exercise Physiology), School of Education, University of Pittsburgh, Pittsburgh, Pennsylvania*

Introduction

David M. Orenstein

WHAT IS CYSTIC FIBROSIS?

Cystic fibrosis (CF) is a life-shortening, inherited disorder that affects the way in which salt and water move into and out of the body's cells. The most important effects of this problem are in the lungs and the digestive system (especially the pancreas), where thick mucus blocks the small tubes and ducts. The lung problem can lead to progressive blockage, infection, and lung damage, and even death if there is too much damage, while the pancreatic blockage causes poor digestion and poor absorption of food, leading to poor growth and under-nutrition. The sweat glands are also affected, in that they make a much saltier sweat than normal. Anyone reading this book has probably heard about the sweat test used to diagnose CF. Most parts of the body that make mucus are also affected, including the reproductive tract in men and women with CF.

ARE ANY PARTS OF THE BODY *NOT* AFFECTED BY CF?

The list of body parts affected by CF can seem overwhelmingly long. But CF does *not* affect the brain and nervous system (it does *not* cause mental retardation); it does *not* affect the kidneys; it does *not* directly affect the heart; it does *not* affect the muscles; it does *not* affect the blood; and, except in the lungs, it does *not* interfere with the immune system (the body's ability to fight infection).

WHAT CAUSES CYSTIC FIBROSIS?

Cystic fibrosis is an inherited disorder that is present from birth, although signs and symptoms of it may not show up for weeks, months, or even years after birth. Although it is inherited, the parents of a child with CF do not have CF, and most often there is no history of it in the family. We all have two CF genes that determine whether or not we have CF. Both of these CF genes need to be abnormal for us to have CF, and CF is inherited by receiving one abnormal CF gene from each parent. Each parent usually has only one abnormal CF gene, and thus has no sign of CF at all. Cystic fibrosis is very common among white people, and is the most commonly inherited profoundly life-shortening disease, affecting 1 in every 2500 live babies born. One in 25 people carry a mutation of the

CF gene. CF is not caused by anything the parents did — or did not do — during the pregnancy. The only way to get CF is to inherit one abnormal CF gene from each parent. You cannot "catch" CF; it is not contagious.

HOW LONG DO PEOPLE WITH CYSTIC FIBROSIS LIVE?

It is impossible to predict how long a single patient will live. It is possible to give some overall statistics. Just a few decades ago, nearly all children with CF died before they reached two years of age. By 2001, the average survival had improved to over 32 years, with many people surviving into their 40s and beyond. A recent analysis predicted that for someone born today with CF, the average survival would be closer to 40 years. Some children do still die with CF, but this is much less common than in past years. For one recent year, the death rate among CF patients under one year old was 0.007 (meaning a rate of seven babies dying out of every 1000), for children aged six to seven years, it was 0.004 (a rate of four children dying out of every 1000), for 14- to 15-year-olds, it was 0.015 (15 of 1000), and for 23-year-olds, it was 0.048.

There are several important factors that explain the tremendous improvement, and that explain why the outlook continues to improve almost year by year. First, CF is a newly recognized disease. (It is not a *new* disease, as is related in Appendix E, but a newly *recognized* disease.) It was not until 1938 that Dr. Dorothy Andersen wrote the first medical paper describing a number of children who had died with digestive problems and lung problems. She was the first to recognize that this was not just a coincidence, but represented a single disease, which she called "cystic fibrosis of the pancreas," because the children she examined after they died all had *cysts* (fluid-filled sacs) and scar tissue (*fibrosis*) replacing almost all the normal tissue of their pancreas. The name has been shortened to cystic fibrosis, but her description helped to lay the foundation for recognizing the disease, and therefore treating children who had it. Around this time, antibiotics were becoming available, and lung infections could be treated to a degree. In 1964, Drs. Carl Doershuk and LeRoy Matthews and their colleagues from Cleveland reported the results of 5 years of a comprehensive treatment program. These results were very much improved over previous results, and most modern treatment programs use the same basic principles which these pioneers used.

In the last 40 years, many new antibiotics have become available, making treatment more effective. Further, knowledge of CF has spread widely, so that now most pediatricians and family doctors are able to recognize the signs and symptoms of CF and are able to give children treatment while it can still be helpful, that is, before there is too much irreversible lung damage. Very importantly, a nationwide network of CF Centers has grown up, where CF experts deliver state-of-the-art care.

The point here is that the medical world has had good comprehensive treatment programs for patients with CF for only a little more than 40 years. This means that there are virtually no patients with CF who are 40 years old *and* were started on a treatment program in the first year of life. There are more and more teenagers and people in their 20s and 30s who were started on treatment programs early in life, before their lungs were in bad shape, and many of these young adults are doing extremely well. Therefore, there is every reason to be very optimistic about the future of a youngster diagnosed and started on treatment today. Certainly, while an average survival to age 32 years reflects a tremendous improvement, it is not something to be satisfied with; but this situation is continually improving.

CYSTIC FIBROSIS CARE

Medical care of patients with CF is best carried out at one of the 117 CF Centers accredited by the Cystic Fibrosis Foundation, in conjunction with your own pediatrician, family doctor, or internist. Doctors are becoming better informed about CF, but it is important to be in touch with the CF experts who stay up-to-date with the quickly changing field that CF has become. These experts are found in CF Centers, and there are also many specially trained professionals (nutritionists, social workers, nurses, respiratory therapists) at these centers with extensive knowledge and experience taking care of people with CF. The record is fairly clear that CF patients whose care is coordinated by a CF Center live longer than those who do not attend a center. With the health care system changing, it may be more difficult to get a referral to a CF Center, but it is important to insist on it.

It is also important to continue to have care from a general pediatrician or family doctor, who can be very helpful with the non-CF health issues that arise in everyone's life.

RESEARCH AND THE BASIC DEFECT

When the first edition of this book was published just a few years ago, the basic defect in CF was not known, and the gene was not yet discovered. Much was understood about the kind of problems people with CF have, how to prevent many of those problems, and how to treat the problems that cannot be prevented. But at a very basic chemical level, no one knew exactly what went wrong within the cells of the body to cause the problems that occurred. What this meant for treatment was that the medications and therapies were all directed at *secondary* problems (problems that are themselves caused by the basic defect) and not at the underlying problem itself. Another way of putting it is that there was no *cure* for CF.

Much has changed in the past few years, and our understanding of what goes wrong within and outside the cells of people with CF has increased tremendously. The gene for CF has been found and cloned (produced in the lab); there is now a "CF mouse," created through genetic engineering, while previously no non-human animal had CF, and we know infinitely more about the alterations of cell functioning caused by CF (the basic defect is discussed in Chapter 1). There are even some experimental treatments that have been designed to try to get around the basic problem with the abnormally functioning cells, and gene therapy trials are under way in centers around the world. However, there still is not a treatment that successfully (and safely) undoes the basic defect, and therefore, there is still no cure for CF.

The situation is similar to that of diabetes. It is known that people get sick with diabetes because they don't have enough insulin to control their blood sugar. These people can lead normal lives by taking daily insulin shots, but they still have diabetes and will have it until scientists discover and eliminate the cause of inadequate insulin production.

When the second edition of this book was published just a few years ago, there was no national network to coordinate clinical research on new CF treatments. Such a network was not really needed then, because the increased knowledge about the basic defect in CF cells had not yet led to possible treatments. How different the story is now! Tremendous progress has been made in the search for the ways to undo or get around the basic defect in CF. This is a very exciting time in CF research, because nearly every month an important piece of the puzzle is discovered and new experimental treatments come to light and enter into collaborative clinical studies. The prospects for ever better treatment in the upcoming years are very bright.

A WORD TO NEWLY DIAGNOSED PATIENTS AND FAMILIES

If you are reading this book because you (or, more likely, your child) have (has) just been diagnosed with cystic fibrosis, this is a hard time for you. Many people in your situation feel panicked, numb, or "spacey." You may be angry, frightened, disbelieving. For some of you, along with the bad feelings, there may also be a sense of relief at having a diagnosis, particularly if you've known something was wrong but couldn't get your fears taken seriously, or couldn't get your questions answered. This may be a time when you don't want to hear any more information, or it may be a time when you want to learn absolutely everything there is to know about CF. However you are feeling, it may be a little hard to take in a lot of new information. And however you are feeling, you can be certain that there have been many, many people who have experienced these same feelings. It may be helpful to talk about how you're feeling with people in the CF Center, and in some cases with other families who have been through what you're going through now. The people in the Center can help you find such people if you're interested. As you learn more about CF, and get used to the idea that you (your child) have (has) it, and as you see that in most cases people can live quite a normal childhood, adolescence, and beyond, your emotions will become less raw and times will be less hard.

HOW CAN PEOPLE LEARN ABOUT CYSTIC FIBROSIS?

The purpose of this book is to help you learn about all aspects of CF, including how it is inherited, the problems it causes, how it is treated, and current research. Cystic fibrosis centers and the Cystic Fibrosis Foundation can provide information also. Some of you will want to plow through the book cover-to-cover now, while others may not be able to face even the first chapter just yet. But the book will be here when you're ready for it, and can certainly be referred back to when a new question comes up, or if you find you've forgotten something. Encyclopedias and many general medical books are *not* a good source of information, since they are likely to be outdated. Newspapers, especially the tabloids we all see in the checkout line in the grocery store, are also not good sources, for they are likely to announce the discovery of a cure that bears little relation to medical truth. Even if you hear something that sounds encouraging on a national TV news show, be sure to check it out with your CF Center, or someone who is knowledgeable and up-to-date on research developments.

There have been several instances of incorrect information — even dangerous information — being reported as medical truth on supposedly reputable news shows. In one of these instances, it was announced that CF was caused by a deficiency of *selenium* (a mineral we all need, and one that most of us — CF or no — get plenty of in the diet), and that a cure existed in taking huge doses of selenium. Several babies died as a result of that report, after being given massive overdoses of selenium. Usually, information about CF that appears in the news is not harmful, and is even fairly accurate. But it is wise to be cautious about "dramatic breakthroughs" that are announced. Most often, medical progress is made not by dramatic breakthroughs but rather by tiny steps, with one group of scientists building upon the work of previous researchers. Your CF Center and the CF Foundation are informed of all the reputable work in the field worldwide and will be happy to provide you with this information.

The World Wide Web has many sites related to CF, some of them excellent. But anyone who has had any experience "surfing the net" knows that alongside superb sources of information, there can be not-so-reliable (and sometimes even "wacko") sources. This rule holds true for CF-related sites as well. In Appendix F, *Bibliography,* you can find a number of web sites that should be reliable. As with any other information source, be sure to check any new information you're not sure about (and maybe some that you *are* sure about) with CF Center staff.

ORGANIZATION OF THE BOOK

The goal of this book is to cover all the important topics that concern people with CF and their families. The opening chapter discusses the basic defect in the cells of people with CF, going over some amazing discoveries that have been made just within the past few years. (My co-author on this chapter, Dr. Ray Frizzell, is responsible for a lot of the exciting research that is unlocking the secrets of the cellular abnormalities in CF.) Next comes a short chapter summarizing how the diagnosis of CF is made. The respiratory system (lungs), how it normally works, the changes brought about by CF, and the treatment of the lung problems are the subject of Chapter 3. Chapter 4, on the digestive and gastrointestinal system, also reviews both normal functioning and that affected by cystic fibrosis. After these sections, there is a brief chapter on the other body systems affected by cystic fibrosis. Then follows a chapter on nutrition.

Chapter 7 discusses hospitalization and other types of elaborate treatments, and is followed by a long chapter on organ transplantation for CF (mostly about lung transplantation, and a bit about liver transplantation), and then a short chapter dealing with various aspects of daily life including daycare, school, sports, home responsibilities, and travel. Exercise is considered separately in the following chapter. Next is a chapter on the genetics of CF, which describes the manner in which CF is inherited, and a lot of the very new information about molecular genetics, how they determine the abnormalities seen in CF, and even prospects for gene therapy. (My co-author on this chapter, Dr. Garry Cutting, is one of the most prominent exerts in CF genetics.)

We then switch gears for a chapter that deals with emotional and psychological issues (growing up with CF, effects on the family of a child with CF, etc.). Teenagers get their own chapter — Chapter 13. The special problems of the adult with cystic fibrosis are discussed in Chapter 14 (my co-author for this chapter, Dr. Michael Knowles, is renowned as a CF researcher and as one of the earliest pulmonologists to take care of adults with CF). The next chapter discusses the difficult issues surrounding dying with CF.

Research—past, present, and future—and some speculation about future treatments are the subjects of the next chapter (co-authored by Dr. Preston Campbell III, the Executive Vice President for Medical Affairs of the Cystic Fibrosis Foundation) . The national Cystic Fibrosis Foundation is discussed by its President and Chief Executive Officer, Dr. Robert Beall, in the final chapter.

The volume includes several appendices: a glossary of technical terms; a listing of commonly used medications, giving brand names and generic names, uses, and side effects; diagrams illustrating the proper techniques for performing chest physical therapy, and discussions of other airway clearance techniques; a short but chubby group of high-calorie recipes; a brief appendix on major historic landmarks in CF; a list of CF Centers in the United States; and a list of CF Centers worldwide. Finally, the last appendix is a brief bibliography of outstanding readings (mostly technical) on CF and listing of web sites on the Internet dealing directly or indirectly with CF.

A FINAL NOTE ON THE ORGANIZATION AND CONTENT OF THIS BOOK

Each of the chapters starts with a section labeled The Basics, which includes a few of the most important points of that chapter. Some chapters are very long and have much more detail than you'll need or want at any one time. Some of the science presented — particularly in Chapter 1 (*The Basic Defect*) and in parts of Chapter 11 (*Genetics*) — is *very* difficult to understand, and can be daunting, especially the first time 'round. Try not to be intimidated by it, but keep in mind that it's been hard even for most physicians to keep up with the torrid pace of CF research, and it's taken some of us months or years to become comfortable with these concepts.

For each chapter, The Basics may give you an idea of what's there, and you can skim the chapter for what you want to get out of it. The details will be there when you want them.

Preface

I wrote this book (with a lot of help) for everyone with an interest in cystic fibrosis, whether they be patients, the friends and family of patients, or health professionals who work with patients and their families. It is designed to be of particular use to parents in the initial months that follow their child's diagnosis of cystic fibrosis. It is also written with the intention that it serve as a "refresher" course for people to review areas of treatment and physiology that they may have forgotten. The relatives and friends of a patient may also benefit from this introduction to cystic fibrosis.

An important group for whom this book is written is teenagers who were diagnosed in infancy. While teenagers grow up knowing a lot about cystic fibrosis, they seldom receive the in-depth explanation that their parents received immediately upon diagnosis. I hope that teenagers will use this book to learn more about cystic fibrosis. A final goal of this volume is to provide a foundation for understanding cystic fibrosis that will enable patients and families to understand more fully the advances that are being made so rapidly in this field.

I've tried to stress throughout this book that cystic fibrosis is a serious disease, yet it is one that can be effectively controlled for long periods of time in most patients. It is a life-shortening disease, yet it is also one in which the outlook for patients' length and quality of life has improved dramatically in a relatively short time and continues to do so. It is a disease for which there is currently no cure, yet it is one for which treatment is very effective. It is a disease that creates demands on patients and families for daily treatments; it is also one in which the efforts of patients and families can greatly influence the health and quality of life of the patient. It is a disease that is commonly accepted as inhibiting normal life, yet the reality is that most patients go to school, play sports, and grow up accomplishing all the tasks, and experience all the joys and sorrows of childhood, adolescence, and young adulthood. It is my hope that patients and their families will find this volume to be of help in all these stages of life.

Many patients, families, and health professionals have responded generously to the first two editions of this book, and have made suggestions that I've tried to incorporate in this edition to make it more useful. I've been extremely fortunate (and honored) to have been able to convince several of the leaders in the fields of CF research and clinical care to help with this edition. It is the hope of all of us that patients, families, and health care workers will find this volume useful.

David M. Orenstein, M.D.

Acknowledgments

Many wonderful people helped make this book possible. I am indeed fortunate that fate put me in Cleveland from 1969–1981 and enabled me to be introduced to cystic fibrosis by five of the most outstanding physicians, teachers, and human beings—LeRoy Matthews, Carl Doershuk, Bob Stern, Tom Boat, and Bob Wood. That they would then accept me as a student, resident, fellow, and finally as a partner, is among the most wonderful things that one could imagine. They taught me reams about CF and life; they helped show me the importance of communication, and helped me develop my skills in the use of the written word; and they showed me what dedication and compassion are. I am forever grateful to them.

Many patients and their families taught me, too, and have given me so much more than I could ever give them. Quite a few have given generously of their time to make suggestions for the first two editions of this book. I thanked most of them in the previous edition, and am happy to be able to acknowledge the helpful comments of Mr. David Brownstein, whose name was somehow omitted from the last edition.

I am especially grateful to the patients (and colleagues) from across the country and overseas who have been kind enough to let me know that the previous editions have been helpful to them. I hope the same will be true for this edition.

Colleagues within the Antonio J. and Janet Palumbo Cystic Fibrosis Center at Children's Hospital of Pittsburgh have also continued to make my work rewarding, and even joyful. Louise Bauer, Nancy Smizik, and Jenny Haglund made particularly helpful suggestions for this edition, as well as being trusted and admired colleagues. Drs. Joel Weinberg and Joe Pilewski continue to amaze me with their wisdom and excellence in their care of our adult patients. Liz Hartigan, Lori Holt, Sandy Hurban, and Kathy Godfrey make every research project and clinic fun. I'm convinced that Judy Fulton, Beth Lytle, and Iris Murdoch are the best CF dietitians anywhere. Donna Wilding has guided me (and our center) through the tricky shoals of a large institution, and unpredictable tides, with humor, an amazing memory, and a few tricks here and there. Janet Palumbo's vision and generosity have helped make it possible for me to continue to devote my energies–and that of our entire center—to CF.

My parents taught me the pleasures of language and humor, and showed me their gentle, loving way with people. I was blessed with the best siblings on earth, who have provided me with the best nieces and nephews in the southern (brother) and northern (sister) hemispheres. Then, unexpectedly, Alex came along and brought me–and continues to bring me—profound happiness. She also contributed some pretty terrific siblings, nephews, and nieces, all in the northern hemisphere. Finally, there aren't adequate words to describe the joy and wonder that are ours each day because of Jacob Atticus An Toan Orenstein.

Cystic Fibrosis

A Guide for Patient and Family

Third Edition

1

The Basic Defect

THE BASICS

1. The main problem with the cells that make up the lungs, pancreas, and sweat glands in people with cystic fibrosis (CF) is that chloride (part of what makes up common table salt) cannot pass through the cells normally.
2. Another problem is that sodium (the other part of salt) may be pumped through the cells more than normal, at least in the lung.
3. Both of these problems probably cause lung and pancreatic mucus and fluid to be drier and stickier than normal, and sweat to be saltier than normal.
4. The cells work abnormally to different degrees in people with CF, depending on which CF gene mutation they have.
5. Possibly, new treatments can be designed to get around these cell abnormalities.

Until recently, it was not known what caused the various problems that people with cystic fibrosis (CF) have. One fact almost explained all of the problems: Examinations showed that extra thick and sticky mucus seemed to be secreted by most of the organs of the body affected by CF: Thick mucus clogged bronchial tubes in the lung, blocked ducts and tubes leading from the pancreas or liver to the intestines, and sometimes blocked the intestines. One of the most noticeable abnormalities in patients with CF is their salty sweat. The salty sweat is why the sweat test is still the best test to diagnose CF, even though it has been around for 40 years. [In the sweat test, as most people reading this book already know, sweat is collected from a patient and is then analyzed for its salt (sodium and chloride) concentration: A "positive" sweat test is one in which the saltiness of sweat is more than three times higher than normal.] Mucus—thick or thin—has nothing to do with sweat glands, and so can't be blamed for this part of CF. When CF doctors used to try to explain CF, there was always that little stumbling block: "All the problems are caused by thick mucus: the lung problem, the pancreas and digestive problem, the intestine problems, and so on. . .Oh, and by the way [we'd say softly], there's the little matter of the sweat glands that seems different."

ELECTRICAL CHARGES IN THE NOSE!

In the 1980s, researchers in North Carolina made important discoveries that for the first time, seemed to tie together all the abnormalities in CF. These researchers happened to be interested in measuring the electrical charge in people's noses. They measured what we now refer to as the nasal potential difference (PD), or simply the electrical charge across the mucous membrane in the nose. As it turns out, everyone has a negative electrical charge across these mucous membranes. In almost everyone, this is a small charge (−5 to −30 millivolt [mV]), but virtually everyone with CF has a much larger PD (−40 to −80 mV). The measurement of nasal PD is somewhat difficult to do correctly, but if experienced people perform the measurements, the PD result distinguishes people with CF from those who do not have CF at least as well as—and maybe even better than—the sweat test.

At the same time as the discovery of the PD in the nose, other researchers in California found the same elevated electrical charge across the cells lining the sweat glands of people with CF. Not long afterward, the cells making up the lining (the epithelial surface) of the intestines and pancreas were also found to have similar changes in their electrical properties. For the first time, all the organs that are affected by CF were found to have a single abnormality: The electrical charge across the cells making up their epithelial surfaces was much greater than the electrical charge seen in these glands in people without CF.

One of the things that made these discoveries, taken together, even more exciting than they might have been individually was that they appeared at about the same time as molecular biologists were discovering the CF gene (more about this in Chapter 11, *Genetics*). The scientists who discovered the CF gene predicted that the protein produced by this gene was like a number of previously discovered proteins that direct the traffic of various chemicals across cell membranes. The electrical charge across membranes has much to do with the speed of sodium (positive charge) and chloride (negative charge) movements across these membranes. Sodium and chloride make up salt, and we're back to the salty sweat. In the next section, we give a few more details about what we've now learned about salt traffic across cell membranes in the organs affected by CF.

MOVEMENT OF SALT AND WATER ACROSS CELL MEMBRANES

The protein whose production is directed by the CF gene has been called CFTR (for *cystic fibrosis transmembrane conductance regulator*), and, as you might guess by its name, this protein is extremely important in regulating how much salt (sodium and chloride) gets across cell membranes.

Here's what seems to happen: For the proper functioning and cleansing of the lungs, there needs to be a certain amount of fluid and mucus lining the airways. This fluid comes from within the cells that line the smallest bronchi, far out in lungs, and the mucus comes from the specialized mucus-secreting cells that lie along the airways. The cells lining the smallest bronchi secrete fluid, that is, they push fluid out onto the airway surface. Although each of these airways is very small and does not hold much fluid, the total amount of fluid in all the thousands of small airways is tremendous, and is as much as 4,000 times greater than the volume of the larger airways. (This is because there are fewer of the large airways.) Since the fluid is constantly moving upward toward the trachea, eventually reaching the back of the throat, this means that the cells in the larger bronchi are required to absorb the fluid in order to keep the layer of fluid lining all along the airway. If the fluid layer becomes too deep, the fluid cannot be moved properly out of the airways. Therefore, mucus builds up.

The way healthy bronchial cells secrete fluid (Figure 1.1) is that they allow chloride to pass out through the luminal membrane of the cells (the part of the cell's membrane that lies on the airway surface, where the air flows). There are several different channels in the cell's luminal membrane through which the chloride can flow. One is opened by increased calcium in the cell, and is called the *calcium-dependent chloride channel*; it may provide an alternative pathway for chloride flow to the one that is missing in CF. But the main one for chloride flow onto the airway surface is CFTR itself. Remember its name ends with "*t*ransmembrane

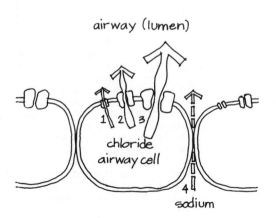

airway (lumen)

chloride
airway cell

sodium

Figure 1.1. Healthy cell chloride secretion. Chloride is secreted out of the cell into the airway lumen through several channels. The main chloride channel is CFTR (cystic fibrosis transmembrane conductance regulator) (*3*). Another channel shown is the *calcium-dependent channel* (*2*). Yet anoher channel (*1*), called the outwardly rectifying chloride channel, is also present. When chloride leaves the cells, sodium passively follows, in this case probably between cells (*4*), in order to keep the positive and negative charges equal, and (not pictured); where sodium and chloride go, water is pulled, so chloride secretion results in fluid being added to the airway surface.

conductance *r*egulator," meaning that it is responsible for conducting chloride across the membrane. Every little chloride ion carries a negative charge, and since (as in many aspects of life) opposites attract, the negative charge of chloride pulls a positively charged ion with it, namely, sodium. There is a law here—the law of electrical neutrality—that says the number of positive charges in a solution must be the same as the number of negative charges. So, whenever a negative charge (chloride) leaves, a positive charge (sodium) is pulled along with it, and vice versa. Therefore, chloride and sodium are transported *onto* the airway surface when the fluid layer is too shallow and *off* the airway surface when the fluid becomes too deep. No matter; it gets to where it's supposed to go, to maintain a very thin fluid layer, which is needed for moving out the mucus and bacteria. Fluid (water) goes onto or off the airway surface following the sodium chloride. In summary, secreting cells open channels to allow chloride into the lumen; the chloride pulls the oppositely charged sodium with it, and the combination of sodium and chloride pulls in water to form the airway lining fluid. The opposite happens when fluid is removed from the airway surface (see below).

As the fluid moves up the tracheobronchial tree from the small bronchi (see Chapter 3, *The Respiratory System*), the depth of the airway lining liquid is adjusted by salt secretion (Figure 1.1) or salt absorption (Figure 1.2). Because a lot of fluid is produced in the small airways, salt absorption tends to be very important in controlling the volume of the airway lung fluid. As you can see in Figure 1.2, fluid absorption starts with sodium ions being pumped out of the airway fluid across the epithelial cells. As the positively charged sodium ion leaves, it pulls the negatively charged chloride ion, and water, with it. Sodium absorption is a two-step process, where sodium enters the airway cell through a channel (a channel that can be blocked by the drug amiloride), and sodium is pushed out of the other side of the cell into the bloodstream by a protein that functions like a pump. In most circumstances, there's only a small force pulling on chloride to go with the sodium, and because chloride normally moves easily, the electrical charge difference across these membranes is normally small.

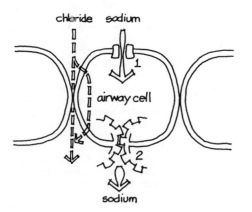

Figure 1.2. Healthy cell sodium reabsorption. Sodium enters the cell from the airway through a sodium channel (*1*). The driving force for sodium entering the cell from the airway lumen is that sodium is actively pumped out the other side of the cell (*2*). Where sodium goes, chloride follows (not pictured). In this case, it is not yet known if chloride passes through the cell membranes or between cells. Once again (not pictured), where sodium and chloride go, water is pulled, so sodium absorption results in fluid being removed from the airway.

Changes in Cystic Fibrosis and the Cystic Fibrosis Transmembrane Conductance Regulator Protein as a Chloride Channel and Regulator of Sodium Transport

This system does not work well in people with CF. As you can see in Figure 1.3, there are problems in both secretion and absorption of salt and water. Both problems lead to less fluid in the airway lumen and drier, stickier contents of the airways, which are harder to move and perhaps more hospitable to bacteria:

1. The secretion problem is that the main channel to let chloride out of the cell is the CFTR protein. *In someone with an altered or missing CFTR protein (because of having two abnormal CFTR genes, as everyone with CF has), this channel is absent or doesn't function correctly: Chloride cannot easily exit from the cell.*
2. Then, the absorption problem is that the sodium channel, which is open to allow sodium to get into the cell and out of the lumen (fluid absorption), is *over*active, so more sodium (and more positive charge) than normal enters

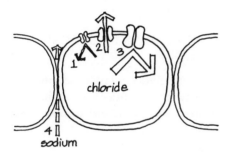

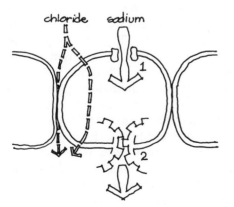

Figure 1.3. Cystic fibrosis (CF) cell secretion and absorption. **A:** Chloride secretion abnormality. With CF cells, the CFTR (cystic fibrosis transmembrane conductance regulator) channel (*3*) is blocked or nonexistent, so chloride cannot exit. A small amount of chloride probably can exit through the calcium-dependent chloride channel (*2*). With limited chloride secretion, there's also limited sodium (*4*) and fluid (not pictured) entering the airway lumen from the cell. **B:** Sodium absorption abnormality. With CF cells, the sodium channel (*2*) is overactive, leading to excessive sodium being absorbed across the luminal membrane (*1*), which also leads to excessive fluid absorption (not shown).

ıd gets absorbed. This makes the electrical charge (PD) across the
er in CF and is the basis of the test for the nasal PD (see the preceding section). This overactivity of the sodium absorption system seems to
be determined—at least in part—by the changes in the CFTR protein that
cause CF.

Together, these problems mean that more salt and water are removed from the
airway lumen and less secretion can occur to replenish that fluid, probably
explaining the dry, thick mucus that we have long observed in people with CF.

WHAT ABOUT THE PANCREAS AND SWEAT GLANDS?

The lungs are not the only organs affected by the abnormal CFTR protein. The
pancreatic ducts are affected in a very similar manner. The CFTR chloride channel is absent or abnormal there, too, and this leads to plugging of the ducts
(because fluid secretion is depressed) and to eventual destruction of the pancreas. In the sweat glands, since chloride (and therefore sodium) cannot be
absorbed out of the gland fluid (see Chapter 5, *Other Systems*), that fluid retains
a high concentration of chloride (and sodium), resulting in salty sweat, a hall-
mark of the disease.

WHAT CAUSES CYSTIC FIBROSIS AIRWAYS TO BECOME INFECTED?

We have long thought that people with CF got frequent bronchial infections
because their airway secretions were drier, stickier, and harder to clear than normal secretions. This is still a likely explanation, and our knowledge about salt
movement across the bronchial epithelial cells lends support to this notion. However, from what we know now, we cannot say that this is the only explanation for
the ease with which the airways of patients with CF become infected. For one
thing, although we are fairly certain about the abnormalities in chloride and
sodium transport, we do not have proof that the airway secretions in people with
CF actually have less water content than in those without CF. If we exclude
patients with bronchial infection and inflammation, this may not be true. Furthermore, there may be factors related to abnormal CFTR protein—other than
the dryness of the airway mucus and fluid—that makes the airways easily
infected. For instance, there's evidence that some bacteria (including
Pseudomonas species) can stick more tightly to mucus and airway cells when the
electrical charge of their proteins is altered. In CF, there appears to be a different type of sugar coat on the proteins (with a different electrical charge) that is
secreted in the mucus or attached to the surface membrane. This could make it
easier for *Pseudomonas* organisms to stick to airway cells. If bacteria stick
tightly to airway cells, they are harder to clear from the bronchi, and it's easier
for them to set up housekeeping. Eventually, these bacteria form organized
colonies called biofilms that are very difficult to penetrate with antibiotics.

Another theory is that normal, healthy lung cells respond in a very localized way to inhaled particles, including bacteria. Perhaps the cell can detect when a foreign invader has landed, and it quickly opens its chloride channel to let chloride out of the cell; sodium and water quickly follow, in tiny amounts, but enough in this very small area to wash away the bacteria or dust particle. If the chloride channel cannot open, the bacteria stay there long enough for the next line of defense, namely, white blood cells, to be called in to fight them off. Unfortunately, as you'll see in Chapter 3, *The Respiratory System,* these white blood cells can damage lung tissue along with the bacteria they attack. Under this theory, the airways don't have to start out as overall drier than normal, but because they can't wash away bacteria at thousands of individual sites, they eventually become damaged and filled with thick mucus and debris from dead bacteria, exhausted white blood cells, and damaged airway cells.

Whatever the exact details, it seems clear at this point that the lung problems are related to the abnormal CFTR and the abnormal movement of salt and water across bronchial cells.

ARE THERE DIFFERENCES AMONG THE DIFFERENT CYSTIC FIBROSIS MUTATIONS?

Chapter 11, *Genetics,* discusses the different ways in which the *CFTR* gene (and the protein it makes) can be abnormal. You will see in that chapter that geneticists think that there are over 1,000 different ways that this one gene can be abnormal! You will also see that there's a lot of interest in trying to find out how (or if) these different changes (mutations) cause different problems for patients. In this section, we will discuss briefly what is known about whether different mutations in the *CFTR* gene and protein affect differences in the basic defect, that is, in how the cells work.

The way the CFTR protein seems to work in healthy cells is shown in Figure 1.4. There are four steps involved: (a) the protein is made within the cell *(pro-*

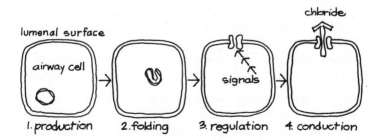

Figure 1.4. The four steps needed for proper functioning of the cystic fibrosis transmembrane conductance regulator (CFTR) protein in healthy cells. (*1*) The protein is made within the cell *(production)*, then (*2*) it has to fold in a particular way so that its shape allows it to be transported to the cell membrane (*folding*), where (*3*) it responds to certain chemical signals that activate it (*regulation*), and it does its job, (*4*) including opening for brief periods to let chloride out (*conduction*).

duction), then (b) it has to fold in a particular way so that its shape allows it to be transported to the cell membrane *(folding),* where (c) it responds to certain chemical signals from the cell that activate it *(regulation),* and it does its job, (d) including opening for brief periods to let chloride out *(conduction).*

Different mutations in the *CFTR* gene can cause it to get "hung up" on its way to the cell membrane or not work correctly, and usually a mutation interferes with one of these four steps. For example,

1. There are quite a few CF gene abnormalities that are known (or suspected) to prevent the CFTR protein from being made at all (defective *production*). These include mutations called G542X, 3905 insT, and R553X. With another abnormal form of the *CFTR* gene, one with the unwieldy name 3849+10kb C→T, CFTR protein is made, but much less of it than normal.

2. The most common CF mutation (ΔF508, pronounced delta F 508) results in the second kind of problem (abnormal *folding*): CFTR protein is made, but it folds into an abnormal shape, and therefore is not transported to the cell membrane to do its work. In the laboratory, when researchers have moved the abnormal ΔF508 CFTR protein into the cell membrane, it has worked fairly well (but not as well as the normal CFTR). Several other mutations seem to have a similar problem of not being delivered to the cell membrane, including ΔI507, N1303K, and S549R.

3. There have been several CFTR mutations that have abnormal *regulation:* The CFTR protein is delivered to the membrane, but is not able to respond normally to the usual chemical signals that should tell it to be active as a chloride channel (this means it doesn't open normally to let chloride pass out through the membrane). These mutations include G551D and several others that are very rare.

4. Finally, there are a few mutations with abnormal chloride *conduction:* These altered CFTR proteins seem to be made and transported to the cell membrane correctly; and under experimental conditions they respond normally to the chemical activating signals. Yet, under usual circumstances, they let a less-than-normal amount of chloride pass through the cell membrane (they open, but either not wide enough or not for a long enough time). The three most common of these mutations are R117H, R334W, and R347P. For the R117H CFTR protein, there's an explanation of its subnormal chloride current: Although this protein-channel opens normally in response to the appropriate signals, it remains open for a much shorter time than normal.

There have not yet been ways identified in which the different CFTR mutations may affect the overactive sodium-reabsorbing channel. It is possible that the changes in sodium transport will be different for each different kind of CFTR mutation.

SO WHAT?

In most cases, the very different CFTR mutations do not seem to make much difference in how the patient is affected: Patients with almost all of these different mutations have identical CF disease. One set of exceptions is that most of the patients with CF with the last type of problem (conduction), caused by R117H, R334W, and R347P, are likely to have relatively normal pancreatic function (see Chapter 4, *The Gastrointestinal Tract*, and Chapter 11, *Genetics*).

What may be even more important one day is that if we know exactly how someone's abnormal CF gene affects his or her cells, there may be very specific ways to correct the problem. One example that may be useful in helping us to understand the situation (but not yet helpful to patients) is with the most common abnormal CF protein, produced by the gene ΔF508. Remember from a few paragraphs ago that this CFTR protein does not escape from the inner portion of the cell to be delivered to the cell membrane, but that if a scientist puts it into the membrane, it can function about half as well as the normal CFTR. What if there was a way to free the ΔF508 CFTR from the cell interior so it could get to the membrane? Again, in the laboratory, there are a couple of ways:

1. In cells growing at normal body temperature (37°C, 98.6°F), the ΔF508 CFTR protein is trapped inside the cell; but, if the cells are grown at a cooler temperature (23° to 30°C; 73° to 86°F), some of the protein escapes and makes it to the cell membrane, where it functions. Now, it is not possible to lower everyone's body temperature 12° to 25°F, but it is helpful and encouraging to know that there's something that can make the protein act closer to normal.
2. There's also evidence that the chemical glycerol can do the same thing that the lower temperature does: The ΔF508 cells grown in the laboratory in the presence of lots of glycerol have some CFTR protein that makes it to the cell membrane. Perhaps one day we'll have a safe drug patients can take to make this happen in their lungs.

For other mutations, perhaps drugs could be discovered or developed that make CFTR protein more responsive to the usual chemical signals that tell it to open to let chloride pass, or to keep a quickly closing channel open a bit longer.

Even before treatments are designed that target the specific CFTR mutations, it might be possible to bypass the cellular problems that virtually all CF cells have: It might be possible to slow down the overactive sodium pump or to "rev up" the non-CFTR chloride channels. In fact, as this book is going to press, there are studies under way looking at drugs to do just that (see Chapter 16, *Research and Future Treatments*). Amiloride is a drug that has been around for a long time and has been used as a diuretic (which makes you lose fluid by increasing the amount of urine made by the kidneys). Amiloride works by blocking the sodium channel. So far, there are conflicting studies as to whether inhaled amiloride is helpful over a several-month period. Another drug, uridine triphosphate (UTP), is being studied for its apparent role in increasing chloride flow through the calcium-dependent chloride channel in the cell membrane (not the CFTR channel).

DOES THE BASIC DEFECT EXPLAIN WHY THE CYSTIC FIBROSIS GENE HAS SURVIVED FOR SO LONG?

You'll see in Chapter 11, *Genetics,* that scientists always wonder how an abnormal gene sticks around, over centuries, instead of dying out. That question is especially puzzling for an abnormal gene that ends up with people dying before they are old enough to reproduce (as was true of CF until just the past decade or so, compared to the thousands of years that CF has been around). In a number of different genetic diseases, there has been something good found out about the mutation in the gene to offset its bad effects. That "good" is usually something that gives an advantage to the people who carry one copy of the abnormal gene. A well-known example is the case of sickle cell disease, a terrible problem afflicting some 1 in 300 African Americans. Like CF, sickle cell disease is a recessive disorder (more about this in Chapter 11, *Genetics*), meaning that to have the disease, someone has to have two copies of an abnormal gene, inheriting one from each parent. The parents almost always have one abnormal gene and one normal gene (as do 10% of African Americans). Having one normal and one abnormal gene for sickle cell disease is called having the "sickle trait," and people with sickle trait are quite healthy. As it turns out, not only are they healthy, but having sickle trait *protects* them from the ravages of malaria. So, if whole villages were being wiped out by malaria, someone with sickle trait had a survival advantage and would be more likely to live through the malaria epidemics and *continue to pass on the abnormal gene.*

For CF, a number of different advantages for carriers (parents of patients with CF and others who carry only one abnormal *CFTR* gene) have been guessed at over the years. Within the last few years, researchers working with CF mice (see Chapter 11, *Genetics*) found that carrier mice (those with one normal and one abnormal *CFTR* gene) were protected from having the terrible diarrhea that comes with being infected with cholera. Cholera causes severe illness and death in many places around the world. Its damage is done by a chemical made by the cholera bacteria ("cholera toxin"), which makes the intestines secrete chloride in huge amounts. As we have seen above, when cells secrete a large amount of chloride, sodium and water will follow. Airway cells secrete into the lumen of the lungs' airways; intestinal cells do the same thing into the lumen of the intestine. A large amount of chloride, sodium, and water pouring into the intestinal lumen creates a watery diarrhea. So people with cholera become dangerously—often fatally—dehydrated. It now appears that the intestinal cells of CF carrier mice do not secrete as much salt and water after they've been exposed to cholera toxin. We know that having two abnormal *CFTR* genes makes chloride secretion very much below normal. It appears that having one normal and one abnormal *CFTR* gene may allow normal, healthy levels of chloride secretion under usual conditions. But under unusual conditions (for example, infection with cholera), perhaps the cells cannot increase their chloride secretion much above the usual level; that is, they can't increase their chloride secretion to the point where they become dangerously dehydrated because of too much fluid lost in diarrhea. Since this is different from the noncarriers (who increase chloride and water secretion dangerously), it is not "normal," but since it protects against fatal dehydration, it certainly is an advantage for the CF carrier. This is an attractive hypothesis: If carriers of the abnormal *CFTR* gene have been protected from cholera or other similar intestinal infections over the centuries, while people with no "CF trait" were being wiped out, that would explain the persistence of the abnormal *CFTR* gene that causes so much trouble. (It is not a *perfect* explanation, though, since the worldwide distribution of cholera is not the same as the distribution of CF. However, the intestinal protection probably extends to other infectious diarrheas, with a geographic distribution more similar to that of CF.)

In summary, the basic defect in CF is becoming better understood. It involves abnormal traffic of salt and water across and through cells that line the airways, pancreas, intestinal tract, and sweat glands. The ways in which the salt and water transport are abnormal may lead to effective new treatments.

2

Making the Diagnosis

THE BASICS

1. The sweat test is the best test for cystic fibrosis (CF) *if* it is done in a laboratory that has a lot of sweat testing experience.
2. Genetic testing can help to tell if a patient has CF.
3. With genetic testing, a "positive" test means the person probably has CF, but a "negative" test does not completely rule out CF.
4. If there is any question about the possibility of a person's having CF, that person needs to be tested.

Making the diagnosis of cystic fibrosis (CF) is one of the most important things that can be done for the health of people with CF. It can clear the way for starting extremely effective treatment that will have a tremendous influence on how healthy they will be and how long they will live. The earlier the diagnosis is made, the sooner treatment can begin, and the better the outlook for the patient. Making the diagnosis will also have a big impact on the patient's family, in several ways. It will have a big emotional impact, perhaps overwhelming at first. For some families, it will actually be a relief or a vindication, since they might have known for a long time that something was wrong, yet they had not been able to discover what. (See Chapter 12, *The Family*, which has more discussion of the emotional impact of CF on patients and families.) It will certainly influence the family's time, finances, insurance, and perhaps even employment (since having good insurance will become a very important part of job considerations).

For these and many other reasons, making the correct diagnosis and making it early are extremely important. Yet in CF centers, many patients are seen who have received an incorrect diagnosis of CF. Some have had negative test results, and their families were told they did not have CF (or CF was never mentioned), when they really did have CF. Alternatively, others had positive test results and were told they had CF, when they really did not have it.

In this chapter, I'll discuss the various ways of making the diagnosis of CF, including sweat tests, newborn screening, and DNA analysis (sometimes called genetic testing). I won't discuss prenatal testing and carrier testing, because these are covered in Chapter 11, *Genetics*.

Before a CF test can be done, someone has to think about ordering one, so I will begin with a brief consideration of who should be tested.

WHO SHOULD BE TESTED?

Not everyone needs to be tested for CF. Anyone with any of the signs or symptoms that are part of CF should be tested for it. The most important of these signs and symptoms are listed in Table 2.1, and are discussed throughout the book.

One other situation where testing is done is in hospitals (and some entire states) that have included CF in their newborn screening programs.

TABLE 2.1. *Reasons to Test for Cystic Fibrosis*

Family History of CF
  Every sibling of a patient with CF should be tested; cousins should be tested if there are signs, symptoms, or worry of CF
Respiratory System
  Upper Respiratory System
    Nasal polyps
    Sinus disease with radiographic findings showing "pansinusitis" (all the sinuses abnormal)
  Lower Respiratory System
    Recurrent or severe bronchiolitis
    Severe or nontypical "asthma"
    Frequent productive cough
    Persistent cough, especially with hard coughing spells
    Coughing up blood
    Recurrent pneumonia
    Throat or sputum culture positive for *Pseudomonas* organisms
    Collapsed lung or partially collapsed lung
Gastrointestinal System
  Meconium ileus (bowel obstruction in the newborn)
  Frequent bulky, loose, oily, foul-smelling stools that float in the toilet
  Failure to gain weight, especially with a big appetite
  Rectal prolapse (see Figure 4.2)
  Liver disease
  Pancreatitis (inflammation of pancreas)
Miscellaneous
  Tastes salty when kissed
  Finger clubbing (see Figure 3.10)
  Male infertility

CF, cystic fibrosis.

WHAT CONFIRMS A DIAGNOSIS OF CYSTIC FIBROSIS?

To make the diagnosis of CF, most experts require a positive sweat test (discussed below) from a reliable, experienced laboratory, PLUS one or more of the following: (a) pulmonary symptoms, (b) gastrointestinal symptoms, (c) family history of CF.

In some cases, genetic testing that shows two abnormal CF genes can substitute for any of the items on the list. In most cases, CF experts will be willing to say that someone has CF if the person has two abnormal CF genes.

In the case of newborn screening, most experts will make the diagnosis on the basis of a "positive" newborn screen and a "positive" sweat test, or a "positive" newborn screen and genetic testing positive for two abnormal CF genes.

Let's now consider the different tests.

Sweat Tests

The sweat test has been the "gold standard" for diagnosing CF for over 40 years, and when it is done in an experienced, reliable laboratory, the sweat test is still the best test for CF. It is a superb test. It is painless, relatively inexpensive, and gives definitive answers within a few hours. There are almost no false positives (people who test positive for CF, but don't really have it) or false negatives (people whose tests say they don't have CF, but really do have it). Furthermore, in almost every case, the result of the test is positive or negative: There are almost no people who have test results in an "in-between" range (or "gray zone" or "intermediate range"). The test can be performed—with accurate results—on patients of any age. Many physicians mistakenly believe that sweat tests are not reliable in young infants. Some young babies may not make enough sweat for the laboratory to analyze, but most will produce enough. If a baby doesn't produce enough sweat on a sweat test, it should be repeated, either the same day or, at most, a week later.

Details on how the sweat test is performed and interpreted can be found in Chapter 5, *Other Systems*. Sweat is collected from the arm or leg and then is analyzed for its salt (sodium chloride) content. To do this, the laboratory measures the concentration of chloride (and/or sodium). A positive test is one in which the concentration of chloride (or sodium) is 60 milliequivalents per liter (mEq/L) or higher. Almost everyone with CF has values between 60 and 110 mEq/L. A negative test is one in which the concentration of chloride (or sodium) is 40 mEq/L or lower. Very few people have values between 40 and 60 mEq/L. (Later in the chapter, we'll talk about what to do with these few difficult cases.) There are very few cases of positive sweat tests caused by rare diseases other than CF. These diseases are readily distinguished from CF. Lists of these diseases can be found in any pediatric textbook.

Once a test result is positive, it is always positive. Sweat test values do not change from positive to negative or negative to positive as a patient grows older.

And sweat test values do not vary when the patients have colds or other temporary illnesses. There is no point in saying, "it was positive now, but the baby was sick; let's repeat it when she feels better." Two rare exceptions to this rule are the child who is undernourished because of psychological deprivation and the adolescent suffering from anorexia nervosa. These children may test positive until they are treated for their emotional or environmental causes of malnutrition, at which time their tests turn negative.

I need to stress again the importance of the experience of the laboratory doing the tests. Most CF centers find that CF has been misdiagnosed in about half of all the patients they see who have been tested by inexperienced laboratory personnel. The mistakes happen in both directions: People who do not have CF are told they do, and vice versa. Sweat test laboratories associated with an approved CF center have passed accreditation by the national Cystic Fibrosis Foundation, and can be trusted. Many other laboratories are also good, but it is harder to know about those that are not in CF centers.

Newborn Screening

Since early diagnosis is so helpful to the long-term health of patients with CF, some states have mandated newborn screening. In states where this screening is not required by state law, some hospitals have taken it upon themselves to offer newborn CF screening as a service to their obstetric patients.

The test used for newborn screening is called the IRT. Those initials stand for immunoreactive trypsinogen, and the test is discussed in Chapter 4, *The Gastrointestinal Tract*. For our purposes here, it will suffice to say that the test is done on a spot of blood that is taken from the baby's heel within the first days of life. Almost every baby with CF has a high level of IRT. Different screening programs use this information in different ways: Some programs get the results of the initial IRT in a week or two, and if it's elevated, they notify the baby's doctor, who calls the family to bring the baby for a repeat test. The repeat test is needed, because many, many babies (not just those with CF) have high IRT levels on the first test. By the time the test is repeated, the IRT levels for most babies without CF will have fallen to normal, whereas most babies with CF will still have high IRT levels. If the level is still high on the second test, sweat testing is needed. In other programs, genetic testing is done on blood spots with elevated IRT levels (more about this in the next section).

This newborn screen has its good and bad features: The good is that very few babies with CF are missed by this test; the bad is that lots of babies who don't have CF have to come back for the second test, and some who don't have CF have to get a sweat test. This means that many families have days or weeks of worrying that their little ones have CF, when it will turn out that they do not. Most families and CF experts now think that the good of getting babies diagnosed and started on treatment early outweighs the bad of some temporary worry for the families whose babies end up getting a clean bill of health.

Gene Testing

Gene testing is discussed further in Chapter 11, *Genetics*.

We all have two CF genes, one from our mother and one from our father, that determine whether we have CF. Both of these genes must be abnormal (have mutations) for us to end up with CF. If one is abnormal, we are said to be a "carrier," meaning we don't have the disease, but we carry the gene and can pass it along to our children. (Then, if we do pass the abnormal CF gene on to our children, whether our children get CF depends on whether they also get an abnormal CF gene from our spouse.)

The CF gene is very large, and there are many sites along the gene that can have changes ("mutations") that cause problems. To date, scientists have discovered more than 1,000 different ways in which the CF gene can be abnormal and can cause CF! A few of these mutations are common and are found in different combinations in most patients with CF; many of the CF gene mutations are uncommon. There are even some that occur in only one family. There are patients with CF whose mutation has not yet been discovered. We can analyze blood or other tissue and see if people have CF gene mutations of a type that has already been described. Most patients with CF have two common CF gene mutations that are identifiable on genetic testing. However, some patients have abnormal CF genes that standard genetic testing won't find because they are rare, and the standard tests look only for the most common mutations. Since the normal structure of the CF gene is known, it is possible to analyze the entire CF gene to see if it is abnormal in any way, including ways that have not previously been recognized. This testing is very time-consuming and is done only at a very few highly specialized research laboratories. Some day soon, testing of the entire CF gene for *any* mutations will be automated, making it much easier to identify all patients with CF from a blood test or cheek brushing

With the testing now available for only the most common CF mutations, if we wonder about the diagnosis of CF and do genetic testing, finding two known abnormal CF genes pretty much tells us the person has CF. But finding one or no known CF mutation doesn't give a definite answer. It may say the chances are a little better that the person doesn't have CF, since most people with CF have two of the abnormal genes we've been looking for, but it doesn't tell us for sure.

Some newborn screening programs automatically test all blood spots, or all samples with elevated IRT, for the most common CF gene mutation (called *ΔF508*, pronounced "delta-F 508"). Finding two of this particular CF mutation (as happens in about 50% of people with CF in North America) pretty much confirms the diagnosis. A few screening programs look for more of the common mutations, thus increasing the chances of finding two mutations if they are present.

There are some unusual situations in which genetic testing might be done instead of sweat testing. These situations might include a patient who does not make enough sweat for analysis or who lives far removed from a reliable sweat testing laboratory. In these cases, it would probably make sense to send a blood sample (or a simple painless cotton-tipped swab rubbed on your inner cheek) for genetic analysis. If the test comes back with two CF mutations identified, the diagnosis is almost certain. If the test comes back with one or no abnormal CF genes found, you won't know whether there's CF or not, and you'll have to go to a good sweat testing laboratory after all, but nothing's been lost.

Other Testing: "Nasal Potential Difference"

A very few specialized laboratories can perform a test called a "nasal potential difference." This test is discussed a little more in Chapter 1, *The Basic Defect*. The test measures the electrical charge (also called the potential difference) inside someone's nose. People with CF have a large electric charge, while people without CF have much lower values. This test is probably even better than the sweat test in separating those with CF from those without. The problem with it is that it is very difficult to do correctly, and very few centers are set up to do this testing.

What About the Unusual Cases?

In some cases, it might be difficult or impossible to make the diagnosis in the usual way. Examples might include a patient who doesn't make enough sweat to analyze or one of the rare individuals whose sweat test results are in the "gray zone"—neither clearly positive nor clearly negative—and genetic testing has been inconclusive. We'll assume that testing of nasal potential difference is not available. In these cases, the physician has to consider the whole picture: What are the patient's lungs like? What germs grow on throat cultures? Does he or she have abnormal sinuses on radiographs (x-ray films)? Are the stools abnormal? Is there finger clubbing? (All these signs and symptoms are discussed in Chapter 3, *The Respiratory System*, and Chapter 4, *The Gastrointestinal Tract*.) Occasionally, the physician and family will decide that the wisest course of action is (a) to accept the fact that for the time being a definite diagnosis cannot be made, and (b) to decide to treat the child *as if he or she has CF*. This makes sense because the treatments are not harmful for someone who does not have CF, but not getting the treatments could be very harmful for someone who does have CF.

3

The Respiratory System

THE BASICS

1. The lungs are the most important part of the body in people with cystic fibrosis (CF), and they cause most of the sickness and more than 95% of the deaths from CF.
2. Thick mucus blocks the bronchial tubes in people with CF, causing infection and inflammation.
3. The lung problem is progressive, meaning it keeps getting worse as time goes by.
4. With very good treatment, the progression of the lung disease can be slowed dramatically, and the lungs can be kept relatively healthy for long periods of time.
5. Regular treatment to keep the airways clear of mucus and infection is extremely important.
6. New or increased cough is usually the first sign of worsened infection and inflammation. If cough increases, you should call your CF doctor for treatment.

The respiratory system is the most important organ system for patients with cystic fibrosis (CF). Problems with this system account for over 95% of the sickness from CF and for more than 95% of the deaths from this disease. In the years since CF was first recognized, treatment of lung disease has improved considerably, resulting in the tremendous improvement in longevity and quality of life that CF patients can now expect.

The three sections of this chapter are devoted to (a) a discussion of the normal anatomy and functioning of the respiratory system, (b) an explanation of how CF changes the functioning of this system, and (c) a review of the treatments that are aimed at preventing, correcting, or minimizing the changes that CF brings about in the respiratory system.

ANATOMY AND FUNCTION OF THE RESPIRATORY SYSTEM

All tissues in the body, especially the brain and exercising muscles, need oxygen to function. It is the task of the respiratory system to bring in oxygen from the air that surrounds us and transfer it to the bloodstream. Once oxygen is in the bloodstream, the cardiovascular system (heart and blood vessels) delivers it to all the parts of the body that need it. It is a further responsibility of the lungs to dispose of excess carbon dioxide, which builds up in the process of normal metabolism. These tasks are essential to life, since all body tissues need oxygen to survive, and if too much carbon dioxide builds up in the bloodstream and brain, it can put someone so deeply to sleep that he or she will not breathe.

The Airways

The actual transfer of oxygen from the air we breathe to the bloodstream (and carbon dioxide from the blood to the air we exhale) takes place deep in the lungs, in the alveoli (air sacs), which are located at the end of a long series of tubes. (One air sac is an alveolus, two or more are alveoli.) At the beginning of these air-carrying tubes, or "airways," are the nose and mouth, followed by the throat, then the larynx (or "voice box," another name given to this area, which includes the vocal cords), and the trachea (also called the "windpipe"). As the trachea enters the chest, it divides into two branches, and each branch leads into a lung. These branches are referred to as the bronchial tubes, or simply, bronchi (Figure 3.1). Each bronchus reaches into its lung where it divides again, and yet again, forming a network of bronchi that extend into the various lobes, or sections, of the lung, and the segments of each lobe, the subsegments of each segment, and so forth. Each time the bronchi branch, they become smaller and are thus able to distribute air to the smallest and farthest reaches of the lungs. [The word "branch" is frequently used to describe the bronchial system, for it does look very treelike. Pulmonary physicians (lung specialists) and anatomists often adapt words used in forestry to describe this bronchial "tree."]

The bronchi divide, or branch, approximately 20 times before they reach the alveoli. It is in these air sacs that oxygen finally leaves the inhaled air and enters the bloodstream. Throughout most of this branching network, the bronchial tubes are referred to as "bronchi," or, for the smaller ones, "small bronchi" (how *do* they come up with these clever names?). Toward the very end of this network, the bronchi become quite small and are referred to as *bronchioles*. Bronchioles are the last segment of tubes through which air passes before it reaches the alveoli.

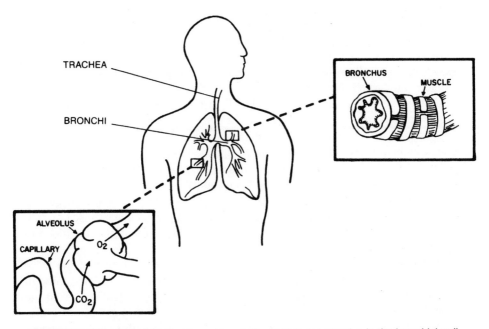

FIGURE 3.1. The lungs, including bronchi and alveoli. Note the muscles in the bronchial wall. Oxygen enters the bloodstream by passing from the inhaled air through the wall of the alveoli and into the blood cells in the capillaries.

The difference between bronchi and bronchioles, aside from their size, is that bronchi have cartilage in their walls and bronchioles don't. Both bronchi and bronchioles need something to stiffen their walls so that they maintain their shape and, particularly, so that they stay open. In healthy lungs, there is a tendency for the bronchi and bronchioles to enlarge slightly as the chest expands with each breath inhaled, and to narrow with each breath exhaled. If breathing is particularly strenuous, or if the support of the bronchial walls is not very strong, the bronchi and bronchioles can collapse during exhalation, making it difficult for the proper amount of air to leave the lungs.

In addition to cartilage, other tissues help support the bronchi. One of the most important is muscle: The bronchi and bronchioles have bands of muscle running around their walls. If a dangerous substance threatens to enter the lungs (such as a chemical with toxic fumes), these muscles can contract, squeezing down and making the bronchial opening much smaller than normal. With the bronchial passage blocked in this way, it is difficult for anything to get deeply into the bronchial tree. This action protects the lungs only if it happens briefly, and only if it happens when there is a true danger. However, this "protective" mechanism can actually be harmful if the bronchial muscles squeeze down at inappropriate times.

Gas Transfer and Delivery

The transfer of oxygen from the inhaled air to the bloodstream takes place at the alveoli. Running past each alveolus is a tiny blood vessel called a *pulmonary capillary*. The walls of the alveoli and the capillaries are membranes, so thin that oxygen and carbon dioxide can pass directly through them. It is through these walls that oxygen passes from the alveoli to the bloodstream and that carbon dioxide passes from the bloodstream to the alveoli. There are 20 million of these tiny air sacs in a newborn infant's lungs, and 300 million in an adult. The enormous extent of these figures can be better grasped by imagining that, if you were to lay out the working surfaces between the alveoli and capillaries side by side, they would span an area the size of a tennis court.

After the oxygen has been supplied to the blood, the task remains of getting the blood to the tissues that need the oxygen (the brain, exercising muscles, etc.). Fortunately, an excellent system accomplishes the task of pumping the blood to where it is needed. The pump, of course, is the heart.

Actually, the heart is a muscular double pump. The right side of the heart pumps blood through the lungs, where the blood becomes oxygenated through the process just described (and where the carbon dioxide is dumped out of the blood). After the hemoglobin molecules, which are the oxygen-carrying elements in the blood, are loaded with as much oxygen as possible (that is, they are fully saturated with oxygen), the blood flows back to the heart. It then enters the left side of the heart, where it is pumped to the rest of the body. Oxygen is removed from the blood by the tissues that need it. The deoxygenated blood then returns to the heart through the veins, and enters the right side of the heart. The heart then pumps the blood back to the lungs, where it is loaded with oxygen once again. At rest, an adult's heart will pump 4 to 5 liters (L) of blood per minute (1 L is approximately equal to a quart). During heavy exercise, that amount can increase to 25 or even to 30 L per minute.

The condition can arise in which the oxygen levels are too low and the carbon dioxide levels are too high. This is called *respiratory failure*, and can result from several circumstances. If someone with normal lungs is paralyzed in a car crash, for example, the breathing muscles (see section, *The Respiratory Muscles*) could also become paralyzed and thus be unable to accomplish the work of breathing. Brain injury or brain disease or drug overdoses may also result in respiratory failure by damaging the brain's ability to direct the muscles to move the chest, in which case breathing will not occur. Serious lung disease can also cause respiratory failure if oxygen cannot be brought into, or carbon dioxide removed from, the bloodstream.

Control of Breathing

Among the many amazing things our body can do without our awareness is regulating how much we breathe. The main job of the lungs is to bring in the right amount of oxygen and eliminate the right amount of carbon dioxide that has been produced. This balancing act is controlled with astounding precision.

In general, the more we breathe, the more oxygen we bring into the body, and the more carbon dioxide we breathe out. When we exercise, our muscles use as much as 10 to 20 times as much oxygen as when we're resting, and even more carbon dioxide is formed, which needs to be eliminated. During strenuous exercise, we breathe five to ten times as much air as when we're resting, and our heart pumps five or six times as much blood each minute, yet all the while the levels of oxygen and carbon dioxide in the bloodstream remain almost exactly the same! You'd think that a little extra oxygen would come in, or not quite enough, or that a bit too much carbon dioxide would be breathed out, or not quite enough, but this doesn't happen. In healthy people as well as in most people with lung disease (including those with CF), the blood levels of oxygen and carbon dioxide remain steady, regardless of what the person is doing.

This tight control is achieved by the brain's response to the two gases that the lungs manage—oxygen and carbon dioxide. Carbon dioxide is usually the more important regulator. If the breathing slows down (as it does in all of us now and then), less carbon dioxide will be breathed out and it will begin to build up in the body. As soon as this happens, the brain senses the buildup and sends the signal to the breathing muscles to breathe more, until the carbon dioxide level is back down to normal. The opposite occurs also: If the carbon dioxide level gets too low, the brain sends out the signal to slow down the breathing. Most of the time this is very fine-tuning, requiring such small changes in breathing effort that we are unaware of the adjustments that are being made.

If the lungs are severely affected by disease and are not able to eliminate carbon dioxide effectively, the carbon dioxide level will build up and the brain will "instruct" the body to increase the rate and depth of breathing. After a while, however, the brain acts as though it has "gotten tired" of the message that the carbon dioxide level is too high, and it ignores the message. In its place, the brain will respond to another signal that regulates breathing—the oxygen level. It notices that the oxygen level is too low, and continues sending the message to the breathing muscles to increase breathing more. It is in this way that severe lung disease (from whatever cause) may alter the way the brain controls breathing patterns. Various drugs may also affect breathing patterns, either by making us breathe more, or by making us less sensitive to breathing commands, and therefore breathe less.

The Respiratory Muscles

Once the message to breathe is sent, it must be carried out. The work of breathing is done by the respiratory (or ventilatory) muscles. The most important ventilatory muscle is the diaphragm, which separates the inside of the chest from the abdomen. Since the chest wall (ribs, chest muscles, skin, etc.) is relatively firm, when the diaphragm contracts and moves downward, it leaves more space inside the chest for the lungs to expand. This action creates a vacuum inside the chest, and air rushes into the trachea and bronchi (through the nose and/or mouth) and fills that extra space. When it is time to breathe out, most of the force comes as the lungs and chest wall just naturally spring back into their usual resting size. With hard breathing, exhalation gets a boost from the expiratory muscles, which include the abdominal muscles, the muscles between the ribs, and some muscles in the neck. During very hard breathing, inhalation gets extra help, too (even the tiny muscles that widen the nostrils contribute to inhalation). All of these muscles are called the **accessory muscles** of respiration, since they are helpful, but are not absolutely necessary, for normal quiet breathing. It is possible to see these muscles at work during hard breathing: When the muscles between the ribs (the **intercostal muscles**) are used, the skin seems to sink in between the ribs (this is called *retracting*), and when the neck or abdominal muscles are used, they stick out prominently. If the nose muscles are pitching in, you can see the nostrils widening, a sign called "nasal flaring," or simply "flaring."

Lung Defenses

The air we breathe has an abundance of potentially harmful elements in it (in addition to the good), such as cigarette smoke, pollution, dust, bacteria, viruses, and other germs. Yet, in most people, the lungs stay fairly clean, remaining unclogged by these substances and free from infection. This is the result of a very efficient lung protection system at work.

The Nose and Mouth

The defense of the lungs begins in the nose and mouth. Many of the largest particles breathed in get trapped here, especially in the hairs of the nose.

However, some of the smaller particles do make it past the air conditioning and filtering system of the nose and mouth, and reach the trachea or bronchi. When they reach the bronchi, they get stuck in the mucus that lines the airways. Fortunately, the lung defenses are very active in these lower airways, and can remove small particles through coughing, and the action of the **mucociliary escalator**.

Cough

A cough is an explosive release of air from the lungs. It is something we can do voluntarily, but it can also happen without our conscious control. The steps to producing a cough begin with the stimulation of nerves in the nose, throat, trachea, bronchi, or diaphragm. Some of these nerves can be triggered by pressure, others by noxious chemicals, and others by being touched by inhaled particles. Once the cough signal is sent out, there is a deep breath in, followed by a sudden forcible attempt to breathe out at a time when the upper portion of the airway (around the vocal cords) is tightly shut. Since air cannot get out through this closed door, pressure builds up within the lung. Then, after about one fifth of a second, the upper airway suddenly opens and the air bursts out, at a speed reaching 600 miles per hour! This burst of air is very effective in carrying mucus (with its trapped particles of dirt or bacteria) to at least as far as the back of the throat, where it can be spit out or swallowed into the stomach. This tremendous air force is only effective in the largest bronchi and trachea, for the air moves much more slowly in the smaller bronchi farther out in the lungs. Coughing is therefore not an effective method for mucus clearance in the smaller bronchi, and another action is used, which involves the mucociliary escalator.

The Mucociliary Escalator

Many of the cells lining the trachea and bronchi have tiny hairlike projections, called cilia. A thin layer of fluid bathes these cilia and reaches part way up their length, but not to their tips (Figure 3.2). Resting atop the cilia—and atop the fluid layer—is a blanket of mucus, which has been produced by special glands within the bronchi and bronchioles. This layer of mucus protects the airways by trapping substances that might be harmful to the lungs, and removing them through the action of the cilia. The cilia beat approximately 1,200 times per minute in a coordinated action that sweeps the mucus (and everything trapped in the mucus) toward the largest bronchi. When the mucus reaches the large central bronchi, it is carried up the trachea in a movement that is similar to that of an escalator. Hence, this system is sometimes referred to as the mucociliary escalator. When the mucus reaches the top of the trachea (the back of the throat) it is swallowed, usually without our being aware of it. This amazing escalator clears about 2 tsp of mucus each day. Cigarette smokers and others with extra mucus are often aware of the mucus that has been carried to the back of the throat. If there is an especially large amount, or if it is particularly thick, it may be

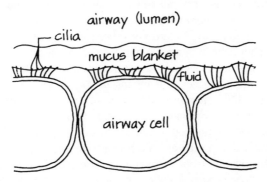

FIGURE 3.2. Cilia project into the airway from atop airway cells. The cilia are bathed in airway fluid almost—but not quite—to their tips. Above the fluid, and just at the tips of the cilia, is a blanket of mucus and trapped inhaled particles.

coughed up once it gets to the large central bronchi. Once it is coughed up, it can be spit out, or it can be swallowed down into the stomach, sending it on its way through the digestive tract, where it will do no harm. The functioning of this wonderful airway-cleaning escalator depends in part on the composition of the mucus, in part on the composition of the fluid layer, and in part on other factors. If the mucus is too thick and sticky, it may be hard for the delicate cilia to move. If the fluid layer is too deep, the tips of the cilia may not reach the mucus, which is now floating above them. If the cilia don't reach the mucus, they can't grip the mucus blanket to move it. On the other hand, if the fluid layer is too shallow, the cilia may not have enough support to be effective. As you've seen in Chapter 1, *The Basic Defect*, the composition of the fluid lining the airway is controlled in part by the cystic fibrosis transmembrane conductance regulator (CFTR) protein made under the direction of the CF gene. This protein helps regulate secretion of fluid and salt from the airway cells into the airway and absorption of fluid and salt from the airway back into the cells. Abnormal CF genes—as everyone with CF has—make for defects in this CFTR protein, which in turn makes for abnormal secretion and absorption of salt and water by these cells, almost certainly leading to abnormal fluid, and very likely interfering with the functioning of the mucociliary escalator.

Other Protection Against Lung Infection

It is thought, but not yet proven, that airway cells may be able to sense when they are touched by inhaled particles (including bacteria). The theory goes that when they sense an "invader," they suddenly secrete a burst of fluid that washes it away. If this doesn't happen (for example, if there is a defect in the ability of the cells to secrete fluid—as seems to be true of CF airway cells), bacteria may not be removed immediately, or not completely, by the mucociliary route. When this happens, further steps are taken to protect the lungs. One such step is the delivery of **white blood cells** to the area where there are foreign substances and bacteria. These blood cells work in two ways: They can surround the bacteria and other particles, capturing them within the blood cells. Then, when the blood cell is removed from the lung, the bacteria or other particles are removed also. They can also release chemicals that attack and destroy the bacteria. These are potent chemicals, some of which degrade structural proteins of the bacteria, and are called *proteases* (the "*-ase*" ending means *breaks down*). A particular one of these proteases is called *elastase*, and its main target is *elastin*, an important structural protein. It is unfortunate but true that these proteases can also attack proteins that make up airway cells—not just bacterial protein. The lungs have a finely tuned system that produces antiproteases to keep the proteases in check and to prevent degradation of proteins that are important for the structure of the airways.

There are certain proteins in the blood that also protect the lungs against infection. These are the **immunoglobulins** (gamma-globulin is one such protein).

Immunoglobulins are part of a system that recognizes materials that are foreign invaders in all parts of the body, and produces antibodies that attack the foreign substances.

Another factor that influences infection in the airways is how tightly bacteria stick to airway cells. The stickiness of these cells seems to be related in part to the electrical charge on the surface of the cells.

THE RESPIRATORY TRACT IN CYSTIC FIBROSIS

The Upper Respiratory Tract

There are two major differences between the normal upper respiratory tract and that in people with CF. The first difference is in the condition of the **sinuses**, and has relatively little to do with the person's health or day-to-day comfort. The second difference is the presence of **nasal polyps**, which affects only about 20% of people with CF.

The Sinuses

The sinuses of people with CF usually look abnormal on radiographs (x-ray films). On the radiographs, the sinuses appear as though they are badly diseased, indicating a condition called pansinusitis (*-itis* meaning "inflamed," *pan-* meaning "all"; thus, "all the sinuses are inflamed"). It is useful to understand the meaning of the appearance of pansinusitis on sinus radiographs for several reasons. First, because it is very unusual to find in children, except in children with CF, the appearance of pansinusitis on the sinus radiographs may help make the diagnosis of CF. Second, the appearance of the radiographic image will suggest that problems exist such as sinus headaches. However, in children with CF, this is rarely the case. There may be some sinus infection, but this, too, is relatively uncommon. (Sinus infections are discussed in more detail below, *Infections of the Upper Respiratory Tract.*)

At some point, a child may have skull radiographs taken, and if the child has CF, the radiograph will most likely show abnormal sinuses. It is important for parents to know that the appearance of sinus abnormality is primarily a problem with the radiograph, that (in the absence of symptoms) it is not something that bothers the child, and that nothing needs to be done about it.

Typically, treatment is not needed for the sinuses in people with CF. Some patients—particularly adults—with CF may have sinus infections that actually cause discomfort. In these cases, antibiotics might be helpful, but this is relatively uncommon. In rare cases, patients with CF with repeated or persistent sinus problems may benefit from surgery to help the sinuses drain better. However, there is little evidence that sinus surgery is of any use to most patients with CF. If a specialist who is not very experienced with CF suggests surgery for the sinuses, a second opinion should be sought.

The Nose

About 20% of patients with CF at one time or another will have **nasal polyps**. Polyps are growths of extra tissue that form in various parts of the body. The formation of polyps in the nose occurs much more commonly in patients with CF than in people who don't have CF. In fact, this can be another diagnostic clue: If a child has a nasal polyp, this is a strong indication that she or he has CF. Nasal polyps are also found in people who don't have CF, especially in those who have many allergies. In children, however, it is very uncommon to find nasal polyps, except in those with CF.

Generally, having a nasal polyp is not a major problem. It is never life-threatening, and it never becomes cancerous the way other polyps can in people without CF. What it may do is block up one side of the nose. When there is one polyp, there are often others, and both sides of the nose may become blocked. Rarely, they can become so large that they can protrude from the nostril. In either of these cases (when the polyp blocks the nose or sticks out of the nostril), it is a nuisance but not a threat to the person's health. Since it is usually a significant nuisance at this point, it is advisable to have the polyps removed. One other instance in which it is wise to remove polyps is when, after some time, the bridge of the nose grows wider in response to the increasing size of the polyps inside the nose.

It is not yet known why 20% of patients with CF do get polyps, why most people without CF don't get polyps, or why some patients with CF get a polyp once, while others get them often.

Treatment of Nasal Polyps

Polyps are strange growths that have a mysterious course of development. They frequently get larger or smaller without treatment, making it difficult to tell if medications are effective. If a polyp gets smaller after medication, one can't be sure that it wouldn't have gotten smaller on its own. Nonetheless, some medications may help shrink polyps. These medications are steroid sprays, such as beclomethasone (see Appendix B, *Medications*).

If the medicines don't work, and if the polyp is completely blocking one or both nostrils, or protruding from the nostril, or is widening the outside of the nasal bridge, then surgery to remove the polyp or polyps (polypectomy) is advisable. This surgery is best done by an ear, nose, and throat surgeon, in the hospital, and under general anesthesia. Simple polypectomy (just removing the polyps the surgeon sees in the nose) or a more extensive procedure called FESS (functional endoscopic sinus surgery) can be done. With the FESS, the surgeon uses an endoscope [a tube for looking (*-scope*) into (*endo*) things] to see further into the sinuses, to get at the roots of some of the polyps. It is not clear yet if the more extensive procedure actually gives better results. In most cases, a very short (overnight) hospital stay is all that is needed for either procedure. After the surgery, the nose is packed with gauze for several hours to make sure the bleeding has stopped, and once the gauze is removed, the patient can go home. In older patients, the simple polypectomy procedure may even be done in the surgeon's office, with local anesthetic. Most often, CF physicians, surgeons, patients, and families feel more comfortable if the surgery is done in the hospital, while the patient is asleep under a general anesthetic.

Surgery is very effective in removing the polyps, and once they are gone, they may never reappear. In some people, though, they may come back, once, twice, or many times.

The Lower Respiratory Tract (the Lungs)

More than any other factor, the lungs determine the health and life span of the large majority of patients with CF. In little more than one generation, the greatly improved treatment of the lungs has transformed the outlook for infants with CF from one consisting of a few difficult months to one entailing many bright years. Infants with CF are born with lungs that appear normal, but, at varying times after birth, they begin to develop problems. In some, these problems may become noticeable within the first weeks, whereas in others, it may take years or even decades before any problems become apparent. Without treatment, lung problems will eventually appear in everyone with CF and the problems will progress. With treatment, this progression can be slowed, in some, almost to a halt.

The problems in the lungs can almost certainly be blamed on the abnormal movement of salt and fluid through the airway cell membranes. This abnormal traffic of salt and fluid, and the abnormal electric charge associated with it (see Chapter 1, *The Basic Defect*) are caused by the abnormal CFTR protein whose production was dictated by the two abnormal CF genes that everyone with CF has. The salt, fluid, and electrical abnormalities lead to inflammation and infection and mucus clogging the smallest airways (the bronchioles). Infection and inflammation of those bronchioles is called *bronchiolitis*. The inflammation then readily spreads to the larger airways, the bronchi (*bronchitis*). If the mucus is too thick to be cleared by the normal mechanisms, such as the mucociliary escalator, it is very easy for germs (viruses and bacteria) to take hold, making it hard for the lungs and body defenses to combat them.

The more inflammation there is within the bronchi and bronchioles, the more swelling there is (Figure 3.3), and the narrower the opening becomes to these airways; or, said another way, the greater the bronchial (and bronchiolar) obstruction. With increasing obstruction, it becomes more difficult for air to move in and out, which forces the respiratory muscles to work harder. Also, when the airways become obstructed, it is difficult to clear them of mucus. Other mucus-clearing mechanisms, especially cough, are then used more frequently to force the mucus up and out of the bronchioles and bronchi. *Increased cough is often*

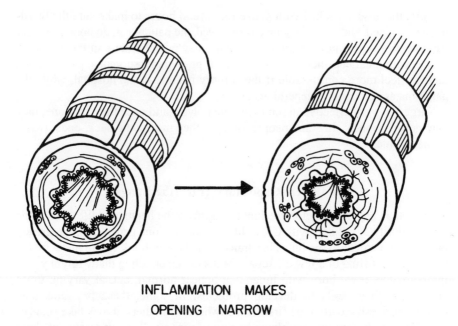

INFLAMMATION MAKES
OPENING NARROW

FIGURE 3.3. Inflammation within the bronchi makes the bronchial opening ("lumen") smaller.

the first sign that the bronchial infection and inflammation are getting out of control.

If the bronchial and bronchiolar infection and inflammation remain out of control for too long, they can damage the bronchioles and bronchi. Bacteria can cause direct damage to the bronchial walls; and the body's response to the bacteria can cause even more damage: You've seen above (*Other Protection Against Lung Infection*) that white blood cells are sent to kill bacteria. These white blood cells release chemicals that cause inflammation to attack and destroy the bacteria. Unfortunately, these chemicals (sometimes called *mediators of inflammation*, including proteases like elastase—see above) cannot distinguish between bacteria and airway tissue, and they can damage the cells lining the airways. In recent years, we've come to understand that this damage from inflammation from our own white blood cells is just as harmful as—or even more harmful than—the harm from the bacteria (which also release chemicals that cause inflammation). If the damage to the airways continues, it can weaken their walls so that they become floppy, and the airways enlarge (**dilate**). The suffix for words describing abnormal dilatation or distention is -*ectasis*, and these changes in the airways are referred to as *bronchiolectasis* and *bronchiectasis*. If the lung damage progresses, it can lead to permanent changes such as infected cysts and scar tissue (*fibrosis*), which are indicated by the name of this disease.

The progression of lung damage is most often very slow and subtle, but it can be relentless. This is why the lung disease of CF is often referred to as "progressive"—if left to its own (and even in most cases with treatment), it gets worse and worse. If this progression of infection, inflammation, and lung destruction continues uninterrupted for too long, it will eventually reach a point where there is no longer enough healthy lung to bring oxygen into the body or to eliminate carbon dioxide.

As a particular episode of increased infection and inflammation develops, or as the lung disease increases over the years, the following progression occurs: First, there is more cough. Someone who usually doesn't cough at all may develop a mild cough for a few minutes in the morning, or someone who coughed only in the morning may now cough during the day or through the night. Morning is a common time for people with CF to cough, since they have been in one position for many hours, making it easier for the lung mucus to stay down in the lungs. During the day, when people are active and breathing harder, mucus is more easily shaken loose and sent on its way out of the lungs.

Along with increased cough (and part of its cause) there is often an increase in lung mucus production and an increase in *sputum* (mucus that is coughed up and spit out of the lungs): The patient is more likely to feel "crud" in the lungs that feels like it needs to come up. The airways now contain mucus made by the bronchial glands and increasingly large amounts of other material. This other material includes DNA (genetic material contained in all cells) that has been released from white blood cells (*neutrophils*) that have died fighting the bronchial infection. There is also a stringy substance called *actin*. The neutrophil DNA and the actin account for a lot of the thickness of CF sputum. There are also numerous dead bacteria and old airway cells that contribute to the thickness and stickiness of CF airway secretions.

With the progression of the lung disease, patients often have decreased exercise tolerance, with quicker tiring and even some shortness of breath (difficulty breathing).

As the particular episode of infection and inflammation subsides—on its own or with treatment—the symptoms also subside, either fully or partly, depending on whether any new lung damage has been caused. The goal of treatment is to get back to the baseline (the condition prior to the onset of the problem) after each episode of worsening (*exacerbation*) of lung infection. This is often, but not always, possible.

Asthma

Asthma affects people with or without CF, and is a condition in which the muscles that surround the bronchi squeeze down readily. This ability of the muscles to tighten and make the opening of the bronchi smaller is basically a protective mechanism (see section, *The Airways*), since it can prevent dangerous substances that have been breathed in (*aspirated*) from getting deep into the lungs. But if bronchial wall muscles go into spasm (*bronchospasm*) when there isn't a real threat to the lungs, the result is that this "protective" mechanism does more harm than good. The bronchi become partly squeezed shut, making it difficult to move mucus out and to breathe air in and out. The airways also become inflamed in people with asthma. When the bronchi are narrowed from bronchospasm and inflammation, there is often a characteristic whistling sound to the breathing. This sound is called *wheezing*, and is heard especially when someone breathes out.

Asthma episodes can be related to allergies, infections, exercise, cold air or to breathing irritating substances such as cigarette smoke or air pollution. In some patients, a condition known as *gastroesophageal reflux* ("GE reflux," simply "reflux," or "GER") can also cause bronchospasm (see Chapter 4, *The Gastrointestinal Tract*). Between 10% and 40% of patients with CF also have asthma.

Infections of the Respiratory Tract

This subject can be confusing since there are many different kinds of respiratory infections (which may or may not present serious problems for people with CF), and it is not always clear which are the potentially dangerous ones and which are merely a nuisance.

Infections of the Upper Respiratory Tract

Sinusitis

Sinusitis is an inflammation of the sinuses, usually caused by infection. This is not often a problem for children with CF, even though sinus radiographs always look as though there is an active sinus infection. Many people attribute their cough (or their child's cough) to sinus problems ("mucus drips down my throat and makes me cough"), and this may be, but much more of the cough in people with CF is caused by lung (bronchial) infection. Some patients—mostly adults—do have bothersome sinus problems, and usually these can be controlled with antibiotics. In a very few patients, sinus surgery may be able to allow the sinuses to drain better and prevent recurrent sinus infections.

Colds

Colds are often referred to as "URIs," for *upper respiratory infections*. Everyone gets colds and has experienced first hand what they are: They are infections of the nose and throat that may produce mucus in the nose, sneezing, and a sore throat. The person with a cold feels generally bad. There may or may not be a fever. Often, there is some cough, and scientists don't agree about the cause of the cough. Some say the cough means that there is inflammation in the trachea and bronchi, as well as in the nose and throat, whereas others say that it results from nose (or sinus) mucus dripping down the back of the throat and tickling the nerves that activate the cough.

Colds are caused by viruses. The main source of cold viruses is other people. People catch colds from other people, who have the cold viruses in their noses and throats. The closer the contact with the infected secretions, the easier it is to catch cold. Sneezing on someone is probably one way to give that person your cold, but the most common way the cold virus is passed around is from one person's respiratory secretions to his or her hand, to the next person's hand, and to that person's mucous membranes in the nose or eyes. Despite what everyone's grandmother has said, *you do not get colds from going out without your galoshes* (or from playing in the snow, or from being outside in cold weather)! In fact, it's probably safer to be outside during cold weather than inside, where there is less ventilation and closer contact with people who might have cold viruses in their noses and on their hands. During the fall and winter seasons, children in day care or school are almost constantly in contact with cold viruses, and are likely to carry those viruses home with them to share with the whole family.

Avoiding colds. Unfortunately, little can be done to avoid catching colds. It is possible to try to avoid colds by staying away from all public places, such as shopping malls, church or synagogue, and school. However, even this will not be effective in avoiding all contact with the cold viruses. While it is probably sensible to avoid snuggling with someone who has a terrible cold, this also won't do the trick completely, since people can have the cold viruses—and pass them on—*before* they feel sick with a cold themselves.

Most colds for people with CF are no worse than colds for other people: You feel miserable, but they do not damage the lungs and they have no long-lasting consequences. Some colds definitely can lead to bronchial infection and can be serious, especially in infants, whose bronchi are tiny and therefore harder to clear of infection. Bronchial infections can be more serious than an infection that stays in the nose and throat, but most often bronchial infections can be successfully treated. In some cases, it may actually be helpful to get a cold. When we are exposed to viruses, our body's immune system produces antibodies that will prevent infections with these same viruses when we are exposed to them at another time. Many infections are more severe later in life, so it's good to get them early and get them over with (mumps and chickenpox are viral infections that are more severe in adults than in children). This doesn't mean that people with CF should try to get as many colds as possible. It just means that it's not worth losing sleep worrying about colds, and no one should disrupt the patient's or family's life in attempting to avoid all colds.

Infections of the Lower Respiratory Tract

Colonization and Infection

Most patients with CF have some bacteria in their lungs most of the time (people without CF do not). Whether the bacteria are merely colonizing the lungs (that is, the bacteria are there and have set up colonies, but aren't causing any inflammation or destruction) or whether there is actual infection (that is, bacteria are present and the body has set up an inflammatory reaction to those bacteria, possibly with tissue damage) may be hard to say at any one time. This question has become even harder to answer now, because recent studies have shown that some patients with CF may have bronchial inflammation even without any bacteria or viruses present.

Bronchiolitis

Bronchiolitis (infection and inflammation of the bronchioles) is most commonly seen during the winter months in babies, with or without CF, and is most often caused by viruses. As many as four babies in 100 without CF will get bronchiolitis in the first 2 years of life. Babies with bronchiolitis may cough and wheeze, become very sick, and need extra oxygen. They may tire to the point of being unable to breathe independently, and require assisted ventilation, also called *mechanical ventilation*. Both of these terms mean that a machine is used to do the work of breathing for the baby by blowing air and oxygen into the baby's lungs. Of course, like most other infections, bronchiolitis can also be a mild disease and can cause just a little cough and wheezing. Many infants with CF have bronchiolitis as the first sign of a lung problem.

Bronchitis

Bronchitis (infection and inflammation of the bronchi) is a term that is often used incorrectly, referring to a cough that has no obvious cause. Many children and adults with CF have true bronchitis, which is caused by bacteria. Bronchiolitis and bronchitis are the main types of infection that affect the lungs of people with CF. It is these infections that, if not controlled, can lead to lung damage and scarring (fibrosis). Therefore, controlling the episodes of increased infection and inflammation in the bronchi is the most important part of the treatment of someone with CF. The more lung damage can be prevented or delayed in someone with CF, the better and longer that person's life is likely to be.

Pneumonia

Pneumonia occurs when bacteria, or the blood cells sent to fight bacteria, get into the air sacs (alveoli) or in the lung tissue between the sets of airways. Bacteria and white blood cells are frequently found in these areas in people with CF, but since the infection starts and is mostly confined to the airways, CF lung infections are most accurately thought of as bronchiolitis and bronchitis, and not as pneumonia. Even if the illness of someone with CF is diagnosed as "pneumonia," it is almost never the dreaded kind of pneumonia that kills elderly nursing home patients.

Causes of Lung Infection in Cystic Fibrosis

Often it is not clear why a particular lung infection occurs, or why it gets out of control when it does. In some instances it is clear, as, for example, when someone has a cold, and a slight cough that develops into a worse cough remains long after the runny nose has disappeared. In a case such as this, the virus infection that caused this cold has thrown off the balance of the lung defenses enough for some of the hardier bacteria in the lung to multiply and cause problems. In someone who has asthma, the asthma may become worse because of pollution, allergies, cigarette smoke, and so forth, and lead to a serious infection (it may be difficult in this case to tell how much of the problem is asthma and how much is infection, and which came first). In some cases, there is no explanation of why a lung infection has gotten worse.

Bacteria, Viruses, and Fungi

Bacteria and viruses are the most important types of germs that cause infection in people with CF; fungi can occasionally cause problems as well.

Bacteria. Bacteria are probably the major cause of bronchial infection (and lung damage) in people with CF. Bacteria are larger than viruses and can usually be killed by antibiotics. Normally, the number of bacteria in the lungs of someone with CF is relatively small, and the body's defenses (immune system) are able to keep these bacteria under control. But, when something happens to offset this balance, the bacteria can multiply and cause inflammation. In this situation, there is bronchial infection and not just colonization.

There are several different bacteria (which seem to change their names as often as some people change their socks) that most often colonize and infect the lungs of people with CF: *Haemophilus influenzae*, sometimes called *H. flu* (not to be confused with the influenza virus); *Staphylococcus*, or "staph"; and *Pseudomonas aeruginosa*. Other bacteria that can be found include *Klebsiella* and *Serratia* species, *Escherichia coli*, *Stenotrophomonas maltophilia* (formerly called *Xanthomonas maltophilia* and before that *Pseudomonas maltophilia*—!), *Alcaligenes xylozoxidans* and *Burkholderia cepacia* (formerly called *Pseudomonas cepacia*). *Streptococcus* organisms, which causes "strep throat," and *Pneumococcus* organisms, sometimes called the "pneumonia germ" because it is the most common cause of pneumonia in people with normal lungs, are not especially common in people with CF.

The most prevalent bacteria affecting people with CF are *Staphylococcus* organisms and the various types of *Pseudomonas*. Over 80% of people with CF eventually have *Pseudomonas* organisms in their throat or sputum cultures. The *Pseudomonas* family has a reputation, which is only partially deserved, of being particularly dangerous bacteria. Although most *Pseudomonas* organisms are harder to kill than other bacteria—especially with antibiotics that are taken by mouth—it is not true that *Pseudomonas* (or any other particular bacteria) are the kiss of death. The important factor is not *what bacteria* are in the lung, but rather *what harm* they are causing. Although it is probably true that —*as a group*—the few patients who never have *Pseudomonas* organisms on their cultures survive longer than patients who do have *Pseudomonas* organisms on cultures, the generalities that apply to groups are not useful in considering individual patients. Many people with CF have *Pseudomonas* colonization of the bronchi for many years and experience little or no trouble. If someone has no cough, no problems exercising, and no trouble breathing, it doesn't much matter if a throat or mucus culture has shown *Pseudomonas* organisms. On the other hand, if someone does have all those problems, and the culture grows only *Staphylococcus*, the person is still sick.

Some years ago, it appeared that *B. cepacia* was an especially dangerous form of bacteria, causing death shortly after colonization, and it does appear that some forms of these bacteria are very serious. It is now clear, however, that this is not always the case, and that some types of *B. cepacia* are no worse than other CF bronchial bacteria, like *Pseudomonas* organisms. The major issues are how much damage they cause and how readily they are killed by antibiotics.

Mycobacteria are bacteria in the tuberculosis (TB) family. There have been cases of patients with CF getting TB (that is, infection with *Mycobacterium tuberculosis*). TB can be serious, but is very uncommon in patients with CF. Much more common in CF is finding a culture that's positive for *nontuberculous mycobacteria* (NTM), also called *atypical* mycobacteria, that is, bacteria in the same family, but that don't cause TB. These bacteria may occur in nearly 15% of patients over 10 years old. The most common NTM are *Mycobacterium avium* complex (MAC), *Mycobacterium abscessus* (formerly known as *Mycobacterium chelonae*), *Mycobacterium fortuitum,* and *Mycobacterium kansasii*. The effect of these organisms on the health of people with CF is unclear. There are some patients who seem to have disease caused by these organisms (sicker when they get positive cultures for these bacteria, better after specific treatment), yet overall, one study showed better pulmonary function among patients with CF who had positive cultures than those with negative cultures! Your physician may want to do fairly extensive testing, perhaps including bronchoscopy and computed tomography (CT) scans, to try to decide if the atypical mycobacteria are causing disease, and need to be treated, or are just present without causing harm. It's an important decision, because the treatment lasts as long as 18 months.

Viruses. Viruses are smaller than bacteria, and generally cannot be killed by medicines. Antibiotics have no effect on viruses. Viruses are the most common cause of upper respiratory infections (colds), and may affect the bronchi as well. Not only can viruses cause infection, but infection with viruses makes it easier for bacteria to take hold in the bronchial tree, perhaps because the viruses interfere with mucociliary clearance. Some 20% of episodes of increased bronchial infection in patients with CF are associated with virus infections (either viruses alone or together with bacteria). Some of the common respiratory viruses are *respiratory syncytial virus* (RSV), parainfluenza virus, rhinovirus, and influenza virus. This last virus, influenza ("flu"), causes epidemics in the winter, afflicting many people with miserable coldlike symptoms. Influenza can cause a very serious pneumonia, which can even be fatal.

Some of the common childhood illnesses, such as chickenpox, measles, mumps, and rubella (German measles), are caused by viruses. On rare occasions, measles can cause a very serious pneumonia. This is true of chickenpox (varicella) as well, although chickenpox pneumonia is extremely rare in people with CF.

Fungi. Fungi, especially the fungus *Aspergillus fumigatus*, are sometimes found in the bronchi of patients with CF. They can cause trouble, but not usually in the same way as viruses or bacteria. The problem with *Aspergillus* organisms is not infection with tissue damage, but rather an allergic reaction (*allergic bronchopulmonary aspergillosis,* or *ABPA*), which induces swelling within the bronchi. This can cause cough, wheeze, and worsened pulmonary function. In many patients with CF, *Aspergillus* organisms may be present and cause no problems at all. As many as 80% to 90% of patients with CF have *Aspergillus* organisms in their airways at one time or another, and only 2% to 3% of patients have ABPA in a given year. It can be difficult to tell the difference between the symptoms of ABPA and those caused by bacterial infections. One of the main ways to diagnose ABPA is by checking the level of *IgE* (immunoglobulin E—a protein whose level is elevated in allergic conditions and *very* elevated in ABPA) in the bloodstream.

Treatment of the Lungs in Cystic Fibrosis

Since the main problems in the lungs are obstruction of bronchioles and bronchi and the resulting infection and inflammation, treatment is aimed at relieving bronchial blockage and fighting infection and inflammation. There are also some general principles to be observed.

General

CF is unusual in how very much of the outcome (how healthy someone is, indeed, how long people live) can be influenced by what the patient and family do for care of the patient's lungs. Being careful not to miss treatments (or to miss as few as possible), getting adequate rest and exercise, paying attention to good nutrition, avoiding cigarette smoke, and having regular CF clinic visits all have been associated with better outcomes.

Cigarette Smoke

Everyone knows that smoking is not good for the smoker. More and more people are beginning to realize that it's also harmful for "innocent bystanders," who breathe the smoke coming from the end of the cigarette (*sidestream smoke*) or the smoker's exhaled smoke (*secondhand smoke*). This has been shown very clearly for patients with CF: Those who are exposed to smoke in the home have worse lungs than those who aren't. Period. So, parents who smoke should not, or—at a minimum—should not smoke in the house (even from another room, the smoke can get to where it can do harm) or in the car. Parents who have thought about quitting for their own health but haven't been able to are often able to stop for their children's health and life. (In many cases, the drive to protect our children is even stronger than the drive to protect ourselves.) Certainly, teenagers and adults with CF who feel peer pressure to take up smoking should resist that pressure.

Medical Care

Regular checkups with your CF physician are extremely important for detecting small signs of lung infection and inflammation before these problems have caused irreversible damage. When someone appears to be doing well, it is very tempting to put off a time-consuming (and perhaps expensive and anxiety-producing) visit to the CF center, but these visits are important. One study showed a clear difference in actual patient survival between centers that saw their patients frequently (best survival) and those that saw their patients less frequently (worst survival). Visits to your regular pediatrician or family doctor are also important for good health maintenance.

Relieving and Preventing Obstruction: Airway-clearance Techniques

Chest Physical Therapy

A major portion of most treatment programs is aimed at keeping the airways as free of mucus as possible. The methods seem crude, but are quite effective. The most common method is based on a principle taken from everyday life, namely, the "Ketchup Bottle Principle": If you want to get a thick substance out of a container with a narrow opening, you turn the container upside down so that its opening is pointing downward, and then you clap it, shake it, and vibrate it. If the thick substance is mucus, and the container is the various segments of the lungs, the procedure is the same, and may be equally effective: You turn the child (or yourself) in various positions, with each position allowing one of the major portions of the lungs to have its opening pointing downward, and then you clap firmly on the back or chest over that part of the lung, and actually shake the mucus loose (for details on positioning for these treatments, see Appendix C, *Airway-clearance Techniques*). Once it's shaken loose, the mucus can fall into the large central airways, and then be coughed out. This form of treatment goes by many different names, a few of which are *postural drainage*, *chest physical therapy* (chest PT, or just CPT), and *percussion and drainage*. Often, children and families invent their own pet names: "exercises," "clapping," "boom-booms."

CPT treatments are not painful; in fact, they can be very soothing and relaxing in the way that a massage is. Babies who may be crying at the beginning of their CPT are often asleep halfway through the procedure. The treatment can be time-consuming, however (from 1 to 2 minutes for each of ten or 12 positions), and can be a bother to children, adolescents, and adults alike, since it interferes with the day's agenda. It may also keep an older child or adult tied to home, since it is awkward to perform on oneself and may require accommodating to someone else's (usually a parent's) schedule.

There are several pieces of equipment that make these treatments easier to perform at home. The first is the vibrating vest. This looks a bit like a life vest, and it is hooked to high-pressure air hosing that rapidly inflates and deflates the vest, causing a vibrating that helps shake loose airway mucus. Although it cannot be used in the very youngest infants and children, it seems to have been helpful in many adults and children over 3 years or so. There is little scientific proof of its effectiveness, but some families have felt it to be even more effective than manual CPT. It is very expensive (about $17,500). It has the advantage of freeing an adult or adolescent patient from dependence on someone else (parent, most often; perhaps a spouse) for treatments, and the corresponding advantage of freeing that parent or spouse from the time-consuming and sometimes physically challenging job of manual CPT. Another in the category of "devices you wear" is a percussor pack, which you slip on like a backpack. This device has pistons inside the pack pounding on the back. Some patients have found these packs useful. Another device is the mechanical percussor/vibrator. This tool comes in a variety of models, the simplest of which is like an electric jigsaw that instead of a blade has a rod with a firm cushion on it. The cushion is held on the chest and bounces firmly and repeatedly where it is aimed. Most models have variable force and speed; some models are driven by electricity and others by compressed air. The action of some models is a pounding motion, whereas others vibrate; some models can do both, depending on the setting selected. Treatments with the good mechanical percussors can probably be just as effective as those done by hand.

Some children (and adults, too) have a strong preference for the hand, whereas others prefer the machines. Clearly, a treatment by either method is considerably more effective than no treatment at all.

Another device that simplifies treatment is a PT table. Although vest treatments are done entirely with the patient in the seated position, manual CPT requires the patient to be turned in many different positions, which can be awkward. Treatments for infants and small children are done most comfortably with the child on a parent's lap, but when the patient outgrows the parent's lap (either because of size or not wanting to be treated "like a baby"), the table becomes very useful. The person receiving the treatment can sit or lie on the table, which can be set at different angles, thereby making proper positioning easier to achieve.

There are several airway-clearance techniques that do not involve hitting the chest, but seem to be very effective for adults, adolescents, and children old enough to cooperate: The first of these uses the *Flutter* valve. This is a handheld device, small enough to carry around in your pocket, that looks a little like a kazoo. It has a stainless-steel ball in it that vibrates up and down (flutters, you might say) as you blow into the tube. The vibrations are transmitted backward down through the patient's mouth into the trachea and bronchi, where they shake mucus free from the bronchial walls. Many teenagers and adults who had done traditional CPT for years have become "Flutter converts," saying that the Flutter is more effective in helping them bring up mucus, letting them feel when there's excess mucus there, and to know when they've cleared their airways. Like some of the mechanical devices, the Flutter has the advantage of enabling patients to work on airway clearance without help (except perhaps the reminder from a parent that so many children seem to need to do any job). The *Acapella* and *Resistex* are newer devices that work similarly to the Flutter.

Other techniques have had more use in Europe than North America. These techniques include one called a PEP mask (*positive expiratory pressure*). The patient breathes through a special mask that has an exhale valve that requires some air pressure to open. It is thought that this expiratory pressure is transmitted back down the airways and helps to prop them open during the exhalation, allowing mucus to be pushed out along with the air (remember that usually during exhalation, the airways tend to narrow a little bit, so this keeps them wider open than they'd normally be). Another method is called the *active cycle of breathing technique*. This technique has three phases: breathing control (quiet breathing), thoracic expansion (deep breaths in), and forced expiration or huffs (quick, strong—but never violent—breaths out, with the mouth and throat open). Autogenic drainage involves a series of breaths controlled so that some are done with very little air in the lungs, some with a medium amount, and some done with the lungs filled almost to capacity. This technique requires instruction by someone very skilled in its use before it can be effective in mobilizing mucus.

Exercise

Many people believe that vigorous exercise may be helpful to loosen mucus and to keep bronchi clear. Certainly, hard exercise, laughing, or crying often result in a coughing spell that brings up mucus, even in people who do not raise mucus during the traditional chest PT treatments. Since there is not yet any scientific evidence that exercise can successfully replace the time-honored PT treatments, it is best to encourage patients to be very active *and* to do their treatments. Several studies have shown that exercise *plus* CPT treatments clear more mucus than CPT treatments alone. (Exercise is discussed at greater length in Chapter 10, *Exercise*.)

An Important Note on Airway-clearance Treatments

One important point to keep in mind is that a method may be helpful even if it does not result in the immediate expectoration of large amounts of mucus. Mucus might be shaken loose from the smallest bronchioles and started on its way to the central bronchi, but it will not cause a cough until it actually reaches the large, central bronchi. There is good evidence that regular airway-clearance treatments are helpful, even though a single treatment makes little or no apparent difference. In one study, a number of children stopped their CPT for 3 weeks and had a significant deterioration in their lung function (even though they didn't *feel* any different); when they resumed their treatments after the 3-week experimental period, their lung function returned to its previous level. This can be a problem for patients with CF and their families: The treatments are time-consuming, and it is not uncommon to see or feel no obvious results right after the treatments. That means it's easy to convince yourself that skipping the treatments won't hurt. But it will! All too often, people have realized too late that they have harmed their lungs by not keeping up with their treatments. Of course, for many patients with CF, the benefit of the treatments is obvious even during the individual treatment sessions.

Breaking up Mucus

For decades, the idea of somehow breaking up, thinning, or watering down the thick CF airway secretions has been appealing, and numerous attempts have been made to accomplish this end, most of them not very successful. For many years, patients with CF slept all night in *mist tents*, which surrounded them with a dense fog of water. It turned out that this didn't really help. The next approach—still used by a very few patients—was a medication called acetylcysteine (Mucomyst), which is inhaled as an aerosol. When Mucomyst is mixed with CF mucus in a test tube, it does make the mucus thinner and easier to move. However, human bronchi and tracheas are different from glass test tubes, and may react with inflammation when Mucomyst is inhaled. Some people have developed increasing bronchial obstruction because of inflammation, or even bronchospasm, after inhaling Mucomyst. While some people do improve with this treatment, most are neither helped nor hurt by it.

There is now a new era in thinning bronchial mucus, based on our better understanding of what makes CF mucus thick. Remember that DNA that's been released from white blood cells is an important component of CF mucus; it happens to account for some 40% of the stickiness of CF mucus. There is now a genetically engineered medication that breaks down this DNA: DNase (the ending "-ase" refers to enzymes that break down other substances). DNase (*Pulmozyme*) is extremely effective in liquefying CF mucus in the test tube (as was true of Mucomyst). Taken by aerosol, it also seems to be very safe for most patients with CF (with the possible exception of those with very severe lung disease and huge amounts of mucus in their airways—these patients do better if all that mucus is not mobilized all at once). So, it works in the test tube and is safe. Does it work in people with CF and is it effective in helping people get mucus out of their lungs? The answer is yes, for some patients. Studies in large numbers of patients have suggested that breathing in DNase once a day does seem to bring about a small (5%) improvement in lung function as compared to the gradual deterioration that might be expected. Perhaps surprisingly, this benefit is not restricted to patients with a lot of trouble bringing up thick mucus, but seems to help improve lung function even in some patients with mild lung disease. It is not clear exactly how the drug has its effect in patients without obvious problems with large amounts of airway mucus: Is it that there *is* a lot of mucus in the smallest bronchi and bronchioles that affects lung function without causing a lot of cough or other symptoms, and this mucus is mobilized "silently" by DNase, or perhaps that the drug works in an entirely different way?

Whatever its reason for working, it does help many patients. However, not everyone does benefit, and the drug is extraordinarily expensive: about $12,000 a year in 2003. The approach many CF doctors have taken is to have patients try DNase for a month or so, comparing pulmonary function before and after. If the patient feels better, and/or the pulmonary function tests (PFTs) have shown an improvement, then it makes sense to use it. There are some patients who do feel better, without any measurable improvement, and we don't know how to explain this.

It is possible that even better mucus-thinning medications—or combinations of medications—will be developed.

Treating Asthma

When asthma is present in addition to CF, there is increased bronchial obstruction with which to contend. Bronchospasm makes the opening of the bronchi smaller than normal, making it much more difficult to get the mucus out. Several very effective bronchodilator medications that dilate (open) the bronchi are available. These medications can be inhaled as an aerosol, or taken by mouth or injection. The aerosols are delivered by an aerosol machine, which is composed of an air compressor, a length of tubing, and a nebulizer (Figure 3.4). The compressor sends air through the tube to the nebulizer, which holds the liquid medicine. As the air rushes by, it lifts the medicine, breaks it into a mist, and blows it out through the mouthpiece or mask to be inhaled. Some medications are available in handheld metered-dose inhalers (Figure 3.5). These devices deliver a measured amount of medicated mist with each puff. Since the puff of medicine is only available for breathing in for a fraction of a second, the timing of the puffing and breathing in is crucial, and may be quite difficult to coordinate, especially for small children. Extension devices are available that attach to the opening of the inhaler and temporarily trap the medication until the next breath, making the timing less crucial. Some aerosol bronchodilator medications

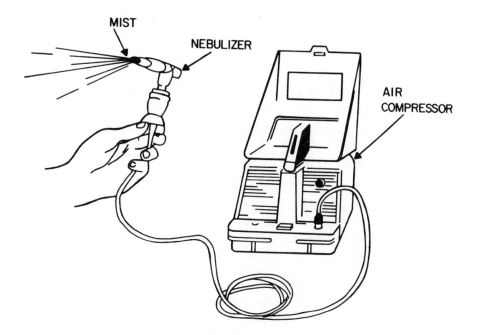

FIGURE 3.4. Aerosol machine. The machine blows compressed air through the tubing, over the liquid medication that is held in the cup of the nebulizer, creating a mist from the liquid medication. The patient then breathes the medicine.

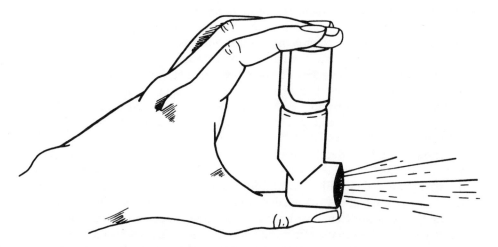

FIGURE 3.5. Handheld nebulizer (also called metered-dose inhaler or MDI). Pushing down the top of the inhaler causes a puff of medicated mist to shoot out into the air, for the patient to breathe.

are albuterol (Ventolin, Proventil) and salmeterol xinafoate (Serevent) (see Appendix B, *Medications*).

Oral bronchodilators include some of the same medications that are inhaled. These are all in the family of β-adrenergic drugs (especially albuterol). They don't work nearly as well as the inhaled drugs, and are more likely to cause side effects. Another family of bronchodilators that can be taken by mouth is the theophyllines. Theophylline is related to caffeine, which is actually a weak bronchodilator. Theophylline comes in the form of a liquid, tablet, or capsule (fast-acting or sustained-release) (see Appendix B, *Medications*).

Reducing Airway Inflammation

Airway inflammation often accompanies infection and/or asthma (see prior section, *The Lower Respiratory Tract*), making the airway opening that much smaller, and possibly damaging the cells that line the airway. Although inflammation is a normal part of fighting infection (see prior section, *Other Protection Against Lung Infection*), if it gets out of control it can do more harm than good. Excessive inflammation appears to be a very important cause of the progressive damage to CF airways; therefore, prevention and treatment of airway inflammation has become an important focus of CF research. Some medications, most notably a group of drugs called *steroids*, can reduce inflammation wherever it occurs, including in the bronchial tree. Within the past few years, prednisone (one of the steroids) has been studied in a number of people with CF and has appeared to be effective in improving their lung function.

Prednisone, however, is a very potent drug that has many possible side effects (see Appendix B, *Medications*). One of the most serious of these side effects is *oversuppression* of the immune response, which makes the body unable to fight infection. Prednisone can also bring out a tendency to develop diabetes, and can interfere with growth. Although the chances of dangerous side effects are much lower if prednisone is given on alternate days (Monday-Wednesday-Friday, etc.), instead of every day, there are still some risks. In fact, in the largest study done to date in patients with CF, prednisone was given on alternate days, and improved pulmonary function, but (after a couple of years) did cause side effects in some patients, so if prednisone is to be used, patients need to be checked fairly frequently.

Steroids have been developed in a form for inhalation, and these drugs have been very helpful in preventing airway inflammation in people with asthma. It is not yet known if they will be helpful for people with CF, although preliminary results are promising. As the inhaled steroids are not absorbed into the bloodstream (or are absorbed in only tiny amounts), side effects from inhaled steroids are much less a concern than from oral or injected steroids. Another inhaled drug called *cromolyn sodium* (Intal) has been known for years to be useful in preventing airways inflammation in people with asthma. Cromolyn sodium has not yet been shown to be helpful for people with CF, but it has barely been studied.

(Unlike most drugs, cromolyn sodium has close to zero side effects.) It has the drawback of needing to be given three to four times a day to be effective.

Other drugs reduce inflammation without interfering with the body's ability to fight infection. These drugs include aspirin, ibuprofen, and related drugs, which are used for people with arthritis. A small study with ibuprofen in patients with CF gave promising results: The drug seemed to slow the rate of decline of pulmonary function over a 4-year period. However, ibuprofen has its own problems, as well. Many (non-CF) patients taking the high doses of ibuprofen needed for the beneficial effects have had bleeding ulcers, while others have had kidney failure. Although these worrisome side effects have not been seen commonly in patients with CF, worry about them has kept many CF doctors from prescribing ibuprofen for their patients. The antibiotic azithromycin has been shown to have some antiinflammatory effects, apart from its bacteria-killing effects, and a recent study showed improved pulmonary function in patients with CF with positive cultures for *Pseudomonas* organisms. Some experts think the improvement can be attributed to reduced inflammation. Studies are currently under way to see if other medications might have antiinflammatory effects without side effects.

Reducing Bronchial Infection

Antibacterial Drugs (Antibiotics)

Antibiotics are probably the most important single factor responsible for the tremendous improvement in the outlook for people with CF, both in terms of length of life and quality of life. Antibiotics are very effective in reducing airways infection, and therefore in preserving lung health. (See Appendix B, *Medications*, for a more complete discussion of antibiotics.) Most CF physicians agree that antibiotics should be used when there is evidence of increased airways infection (such as increased cough and mucus production and decreased exercise tolerance). There is no agreement, however, on whether it is helpful to give antibiotics on a regular basis to *prevent* infection. One large multicenter study suggested that the *preventive* ("prophylactic") use of continuous antibiotics was *not* helpful for young patients with CF.

Oral antibiotics are usually taken when the infection is caused by *Staphylococcus* or *Haemophilus* organisms. (See Appendix B for a review of these antibiotics.) Oral antibiotics may also be helpful for *Pseudomonas* infections, but most often throat and sputum culture results will say that they will not work, and in fact, in many cases they will *not* bring these infections under control. If this is the case, the patient may need treatment with aerosol or intravenous (IV) antibiotics. Compared to oral antibiotics, the aerosol and IV antibiotics are more powerful, more likely to get to the site of infection within the bronchial tubes, or both. IV antibiotics most often require a hospital stay (see Chapter 7, *Hospitalization and Other Special Treatments*).

Preventing Bacterial Infection: "Infection Control"

There is no proven effective method for preventing bacterial bronchial infections. However, in recent years, people have devoted a *lot* of attention and energy to ways of reducing the risks of developing and maintaining bacterial infection in CF airways. Two of the areas that have received the most attention (and that have caused the most emotional upset among patients with CF, families, and caretakers) are (a) *patient-to-patient transmission of bacteria* and (b) the first positive culture for *Pseudomonas* organisms.

Patient-to-patient Transmission of Bacteria: Contact with Other Patients with Cystic Fibrosis and Their Bacteria

The sources of bronchial infection in patients with CF are not completely understood. Some of the bacteria and viruses that cause these infections are all around us, in the air, in soil, and so on. But, we have found out that some of the bacteria can be passed directly from one patient with CF to another. A prime example of this "person-to-person transmission" of CF airway bacteria is *B. cepacia*. As you've seen above, these particular bacteria that have in some cases been associated with an especially serious sickness. Because of dangers from *B. cepacia* for some people, and other bacteria, including *Pseudomonas*—especially those that are resistant to antibiotics—and because of the possibility of person-to-person spread of these bacteria, most experts are now recommending that patients with CF limit their contact with other patients with CF. These recommendations have been carried out in different ways by different individuals; and different CF centers and organizations have all set up different guidelines (or none at all). Nationally and internationally, there has been a lot of attention paid recently to "*infection control.*"

Some typical recommendations for infection control include:

- No direct physical contact (like kissing, or perhaps even hand-shaking) between patients with CF.
- No prolonged close contact between patients with CF (no playing together for young children, no long car rides together, etc.).
- No holiday parties for groups of CF families.
- No CF camps.
- Careful hygiene including thorough hand-washing (especially with the new alcohol-based products like Purell) for patients with CF and their caretakers; cover your mouth and nose during coughing spells, carefully dispose of tissue that has sputum in it, and so forth.
- Changes in procedures in clinic and during hospitalization:
  Clinic: Attempts to prevent prolonged waiting times in crowded waiting rooms. Some clinics have instituted a beeper system similar to what you find in some restaurants: check in, get a beeper, then go wander around until your beeper goes off, letting you know that your clinic room is ready.
  Hospital: Patients can't room together, can't be in the same room during aerosols or CPT; patients wear masks outside rooms; caretakers in some cases

wear masks and protective gowns and gloves when they are in contact with patients in their rooms.

Some hospitals have different guidelines or even strict rules for patients whose cultures have shown different bacteria or viruses. One example of this is an organism known as MRSA (for **m**ethicillin-**r**esistant *Staphylococcus aureus*). *Staphylococcus* organisms that are resistant to the antibiotic methicillin are fairly common among patients with CF, and are no more vicious or damaging than other *Staphylococcus* organisms, but are killed by fewer antibiotics. Because it is killed by fewer antibiotics, MRSA causes some hospital infection control experts to worry and to institute very strict isolation for patients who are "culture-positive" for this organism.

One of the things that makes these new recommendations difficult is that they are not all based on solid scientific proof. Take *masks*, for one example: It seems to make sense that wearing a mask should keep a patient from spreading his or her own germs to others or breathing in someone else's germs, but we don't really know that this is true, in all situations. Masks are different from each other and some are probably better than others; they probably work better right when they're put on, and less well as they get wetter from exhaled humid air. Bacteria are different, and some likely are blocked more effectively by masks than others, etc. In fact, a Cystic Fibrosis Foundation report on infection control released in 2003 concluded that the use of masks by patients with CF in the hospital was an "unresolved issue," and specifically said on this topic: "NO RECOMMENDATION."

Another challenge in this area is that different experts recommend different guidelines, and (as is true of experts in any field), some of these experts put forth their views—which might conflict with other experts' views—as the *only* right ones. Meanwhile, the nonexperts (patients, families, nurses, doctors) have to try to figure out what to do.

This is a very difficult issue to deal with. Patients with CF and their families have always received information, friendship, and a sense of shared experiences from contact with each other, and those patients who have had to spend any time in the hospital have been able to enjoy a fairly free fun time, with access to computers, play rooms, classrooms (okay, so that's not always *fun*) and other patients. It would be a shame to lose all that. It would also be a shame for someone who is relatively well to get dreadfully ill if that could have been avoided. Many patients have taken advantage of the Internet and e-mail to try to get around some of these problems—they can "talk" with other patients without fear of getting or giving someone harmful bacteria. Discuss these issues with your own CF physician. It should be possible to find a safe and humane approach that's right for you and your family.

Treating the First Pseudomonas Culture

This is a very new concern for patients and CF physicians. For decades, the approach in most good CF centers was to use the results of throat and sputum cultures *to help guide treatment, if treatment was warranted by the patient's symptoms or test results* (e.g., PFTs, see later in this chapter), and not to decide whether treatment was needed or not. The only exception to this approach was when *Streptococcus* organisms showed up unexpectedly on culture, meaning the patient had a "strep throat," which is almost always treated. Recently, however, there has been a lot of talk about aggressive antibiotic treatment for patients the first time (or times) *Pseudomonas* organisms show up on a throat or sputum culture. The reasons for this are that (a) it's probably better not to have *Pseudomonas* than to have it, and (b) it *might* be possible to get rid of *Pseudomonas* if its treated soon after it first appears in the lungs. This possibility has come mostly from the experience of patients with CF in Denmark, where CF physicians report that *Pseudomonas* organisms can be eliminated with early antibiotic treatment. Denmark is a country where in general antibiotics are used *very* aggressively in CF care. (For example, in Denmark, patients are admitted to the hospital for 2 weeks of IV antibiotics every 3 months year-round!) What is not yet known is whether the Danish experience can work here and whether there might be more negatives than positives to using antibiotics in patients with no symptoms. The possible benefit is clear: elimination of *Pseudomonas* organisms. The possible negatives include (a) *Pseudomonas* organisms developing resistance to antibiotics, thus making treatment more difficult when it's needed when a patient develops symptoms; (b) side effects from the antibiotics; and (c) expense. At the time this book goes to press, there is a multicenter study being planned to try answer this important question. In the meantime, patients and their physicians will have to act on the basis of their best beliefs and the latest information available.

Fighting Viral Infections

There are very few safe drugs that kill viruses, and, therefore, no safe, effective drug treatment for viral bronchiolitis or bronchitis. One possible exception is ribavirin, which seems to be effective for some very sick babies with bronchiolitis caused by the RSV. This drug is delivered by an aerosol, and must be breathed in for as long as 12 hours at a time. Ribavirin is not effective for infections caused by most other viruses, and specifically, it provides little benefit to people with colds.

Two other exceptions are amantadine hydrochloride and rimantidine hydrochloride, which appear to be helpful in fighting the influenza virus. They are taken by mouth and are used primarily by people who become infected with influenza during an epidemic. People who are at risk for influenza infection, such as patients with CF who have not had the flu vaccine, may also take one of these drugs as a preventive measure, during a community outbreak of influenza.

Preventing Viral Infections

See also *Avoiding Colds*, above.

The most common type of viral infection, namely, the common cold, cannot be effectively prevented (see above, *Infections of the Upper Respiratory Tract*).

There are other viral infections that can be prevented, though, including measles and influenza ("flu"). All children should be immunized against measles, and all children with CF (or other abnormal lung conditions) should receive a flu shot each year. These vaccines are effective and are safe except in people with very severe egg allergy.

There is a vaccine available that is supposed to prevent infection with RSV (see above). *Synagis* is a "monoclonal antibody" (see Appendix B, *Medications*) fairly widely used now for sick and tiny infants. This has to be given by injection once a month. There is no convincing evidence of its effectiveness in CF.

There is a *varicella* (chickenpox) vaccine available, and the American Academy of Pediatrics recommends it for all children. It is safe for children with CF. Another chickenpox-related medication is *zoster immune globulin*, or ZIG. It is not a vaccine, but rather a gamma globulin–like shot that is given to prevent chickenpox. Most CF physicians feel, however, that this is unnecessary for people with CF, since the chances that someone with CF would have lung complications from chickenpox are very small. In addition, a major drawback to ZIG is that once it is given, it has to be repeated every time there is an exposure to chickenpox. Nonetheless, some CF physicians recommend ZIG for nonimmunized patients who have been exposed to chickenpox. Others recommend "chickenpox parties" for children who have not yet had chickenpox. In this way, they will come in contact with a "poxy" child and contract chickenpox in childhood when it's likely to be mild, instead of in adulthood when it often follows a much more severe course.

Treating Allergic Bronchopulmonary Aspergillosis

The standard treatment for ABPA is oral steroids (usually prednisone) to suppress the allergic reaction that the aspergillus has caused. In some patients, it may be possible to decrease the number of *Aspergillus* organisms in the airway with the antifungal drug itraconazole. In these patients, the airway obstruction and symptoms caused by ABPA may be controlled with much lower steroid doses than would otherwise be possible.

Steps in Treating Worsened Lungs

In CF, the lungs get worse from time to time. These periods of worsening, called *pulmonary exacerbations*, are most often caused by increased airways infection and can usually be brought under control if proper steps are taken.

Recognition

In order for pulmonary exacerbations to be treated, they must first be recognized, which is not always easy. The signs that the lungs are worse may be very subtle and may at first escape attention. These signs include more cough than usual, more mucus, decreased energy, poor appetite, difficulty exercising, and shortness of breath. In most people, the amount of cough is the single most important clue. Many people will *not* have lessened activity or shortness of breath, nor will they have fever, so the absence of these clues should not be taken as a reassuring sign. It is important to recognize when there are more signs of infection than are usual for *you*, since everyone is different. For example, if your usual pattern is to cough only a little bit in the morning, but you begin to cough after laughing or crying and find that the cough lasts just a bit longer, then you will know that your condition is not quite as good as it usually is. On occasion, someone else, such as your doctor or a relative who doesn't see you every day, may point a difference out to you that you haven't noticed. Sometimes, however, it may take an x-ray or PFT to show that a change has occurred. For this reason, it is quite important to make fairly frequent clinic visits. It's very tempting to say, "I [or my child] am doing so well that there's no need to go for a checkup." There are far too many patients with CF (usually teenagers) and parents of patients who have used this reasoning, only to return to regular care after irreversible lung damage has been done. Regular visits, which would include physical examinations, throat or sputum cultures, and periodic chest x-rays and PFTs, can often spot a problem while it is still reversible. Since the progression of lung disease in CF is usually very gradual and subtle—and is *not* characterized by sudden dramatic deterioration—it is easy for patients and families to miss signs of deterioration. Your physician may be able to recognize these signs, because a change in the weeks or months since your last visit is easier to detect than small day-to-day changes, and because sensitive laboratory tests (PFTs and x-rays) help clarify your condition.

Once you have recognized that there is a problem, it is important not to wait until you're terribly ill to do something about it. That wait can give the infection and inflammation an opportunity to destroy a small portion of lung, leaving a little scar tissue behind. A little scar tissue with each inadequately treated infection adds up over the years. Scar tissue can never become normal lung tissue, so it's important to prevent its formation. It is impossible to tell at any one time whether bronchial obstruction is because these tubes are filled with mucus and bacteria and white blood cells—that could be gotten rid of—or because of permanent irreversible scarring.

Oral Antibiotics

During a period of worsening, your physician will probably prescribe an oral antibiotic or change the antibiotic if you are already taking one. The choice of antibiotics is based on several factors, including how the individual patient has responded in the past, how sick the person is at the time, and what recent throat or sputum cultures have shown (what bacteria are there and which antibiotics kill those bacteria in the laboratory). The physician may also increase the number of airway-clearance treatments you're doing in order to clear out the extra mucus that builds up with infections.

If an infection does not improve quickly, and certainly if it becomes worse, it is advisable to take the next step of changing antibiotics. This change will be to a more powerful antibiotic, or to one that is better at killing the particular bacteria a culture has shown to be in your system. If a more powerful or appropriate oral antibiotic is not available, or if the physician believes that an oral antibiotic would work too slowly, then he or she may recommend an aerosol antibiotic or even IV antibiotics. Most often, symptoms will improve nicely with oral antibiotic treatment. In fact, patients are often back to their *baseline* (usual state of health) even before the antibiotic prescription has run out. In these cases, it's tempting to stop the medicines as soon as you feel better, but this is usually not a good idea. Infectious disease experts tell us that one of the surest ways to make bacteria become resistant to an antibiotic (not be killed by it) is to give antibiotics for too short a time. So, if your doctor has prescribed 2 weeks of antibiotics, and your cough is gone (or back to your usual) in 1 week, you should take the second week of antibiotics anyway.

Aerosol Antibiotics

Several different kinds of antibiotics can be breathed directly into the lungs as aerosols, using the same kind of machine that we use for bronchodilator aerosols (Figure 3.4). The most commonly used aerosol antibiotics are TOBI (a special high-dose preparation of tobramycin, designed for aerosol administration), gentamicin (used in the nebulizer in its normal injectable form), and injectable tobramycin. There are widely varying dosages of these medications, and you should be sure you know how much your doctor wants you to take.

Intravenous Antibiotics

If these steps do not work, or do not work fast enough, it may be time for IV antibiotics. In almost every case, putting antibiotics into a vein is the most effective way of treating infection, especially if the infection is caused by *Pseudomonas* organisms. Typically, the administration of IV antibiotics requires a hospital stay, at least at the beginning of the course. In recent years, many patients have gotten all or part of their IVs at home. (For more information about IVs and hospitalization, see Chapter 7, *Hospitalization and Other Special Treatments*.)

The length of time to give IV antibiotics should be determined by how the patient is responding to treatment. Patients seldom improve (and may perhaps even worsen) in the first 4 or 5 days on IVs. Thereafter, most people improve for 1 to 3 weeks, and then return to their usual condition or even to an improved condition. On occasion, someone may stop improving without having returned to his or her previous baseline. Studies have shown that the level of lung function achieved after in-hospital IV treatment of a pulmonary exacerbation can be maintained for at least several weeks, but will not continue to improve after stop-

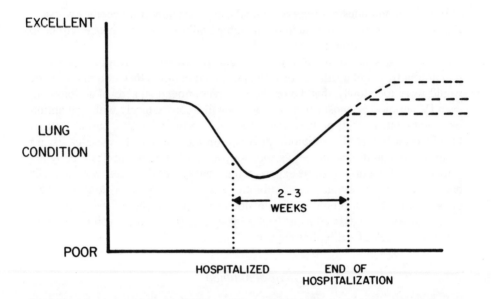

FIGURE 3.6. Timing of hospitalization. When it is recognized that the patient is not doing well out of the hospital, she or he is admitted to the hospital for treatment. Improvement begins within 4 or 5 days. Hospital treatment then continues until the patient has returned to her or his usual state of health. In theory, this same curve could be drawn for timing of intravenous antibiotic treatment, without regard to the setting (in or out of the hospital).

ping the IVs. Therefore, it makes sense to get the most mileage possible from the IV and hospital treatment and not to stop after a predetermined number of days have gone by. Some people will have gotten the maximum benefit from the intensive treatment in as short a time as 10 days, but most people take about 2 weeks, and quite a few people take even longer. Keep in mind that this invest-ment of time can pay off in the long run if it keeps even a small portion of lung from becoming scarred. Figure 3.6 shows a time curve for when someone should enter the hospital and when he or she should leave.

Other Treatments

In some cases, other treatments may be used with IV antibiotics or tried before them. One obvious example is increasing CPT; another (not as obvious) is try-ing medications to decrease bronchial inflammation, like prednisone. Another example is altering antiasthma medications by increasing their dosages or by adding different ones. The best steps to take will differ under different condi-tions.

General Questions About Using Antibiotics

How do we know whether to give antibiotics or not? For individual episodes of increased cough, we will often have the question, "Is this a cold that does not involve the lungs, and therefore shouldn't need antibiotics, or is it a bronchial infection, which definitely should be treated with antibiotics?" And, we can't always tell. Given that we can't tell for sure, we have to base treatment decisions on an educated *guess*, and keep in mind the possible consequences of a *wrong* guess. If we guess this is bronchial infection and it's really only a cold, we would have given unneeded antibiotics. The consequences of that mistaken decision would be: (a) financial (had to pay for antibiotics that weren't needed), (b) small risk of allergic or other reaction to the antibiotic, and (c) small theoretical risk of encouraging the bacteria to become resistant to the antibiotic. If, on the other hand, we guess this a simple cold with no bronchial infection, and we don't give antibiotics, and we've guessed wrong (there really was infection), then the consequences are much worse: possible lung damage, some of which could be irreversible. Given those choices, we'll almost always take the chance of giving antibiotics when they might not have been needed rather than not give them when they might have been needed.

What's too much antibiotics? Will I become "immune" to the effects of the antibiotic? People often worry that they or their bacteria will "become immune" to the antibiotics (or as physicians say, the bacteria become *resistant* to the antibiotics). This *can* happen over time, but not nearly as easily as many people fear. Furthermore, if the choice is between treating an infection that we *know* can cause lung damage—even irreversible damage—or not treating it because of the remotely *possible* development of resistance to a single antibiotic, most experts would go with the treatment every time. In fact, the history of CF has shown this to be the correct approach: We use a lot more antibiotics now than a few decades ago, and there are more resistant bacteria now, but patients live well into adulthood instead of dying before school age. A couple of important studies have shown that the pulmonary health and even survival of patients is better in centers that use a lot of antibiotics than in those that are stingy with their antibiotics.

What if we "run out" of antibiotics that are effective? On occasion, a patient's cultures (see the end of this chapter) may show that one or more of the bacteria in the lungs have become *resistant* to some, many, or even all of the available antibiotics. When this happens, it can be frightening to a patient or parent, for it may signal to them the end of effective treatment for lung infections. While it is undeniably better if the bacteria are all *sensitive* to readily available antibiotics, the problem of *resistance* is not completely straightforward, and therefore not always as bad as a culture report may make it seem. We have known for decades that patients often respond well to antibiotics that *shouldn't* work. Erythromycin, clarithromycin, and azithromycin (Zithromax) are antibiotics that have been used frequently and successfully for CF lung infection, even when cultures showed only *Pseudomonas* organisms that were resistant to these antibiotics. The same is sometimes true for tobramycin. Why should this be so? There are several possible explanations: One (as you'll see at the end of this chapter) is that "resistant" is not an absolute term; that is, although it may sound as though it means that the antibiotic in question has *no* effect on the particular bacteria, this is not the case. Often it means that the antibiotic doesn't kill *all* the bacteria, or that you need a lot of the antibiotic to kill the bacteria. So, *some* killing may be possible. Another important part of the explanation is that the testing for bacterial *sensitivity* or *resistance* takes place in a test tube or culture plate—not in the body. The body has its own defenses, including white blood cells, antibodies, and so on, that help to kill invading bacteria, and these aren't measured in the bacteriology laboratory. Additionally, the bacteria may be in a different form in the laboratory from their state in the body, so it's almost as if the laboratory is testing the effect of antibiotics on different bacteria from the ones in the lungs. Finally, it has become known in recent years that antibiotics have important effects other than their ability to kill bacteria. Erythromycin, for example, has usually been shown in the laboratory to be good for killing *Staphylococcus*, but not *Pseudomonas* organisms, yet it—and its newer cousin, azithromycin dihydrate—has seemed to be effective in improving the lungs of patients with CF whose only cultured bacteria are *Pseudomonas* organisms. Why? Well, we now know that erythromycin and azithromycin have powerful antiinflammatory effects separate from their ability to kill bacteria. Since *Pseudomonas* causes damage largely through inflammation (from the chemicals it itself releases and those released by white blood cells that have come to fight it), lessening the inflammatory response to *Pseudomonas* may do just as much good as killing it. In addition, as suggested above, the *Pseudomonas* organisms in the lung may be different enough from the way it is in the laboratory that it actually *is* being killed in the lung.

What if the culture reports are right, and the antibiotics really don't work any more? This happens occasionally, and is very serious. In these cases, when the antibiotics really seem unable to make a dent in a patient's symptoms of lung infection, the physician may try other means to fight inflammation (for example, steroids). In some unusual situations, physicians have been able to stop antibiotics for a while, and let the bacteria become sensitive to the antibiotics again, so that when the antibiotics are resumed, they are effective once again. This is a risky business, and you should definitely not try it without your doctor's direction, for there is a strong chance that it won't work, and stopping the antibiotics will allow the infection to worsen, without changing the sensitivity pattern of the bacteria.

Finally, there is the helpful fact that the pharmaceutical industry is well aware of the problem of emerging resistance, and is continually at work developing new antibiotics. As with so many other aspects of CF care, there is almost always hope even when things might appear bleak. If you're worried about your (or your child's) culture results and their implications for the future, be sure to let your doctor know.

Complications

There are several problems that can be an indirect result of CF. These problems are often referred to as *complications* of CF. The most important complications related to the lung disease of CF are hemoptysis, atelectasis, pneumothorax, respiratory failure, heart failure, and chest pain. Other complications that relate to the lung disease of CF affect the bones and/or the joints (and are discussed in Chapter 5, *Other Systems*).

Hemoptysis

The literal translation of this term is to "cough up blood" (*heme* is the Greek word for "blood," and *ptyein* translates as "to spit"). Hemoptysis is very uncommon in young children with CF, but as many as 50% of adults with CF will on occasion have some streaks of blood in the mucus they cough up and spit out. A relatively small proportion of patients (3% to 5% of those older than 15 years) will cough out large amounts (more than 10 oz) of blood at a time. This problem, called *massive hemoptysis*, can be fatal, although it rarely is, even in people who bring up very large amounts of blood. In most cases, the significance of hemoptysis is the same as that of an increased cough, namely, both are signs of increased infection. A major difference, however, between having a bit more cough than usual and bringing up bright red blood is that it is very frightening to see the blood, especially the first time it happens. One's first reaction is to panic and to assume that all of one's lungs must be bleeding. This is not the case: It's extremely important to know that *hemoptysis is a fairly common problem that is almost always simple to treat.*

What is happening is that the increased infection in one small area has irritated a capillary or small artery and made a small hole in its wall, causing blood to leak out into the airway. Remember that the size of the working surface of the lungs is about the same as a tennis court; the problem area in someone with hemoptysis is about the size of a little pebble on that tennis court. It helps to keep this in mind if you should see some blood mixed in with mucus sometime. If you see pure blood, you should notify your doctor, because you do need treatment, but there's no need to panic.

In unusual cases, hemoptysis can mean something other than just increased infection. It can indicate a more general bleeding problem. Bleeding problems can be caused by inadequate vitamin K (this would be uncommon in someone with CF who is getting a good diet and taking the prescribed enzymes), advanced liver disease, or rarely, a drug side effect. In some unusual situations, it may be difficult to tell where spit-up blood has come from. Bleeding in the stomach or esophagus can be confused with bleeding in the lungs. Fortunately, bleeding in the stomach or esophagus is not common in people with CF.

Treating Hemoptysis

The treatment required for someone who coughs up bloody mucus, or pure blood, depends on the cause of the bleeding. In most cases, the cause is an increase in bronchial infection that has irritated a blood vessel; therefore, the treatment is the same as the treatment for any increased infection, namely, antibiotics and airway-clearance treatments, such as CPT. There is little or no controversy about the need for antibiotics (or for stronger antibiotics in someone who is already taking antibiotics). Not all CF specialists agree on the usefulness of CPT, and, in fact, some experts recommend stopping CPT treatments in someone who has brought up a large amount of blood. However, in most cases, the clapping and vibrating are very unlikely to cause any bleeding and should be continued.

In some people who bring up blood, a gurgling sensation is felt in the chest (they can sometimes even tell which part of the lung it's coming from) just before the blood comes up. If someone feels a gurgling every time he or she goes into a particular position, the head-down position, for example, then that position should be avoided. In general, though, the treatments should be continued as much as possible, for three reasons: (a) the blood is not good for cilia and should therefore be removed, (b) the blood can make an infection worse by providing a hospitable environment for bacteria, and (c) even if the blood itself is not a problem, one of the underlying principles of treating bronchial infection in someone with CF is to lessen bronchial mucous obstruction as much as possible.

In most cases where a person has brought up a large amount (more than a cup) of pure blood, hospitalization is recommended. In the hospital, IV antibiotics can be given easily, and patients can be watched carefully to make sure the bleeding is under control. If the bleeding is very severe and much blood has been lost, blood transfusions may be necessary, just as they would be if the bleeding were caused by a car crash, for example. It is quite uncommon, however, for a transfusion to be required.

Extra vitamin K is usually given to someone with CF who has hemoptysis, since a lack of that vitamin can cause bleeding problems. If the bleeding is not controlled quickly, it may be necessary to do various tests. These tests would check for a generalized bleeding problem (as might occur in someone with severe liver disease) or examine the possibility that the bleeding is a side effect of a drug or drug combination.

In a few cases of massive hemoptysis that can't be controlled by the above means, methods that are more difficult may be needed. One such method is bronchoscopy, which allows the physician to look into the lungs with a flexible tube that goes through the nose and down the back of the throat or with a rigid tube that is passed directly down the throat. Most physicians, however, doubt that bronchoscopy is very helpful, and a different procedure is more likely to be recommended. This procedure is called *bronchial artery embolization*, and has been helpful in people with massive hemoptysis. An embolus is a clot or other plug in a blood vessel that blocks the circulation in that vessel (*embolos* is the Greek word for "plug"). Emboli are usually harmful, but they can also be helpful when a bronchial artery is leaking. In this case, a radiologist may be able to thread a catheter (a thin, flexible tube) into the artery and inject a plug (typically made of a synthetic substance called *Gelfoam*) or a plastic or metal coil through the catheter that will then seal the leak and stop the bleeding.

Several problems make this procedure less than perfect. The first is that it is not always possible to find the artery that is leaking, even with the sophisticated radiologic technology that is available. The second problem is that, in some people, arteries to the spinal cord may come from the bronchial arteries. If the Gelfoam plug or the coil blocks off the blood supply to a portion of the spinal cord, serious problems could result. Fortunately, with modern techniques, the radiologist can nearly always tell beforehand if the patient has such a spinal artery, and can plan the plugging accordingly. Lastly, a fair proportion of people whose bleeding has been stopped with bronchial artery embolization will bleed again from that spot in the future.

In a very few cases—when there is massive bleeding and bronchial artery embolization cannot be performed or is not successful—surgery may be necessary to remove the lobe of the lung that is the source of the bleeding. There are numerous problems with this approach, a major one being that, although the person will obviously not bleed again from the removed lobe, he or she will also not have the use of that lobe for breathing. In addition, general anesthesia and chest surgery carry their own risks, especially in someone with severe lung disease. Finally, even with the chest open, it may not be possible to identify the lobe that is the source of bleeding with absolute certainty. There are too many cases of patients with CF who have had a lobe removed in a hospital inexperienced in CF care, only to be transferred to a CF center because the bleeding didn't stop. Nonetheless, there *are* some cases in which surgery is necessary and very successful.

Because of the problems and uncertainties with the invasive means of dealing with hemoptysis, many CF experts prefer to treat patients—even those with massive hemoptysis—as conservatively as possible, with antibiotics, CPT, vitamin K, transfusions if necessary, and careful observation.

Pneumothorax

This complication is also called "collapsed lung." The term actually means "air inside the chest," which doesn't sound all that abnormal, since that's where air is *supposed* to be (inside the chest)–isn't air what the lungs hold? But it actually refers to air that's within the chest, but *outside the lung* (Figure 3.7). That is very abnormal, and can be dangerous, since once air gets outside the lung, it can press in on the lung and cause it to collapse. If there is enough air under enough pressure or tension, it can even squeeze the blood vessels (*venae cavae*) that bring

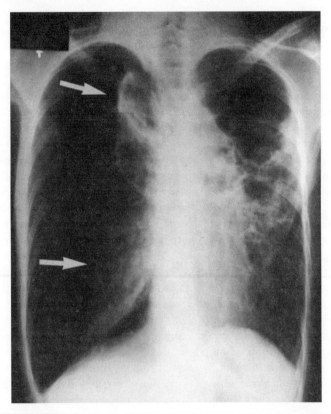

FIGURE 3.7. Radiographic appearance of pneumothorax. The air outside the lungs appears black, while the lungs are lighter in color. Arrows show edge of collapsed lung.

the blood back to the heart. This will mean that there won't be enough blood returning to the heart to be pumped out to the body to keep it functioning normally. This does not usually happen with a pneumothorax in someone with CF. It is unusual for pneumothorax to occur in someone under the age of 10, and after age 10, between 10% and 25% of patients with CF will develop a pneumothorax. Pneumothorax is much more likely to happen in someone with CF if there is relatively severe lung involvement than if the lungs are in very good shape.

Pneumothorax develops when mucus partially blocks a bronchus or bronchiole and functions as a one-way valve or "ball-valve" (Figure 3.8). This kind of blockage allows air to go in only one direction past the blockage. Bronchi enlarge with inhaling and get smaller with exhaling (see *The Airways*). When mucus fills up a portion of a bronchiole, the bronchiole will enlarge enough with each breath that some air can get beyond the mucous plug. But, during exhaling,

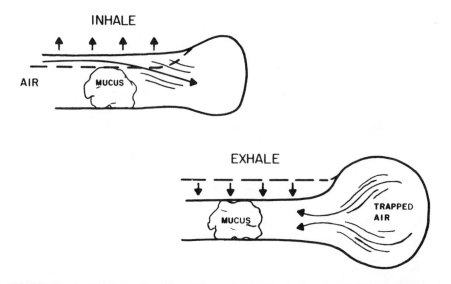

FIGURE 3.8. Partial obstruction of bronchi may cause progressive overinflation of a portion of lung, leading to pneumothorax. The bronchi enlarge slightly when one inhales, allowing air to get into the lungs past the mucus. When one exhales, the bronchi get smaller, trapping the air behind the blockage. With each breath, more and more air can become trapped, leading to progressive overinflation and eventual tearing of the tissue, allowing air to escape from the lung.

the bronchus may collapse to the same size as the plug, so no air will escape. When this happens, the alveoli beyond the blockage will get bigger with each breath in, until, like an overfilled balloon, they finally burst. If these overfilled alveoli are at the edge of the lung (especially at the *apex*, or top, of the lung), when they burst, the air leaks out of the lung.

A pneumothorax usually causes sudden sharp pain in the chest, side, or back, and difficulty breathing (shortness of breath). The only way to tell for certain if someone has a pneumothorax is with a chest x-ray (Figure 3.7). The x-ray will show an area inside the chest that is completely black, rather than the usual combination of white and gray; there will also be a clear outline to the edge of the collapsed lung. Some people "score" pneumothoraces on the basis of how much of the lung is collapsed on the x-ray film. A "25% pneumothorax" means that air outside the lung takes up 25% of the space that the lung normally occupies and that the lung itself has collapsed to 75% of its normal size. If someone with relatively healthy lungs develops a pneumothorax, this can be a useful description. But when a pneumothorax occurs in someone with CF, it's less helpful, since the lungs tend to be stiff in people with CF, and therefore may not collapse readily, even with quite a bit of air outside, under quite a bit of tension. So, what looks like a small amount of air may actually be a lot.

Since pneumothorax needs to be treated, you should let your doctor know if you ever develop sudden chest pain and shortness of breath.

Treatment of Pneumothorax

The treatment for pneumothorax usually requires hospitalization and is directed toward accomplishing three goals: (a) relieving the pressure on the lung by evacuating the air from around the lung, (b) sealing over the hole through which the air has escaped, and (c) ideally, preventing recurrence. There are rare instances in which there is a tiny pneumothorax—just the smallest bit of air outside the lung, with the leak already sealed off by itself—and no treatment is needed. Much more commonly, if there is a pneumothorax, all three treatment goals should be met.

The pressure is usually relieved by a *chest tube*. This is a tube that goes through the skin, between the ribs, and into the *pleural space*, which is the space between the chest wall and the outside of the lung. This is the space where air accumulates if it leaks out of the lung. The tube is hooked up to a vacuum that sucks the air out continuously and allows the lung to expand to its normal size. The system of tubing used to evacuate the air from the pleural space must have a good valving system (most often provided by having the tubes pass through a series of vacuum jars or a water seal) so that air can pass only out of the chest, and not back into it. The physician makes a small skin incision to place the chest tube, then pushes the tube into place and hooks up the vacuum. Placement of the tube can be painful, and having a tube in place is uncomfortable. If the treatment chosen is only chest tube placement, the treatment is often successful in the short run, but very unsuccessful in the long run. Since most air leaks will seal themselves eventually, a chest tube can evacuate the air, the air will stop accumulating, and the tube can be pulled out. Unfortunately, it may take many days for this self-sealing to occur, and during this time, the painful chest tube will interfere with the deep breathing and coughing needed to keep the lungs clear. Even when the leak does seal itself, between 50% and 100% of these pneumothoraces will recur within months or years unless further steps are taken to prevent this from happening.

There are two main approaches to sealing the leak and preventing recurrences of pneumothorax. Both approaches purposely cause inflammation of the pleural surface (the covering of the lung), almost like a burn, so that when the irritated, inflamed surfaces heal, the healing scar tissue will cover over any weak, leaky area. The first approach is called *chemical sclerosing* or chemical *pleurodesis*. For this method, it is necessary to have a chest tube in the pleural space (the space between the lung and the chest wall). An irritating chemical (such as tetracycline, talc, or quinicrine) is sent through the tube once a day for 3 days in a row. When the chemical is pushed through the tube, the patient rotates through different positions, holding each one for several minutes in order to distribute the chemical to all surfaces of the lungs. The head-down position is particularly important, since the weakest spots are usually at the apex (top) of the lung. If the treatment is successful, it causes intense inflammation, and therefore is often very painful. Pain medication before the daily procedure is essential.

Another method of causing inflammation of the surface of the lung is with a surgical operation, during which the patient is asleep under general anesthesia. The surgeon makes an incision between the ribs, spreads the ribs, and examines the lung for weak spots (*blebs*). These areas are then cut out, and the remaining hole is sewn closed. The next step is to strip the pleura off the upper part of the lung, which leaves the lung surface raw and irritated. The side and lower portions of the lung are more difficult to strip of their pleural covering, so the surgeon will take a piece of gauze and rub the surface roughly to set up the same kind of irritation and inflammation. (This whole procedure is referred to as *open thoracotomy, apical pleurectomy, and pleurabrasion*, which means "cutting the chest open, stripping the membrane off the uppermost portion of the lung, and rubbing the rest of the lung surface.")

When the chest is closed, a chest tube must be left in to drain the extra air outside the lung. Usually that tube can come out when the air has been fully evacuated, and when it is clear that the leaks have been sealed. Although this procedure sounds brutal, the patient is asleep and feels no pain. After the surgery, the main discomfort is from the chest tube, which is usually removed within a few days. It is surprising, but true, that most people have less discomfort with the surgical treatment than with the chemical sclerosing. This treatment by an experienced surgeon is nearly 100% successful in preventing recurrences of pneumothorax in the involved lung. In some cases, this time-honored procedure can be accomplished without actually opening the chest. Some specially trained and skilled surgeons can accomplish the pleural stripping and bleb sewing through a *thoracoscope*, a tube that can be inserted into the chest through a small incision in the chest wall. (This is similar to an arthroscope, which has allowed sports medicine orthopedic surgeons to operate on football players' knees without large incisions.) The surgeon looks through the thoracoscope while he or she manipulates special surgical *forceps* through another small hole in the chest wall. These forceps can grasp the pleura, and a similar tube can insert a device to staple over blebs. The surgeon can also inject a chemical (talc, for instance) through the thoracoscope to cause the necessary inflammation. Doing the procedure this way avoids a large chest incision, and greatly speeds recovery.

Treatment of pneumothorax has changed with the advent of lung transplantation (see Chapter 8, *Transplantation*), since the best treatment for preventing pneumothorax (surgery) may make future transplantation much more difficult. The scar tissue that is purposely promoted to seal leaking blebs and prevent future leaks will make it very difficult for a transplant surgeon to remove the lungs in order to put new ones in. Therefore, some physicians recommend a stepwise approach to pneumothorax in a patient who may one day consider transplantation, starting with no special treatment, getting progressively more aggressive, and ending with surgery, if steps short of the definitive surgery do not seal the leak.

Atelectasis

This term is derived from two Greek words (*ateles* and *ektasis*), meaning "incomplete" and "expansion," and refers to different kinds of incomplete expansion of the lung or part of the lung. Like pneumothorax, atelectasis is a kind of collapsed lung, but is very different from a pneumothorax. In someone with CF, atelectasis is usually caused by mucus that completely blocks a bronchus leading to one of the lobes or segments of a lung (much more often in the right lung than the left, and more often in the upper lobe than in other lobes). If the opening to a lobe or segment is blocked, air cannot get into that portion of the lung. Eventually all the air that was in that lobe or segment gets absorbed, leaving the lobe or segment airless. On a radiograph, it will appear white (solid) instead of the usual combination of white and gray (Figure 3.9). About one of every 20 people with CF will develop atelectasis at some point. This problem is more common in infants than older people, probably because their bronchi are smaller and therefore more readily blocked. Usually, atelectasis does not cause any specific signs or symptoms, but is likely to occur during a period of worsened lung infection.

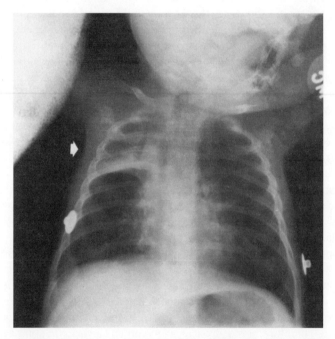

FIGURE 3.9. Radiographic appearance of atelectasis of right upper lobe (x-ray performed as though we are looking at the front of the child, so his right side is on our left). The portion of the lung with more mucus and less air (the atelectatic portion) appears white, while the rest of the lung is darker.

Treating Atelectasis

Since atelectasis occurs when mucus totally blocks the opening of the bronchi in a segment or lobe of a lung, the treatment is similar to the maintenance care designed to keep the bronchi clear on a regular basis. The mainstay of the treatment is airway-clearance techniques, especially CPT and percussion. Once atelectasis is identified, the physician will recommend increasing the frequency of CPT treatments, perhaps to as often as four times a day. Most physicians will also recommend antibiotics, since infection may have caused the bronchial obstruction (by generating more mucus), and may result from the obstruction. Physicians who don't usually advise their patients to inhale mucus-cutting drugs such as DNase (see Appendix B, *Medications*) may make an exception in treating atelectasis. There is little or no information to support its use in this particular circumstance, however.

Bronchoscopy (see above, *Hemoptysis*) with *lavage* (washing out mucus from the bronchi) is often used in treating atelectasis. This is an appealing kind of treatment based on the logic that if mucus is blocking the bronchi, why not just go in and wash it out? Although it is logical, this treatment is seldom successful.

The most inclusive study to examine the results of treating atelectasis with many different methods has shown that the traditional methods of CPT and antibiotics are just as successful as invasive methods such as bronchoscopy. Successful treatment of atelectasis, regardless of the method chosen, may be slow, and it may take weeks or even months before the condition resolves.

Low Oxygen Level

Most people with CF who have any more than the mildest amount of lung disease will have a lower than normal blood oxygen level. In most cases, this causes no problems. If someone lives at sea level, extra oxygen is needed only when the lung disease is very severe. At higher altitudes, the air pressure is so low that it's harder to move oxygen from the air in the alveoli into the bloodstream. At the top of Mount Everest, the air pressure is less than half of what it is at sea level; up there, *everyone* needs to breathe extra oxygen. In Denver (and in the passenger cabins of commercial airliners), the pressure is about four fifths of the sea level pressure. For people with normal lungs, this presents no problems; however, for someone with lung disease, it is likely to mean that extra oxygen will be needed.

With the appropriate treatment, which is simply getting extra oxygen to breathe, it's remarkable how much better a person can feel. The various ways to obtain oxygen are outlined in Appendix B, *Medications*.

Respiratory Failure

As its name implies, respiratory failure is the condition where the job of the respiratory system is not being accomplished, which is usually defined by the blood oxygen level being too low and the blood carbon dioxide level being too high. This problem can occur in different people for different reasons (see *Gas Transfer and Delivery*, earlier in this chapter). Respiratory failure *can* result from nonlung problems (for example, if someone's chest wall muscles are paralyzed or very weak). In CF, if respiratory failure occurs, most often it occurs at least partly because of lung disease. If the lungs are very severely affected by CF, it may be difficult for oxygen to be absorbed into the bloodstream at the alveoli; there will also be airway obstruction, which can be so great that the work of breathing becomes too difficult for the ventilatory muscles. Except in very rare cases, this does not happen suddenly in CF. When respiratory failure does occur in someone with CF, it is in someone who has had severe lung disease for a long time.

Treatment of Respiratory Failure

Respiratory failure is another complication of CF where the best treatment is simply a continuation and intensification of the usual treatments aimed at reducing bronchial obstruction, infection, and inflammation. In many cases, however, respiratory failure occurs only after the usual treatments have failed, and there is so little healthy lung tissue remaining that it cannot sustain the functions of bringing adequate amounts of oxygen into the body and eliminating enough carbon dioxide. If the oxygen level is low enough and/or the carbon dioxide level high enough, this is clearly a life-threatening situation. (You may want to refer back to *Anatomy and Function of the Respiratory System* to review why this is so serious.)

In desperation, physicians and families may consider using a mechanical ventilator to do the extra breathing for the patient. In some special circumstances, this may be effective and may support the sick patient long enough for the lungs to improve, so that independent life is once again possible. These very unusual instances include respiratory failure that occurs suddenly and in a previously well patient, for example, as a result of an automobile crash or, rarely, as a result of a sudden serious viral infection like influenza. Respiratory failure in infants under the age of 1 year is also a special circumstance in which temporary support with a mechanical ventilator may be helpful.

However, in most cases where respiratory failure occurs, it is at the end of a long process, and the use of a mechanical ventilator does not reverse that process. Most patients with CF who are put on mechanical ventilators either die while still on the ventilator or are never able to come off it, despite weeks or even months of very intensive care. In order for a ventilator to work, a patient needs to have a tube in the trachea (either through the nose or mouth, or as a tracheotomy tube, through an incision in the neck). These tubes are uncomfortable, and make it impossible to talk. Ventilator support almost always means living in an intensive care unit, where there is usually little or no privacy, little differentiation between day and night, and constant monitoring by machines and people.

Lung transplantation is a procedure in which a patient's lungs are removed from the chest and a new set of lungs and heart put in their place. By the end of

2001, this procedure had been performed in several thousand people with various kinds of lung problems, including 1,200 with CF in the United States. Some patients have done extremely well with this procedure and have been able to go back to work and resume a reasonably active life, whereas others have had many complications and some have died. As with any new procedure, results are poor at first and improve as more experience is gained with them. This topic is discussed in Chapter 8, *Transplantation.*

Clearly, *the best treatment for respiratory failure is **prevention.***

Cor Pulmonale and Heart Failure

Cor pulmonale literally means "heart disease caused by lung disease or breathing problems." Whenever the lungs are very severely affected (from almost any disease, including CF) or when the blood oxygen level is very low (from any cause), the blood vessels in the lung narrow, and it becomes difficult for the heart to pump blood through these blood vessels. Since it is the right side of the heart that pumps blood through the lungs, the right side of the heart gets a lot more exercise than usual. As with any other muscle, heart muscle will get bigger after it's had a lot of strenuous exercise. People who have had fairly severe lung disease for a period of time will commonly have a thick right-sided heart muscle, a condition called *right ventricular hypertrophy.* Not only will the muscle become thicker, but the whole right side of the heart may also expand. This enlargement is the way the heart adapts to the excess work it's being asked to do. It is most often a *successful* adaptation. Since this is a successful adjustment by the heart to a difficult situation, it is not considered heart *disease.* Although there is an abnormal *shape* and *size* to the right ventricle of the heart, this is quite different from *disease,* which is, by definition, harmful. Right ventricular hypertrophy is the *healthy* adjustment to the abnormally great demands placed on the normal heart by the diseased lungs.

If the lung disease remains too severe for too long, the heart may no longer be able to meet all the demands placed on it. It may not be able to pump all the blood that's necessary, and some fluid may back up. This fluid can sometimes be noticed in the ankles and lower legs, and sometimes a feeling of fullness in the right side of the abdomen under the ribs signifies fluid buildup in the liver. When the heart muscle fails to pump its entire assigned load, we say there is "heart failure," which is a frightening and misleading name for the condition, because it makes one think of heart *stoppage,* which it is not. Heart failure is the failure of the heart to do its *full* job. It is a serious problem, but one that indicates a serious lung problem rather than a problem with the heart itself.

Treatment of Cor Pulmonale and Heart Failure

Once again, the most effective treatment for this complication of CF lung disease is the aggressive treatment of the lung disease itself. In some cases in which there is excess fluid, a diuretic medication may be helpful (see Appendix B, *Medications*).

Chest Pain

Chest pain is a fairly common complication of CF and has many different causes. The major cause is pneumothorax. This is usually a sharp pain that occurs suddenly, is limited to one side, and is accompanied by shortness of breath. Other problems, while not as dangerous as pneumothorax, can be just as bothersome. The musculoskeletal system can be the source of chest pain in CF, especially when someone is coughing a lot: Strained muscles, pulled tendons, bruised or even broken ribs can occur. Infection involving the pleura (the membrane surrounding the lung) can be very uncomfortable, especially with deep breaths or coughs. This problem is called *pleuritis* or sometimes *pleurisy*. Although anatomy books state that bronchi do not have pain-sensing nerves, some CF physicians think that pain may be caused by large mucous plugs caught in small bronchi. Clearly, some patients experience pain that disappears after they have coughed up a large plug of mucus. In younger people, the chest tightness that may accompany an asthma attack or a pulmonary exacerbation may seem like pain. Finally, there are nonpulmonary causes for chest pain in CF (heart attack is not among these): Inflammation of the esophagus from acid reflux (see Chapter 4, *The Gastrointestinal Tract*) can cause "heartburn," which may be accompanied by difficulty in swallowing, and psychologic stress can certainly cause chest pain.

TESTS

Several kinds of tests can give important objective information about the lungs in someone with CF. These tests may be useful to confirm the physician's or patient's assessment of the patient's condition, to guide treatment, to measure the response to treatment, or in some cases to identify a problem before it has become evident to family or physician. Since most problems can be treated best if they are discovered early, many CF centers use these tests on a regular basis, and not just when there is obvious trouble.

Pulmonary Function Tests

PFTs are tests that measure various aspects of lung function. They can determine lung size and presence and degree of bronchial obstruction. They can even give a good idea of which bronchi are blocked (the smallest bronchi or the larger central airways). They can identify asthma in children and adults, and they can measure the amount of oxygen circulating in the blood.

PFTs are sensitive tools for following the condition of someone's lungs, showing subtle changes that might not have been detected otherwise. Since most

PFTs require the understanding and cooperation of the patient, most children under the age of 6 or 7 years are not able to do these tests.

Spirometry

Spirometry ("measuring breathing") is the simplest PFT and is available in most hospitals and clinics. In this test, the patient breathes in and out through a tube while the machine records the amount of air breathed and the speed at which it is blown out.

Figure 3.10 shows two kinds of graphs that the spirometer can produce. The first (Figure 3.10A) records the amount (volume) of air blown out after the largest possible inhalation and the time it takes to exhale it forcefully. Most of the air is exhaled in the first second, and all of it by 3 seconds. The most basic measurement from this curve is the *forced vital capacity* (FVC), the volume of air that is blown out in a single maximum exhaled breath. The next most commonly used measurement is the *forced expired volume in 1 second* (FEV$_1$), since this is a good indicator of whether there is blockage, and how much, particularly in the large central bronchi. The more obstruction there is, the more difficult it is to get air out of the lungs quickly, and the smaller the FEV$_1$. This is illustrated on the graph, where the solid line is from someone who has CF and normal lung function, and the dotted line is from someone who has CF and a moderate amount of obstruction.

The *maximum voluntary ventilation* (MVV) is similar to the spirometric tests just discussed. It calculates the maximum amount of air that someone can breathe in and out in 1 minute. The test doesn't last a whole minute, though. In most laboratories, the technician cheers and yells and vigorously encourages you to "Blow! Blow! Blow!" for 12 or 15 seconds. The volume of air you've been able to breathe is then multiplied by 5 (for a 12-second test) or 4 (for a 15-second test) to give a value for 1 minute's worth of all-out effort.

These tests (FVC, FEV$_1$, MVV) are useful, but they have one important drawback, namely, they are very "effort-dependent," meaning that a half-hearted breath will give worthless information. Experienced technicians can very often tell from the shape of the curve whether the patient has given as good an effort as possible. Newer machines may print out numbers for the FVC and FEV$_1$, rather than a curve. With these machines it is extremely difficult to evaluate the information, since it is difficult to determine how reliable the effort was that went into the breath.

Another way of looking at the information from spirometry is the *flow-volume curve* (Figure 3.10B), which shows how quickly air flows out of the lungs at different points during a maximum expiratory effort. This gives valuable information because air comes out much faster at the beginning of a breath, when the lungs are fully inflated, than it does later on in the breath, when the lungs are nearly empty. The flow-volume curve relates the flow rates to precise portions of the breath. For example, the MEF$_{25}$ is the maximum expiratory flow rate at 25%

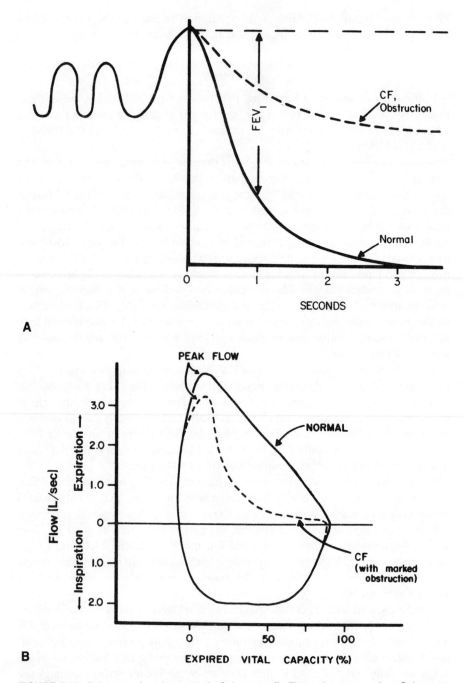

FIGURE 3.10. Pulmonary function tests. **A:** Spirometry. **B:** Flow-volume curve (see Spirometry for discussion).

of vital capacity, meaning it is the rate at which air flows out of the lungs during a maximum effort at the point when exactly 75% of the breath is gone (and 25% remains in the lungs). Another reason this information is so useful is that the flow rates during the second half of a breath out depend very little on how hard a breath is taken; that is, these flow rates are relatively effort-independent and are therefore valuable even in someone whose cooperation is less than perfect. Finally, the flow rates at the end of a breath seem to be a good reflection of the amount of obstruction in the smallest bronchi: During the first part of the exhalation, the air quickly empties out of the larger bronchi, and during the last half or quarter of the breath, the air empties out of the smallest bronchi. Therefore, a slower than normal second half of a breath can indicate some blockage in the smallest airways, even when the larger bronchi are unobstructed and the first half of the breath is perfectly normal.

Lung Volumes

Lung volumes are measured by two different methods and require complex machinery, which may not be available in every physician's office or hospital. Yet, they can give valuable information that cannot be obtained with spirometry. Spirometry measures the air that moves in and out of the lungs, but indicates nothing about the actual size of the lungs or the amount of air left inside the lungs after a person has finished blowing out.

The *helium dilution* method for measuring lung volumes uses the "Iced Tea Principle." If you place a teaspoon of sugar into a full glass of iced tea, and mix it thoroughly, the sweetness of the tea will depend on the size of the glass. Clearly, an 8-oz glass will be much sweeter with a teaspoon of sugar than a quart jar. Another way of saying this is—the smaller the glass, the greater the concentration of sugar. In fact, if you had tools precise enough to measure the exact sweetness or the exact concentration of sugar, and you knew the exact amount of sugar you put in (1 tsp, in this case) you could calculate the size of the glass.

For measuring lung volumes, the sugar-substitute is helium, a gas that is very safe to breathe in and that is not absorbed into the bloodstream. If you breathe in a known amount of helium for a few minutes, until it is thoroughly mixed with the air in your lungs, the concentration of helium in the air you breathe out can tell the size of your lungs. This method works fairly well for determining the size of your lungs at their largest (with the biggest breath in), and at their smallest (after you've breathed out all you can). These are the *total lung capacity* and *residual volume*, respectively. The method is not perfect because it requires that all of the bronchial tubes be open so that the helium can mix completely with all areas of the lung. If a portion of one lung is blocked off, the helium won't mix with the air in that part of the lung, and it will seem that the lungs are smaller than they actually are. What is measured by this method is the volume of lung that freely communicates with the mouth; that's the same as the total lung volume if the airways are healthy, but in obstructed lungs the volume will be underestimated.

The "body box" (*total body plethysmograph*) solves the problem of obstruction. It is an expensive piece of equipment that looks something like a space capsule. Not many hospitals are equipped with body boxes suitable for testing children. The person being tested sits inside the box and breathes through a tube. When the box is shut, it is completely airtight, which allows changes in pressure within the box to be measured very precisely while the person breathes. The changes in pressure reflect the changes in chest size. A mathematical formula is then applied that translates the pressure changes into accurate lung volume calculations, which include all of the lung volume, whether the bronchi are blocked or open. If someone does have bronchial obstruction, the total lung capacity will not be affected very much, but since obstruction (especially of small airways) makes it difficult to empty the lungs, the *residual volume* (the amount of air left in the lungs after a maximum exhalation) will be larger than normal. Normally, the residual volume is less than 25% of the total lung capacity, but in someone with severely blocked small airways, it can be as much as 70% of total lung capacity.

Asthma Testing

Asthma is a condition in which bronchi are blocked because of inflammation within bronchi and contraction of the muscles in the bronchial wall (this contraction of bronchial wall muscles is sometimes called *bronchospasm*). While the flow rates and lung volumes from the tests just described can tell if an obstruction is present, they can't tell what has caused it. However, if someone inhales a fast-acting bronchodilator, the bronchial muscle quickly relaxes, and the obstruction decreases. If the PFTs are repeated, the flow rates will show dramatic improvement within a few minutes. Since it's important to know how much obstruction is reversible, many laboratories will automatically schedule a bronchodilator inhalation and repeated spirometry as part of routine PFTs.

Some laboratories may go one step further, and try to identify people whose bronchi aren't yet blocked by bronchospasm but are susceptible to such blockage. These are people with *reactive airways* (sometimes even called *hyperreactive airways*), which is another term for asthma. These people may have completely normal pulmonary function at a given time, but if they inhale certain chemicals, their bronchial muscles may contract much more readily than the bronchial muscles of someone with normal airways. To test for this, people may be asked to breathe in these chemicals (methacholine is the one most commonly used in this country; histamine is another), starting with a very dilute solution, increasing step by step to a stronger solution, and repeating the spirometry after each new challenge. The test is completed when the PFTs worsen. Someone has reactive airways disease if his or her PFTs get worse with a dilute (weak) solution of the chemical. The tests that measure airway reactivity are called *bronchial provocation or inhalation challenge tests*. Other bronchial challenge tests involve PFTs before and after exercise or before and after inhaling cold dry air.

Blood Gases

Since the major job of the lungs is to bring oxygen into the bloodstream and to eliminate carbon dioxide, it may be important to know the blood oxygen and carbon dioxide levels. To find this out, a blood gas test is performed by inserting a needle into an artery and drawing out blood. Since a needle inserted into an artery can be much more painful than one inserted into a vein, a small amount of Xylocaine may be injected into the skin first, or the skin may be prepared with EMLA cream, which numbs the skin and makes the test more tolerable.

Oximetry

Over the past few years, painless, noninvasive monitors that decrease the need for arterial blood gases have been developed. These monitors are called *oximeters* (either ear oximeters or pulse oximeters), and they work through a computerized method: A light is shined through the fingertip or earlobe to a sensor on the other side of the finger or ear; the amount of light that can pass through the tissues is determined partly by the amount of oxygen that is in the blood in those tissues. The oxygen saturation of the blood is calculated almost instantaneously by computer and is indicated on a digital display.

Exercise Tests

Standard PFTs measure lung function while a person is resting. It may be useful in some situations to see how the lungs (and heart) function when they are put under some stress, as with exercise. Exercise tests can range from the very simple (listening to someone's lungs after he or she has been running in a hallway) to the very complex (measuring the precise amounts of oxygen consumed, carbon dioxide produced, oxygen exhaled, time it takes to inhale and exhale, rate of breathing, heart rate, etc.). Many physicians believe that the exercise test is more successful than regular PFTs in detecting mild problems. This is because a mild problem will not present itself unless the system is stressed, as when people exert themselves to the limit. For most exercise tests, the person being tested pedals on a stationary exercise cycle or walks/runs on a treadmill. The test begins with an easy pace, and gets increasingly difficult. While the test is going on, you may have to breathe through a mouthpiece like a scuba diver's, so that the air you breathe in and out can be analyzed. In other tests, you may have electrocardiogram (ECG) electrodes taped on your chest. In some tests, oximeters may be used, with a light taped to your finger or ear. In very special tests, there may even be a small plastic tube placed in the artery at your wrist. In other tests, none of those monitors may be used.

Exercise tests can show how physically fit a person is, and one study has shown that fitness level (as measured on an exercise test) was the test that correlated most closely with the likelihood of a patient with CF surviving the next 8 years or more.

Chest Radiographs (x-rays)

X-rays are generated by a machine that functions similarly to a camera. The x-ray machine is directed at the object to be studied, and generates x-rays, which pass through that object, in varying amounts and intensity. The x-rays then strike and expose photographic paper, which is situated behind the object. When there is no object in the way, and the x-rays hit the photographic paper directly, it becomes completely black. When an object such as lead is in the way, which totally blocks all the x-rays, the paper becomes completely white. The thicker or more dense a material, the more rays it absorbs, and the whiter the image of that material on the resulting x-ray film. When the object in question is a person's chest, there will be recognizable white/black/gray patterns determined by the bones, lungs, heart, and so forth. The bones are quite dense, and therefore will appear white on the final x-ray film (radiograph). The heart, because it consists of thick muscle and is filled with blood, also appears fairly white. The lungs are much less dense, since they are relatively delicate tissues largely filled with air, and therefore appear much blacker, or at least a darker shade of gray. The lungs do contain some dense tissue, including blood vessels, so they are not totally black. The diaphragms mark the lower edges of the lungs, and are white because they are fairly solid muscle.

Chest radiographs can give important information about the condition of the lungs. If, for example, a lobe of the lung is collapsed because it is filled with mucus, that lobe will appear much denser (whiter) than normal. If thick scar tissue has replaced healthy lung tissue, that too will be whiter than usual. Bronchial walls swollen by fluid or inflammation may have a similar appearance. In many cases it is possible to see "increased markings," meaning more white (dense) markings than normal, but it is not possible to tell if the increased density is caused by inflammation or mucus (which can get better) or by scar tissue (which cannot get better).

A pneumothorax, in which air has escaped through a leak in the lung but is still within the chest, will show up on the radiograph as a totally black area outside the lung, while the lung itself will be whiter than normal (Figure 3.7). The totally black area is air, and the lung will appear denser (whiter) than normal because it is partly collapsed, with the solid parts of the lung closer together than normal.

Lungs that are obstructed and difficult to empty will be larger than normal and will push the diaphragms downward (Figure 3.11). These overinflated (*hyperinflated*) lungs may not only push the diaphragms down into a flattened shape (compared with the normal dome shape), but may actually push the sternum (the front of the chest) forward. This is called *sternal bowing* (since the shape of the sternum comes to resemble an archery bow).

Cultures and Sensitivities

It is important to know what bacteria are in the bronchi of someone with CF in case antibiotic treatment becomes necessary. To identify bacteria, small sam-

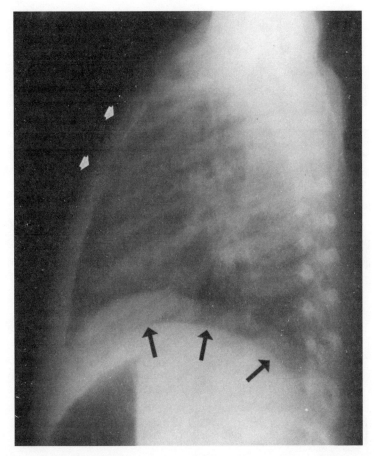

FIGURE 3.11. Radiographic appearance of overinflation of lungs. These are lateral (side) views of the chest of two different children with CF. **A:** Normal lungs, with nicely domed diaphragms (*black arrows*), a normally straight breast bone (sternum, *white arrows*), and little air directly behind the sternum. *(Continued on next page)*

ples of mucus are sent to a bacteriology laboratory where they are placed in different substances called *media*. Some media are good environments for all types of bacteria to grow in, and others will allow only certain bacteria to grow. After the bacteria have grown, they are analyzed and identified, with the entire process taking several days.

Once the bacteria are grown and identified, the task remains of determining which antibiotics are the most effective in killing those bacteria. To find this out, various antibiotics are added to the cultures and their effects are observed. One method of introducing antibiotics is through paper discs that have been soaked with the antibiotic. These discs (called Kirby–Bauer) are placed at intervals around

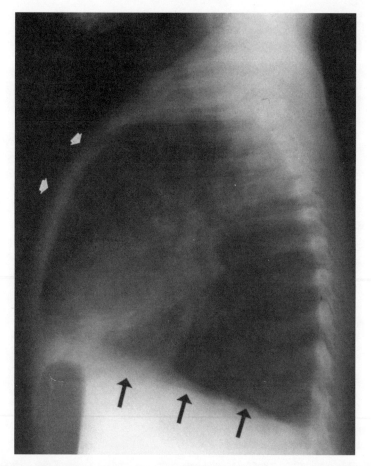

FIGURE 3.11. *(Continued).* **B:** In contrast to **(A)**, this figure shows severe overinflation of the lungs, with the diaphragms pushed downward and flattened (*black arrows*), the sternum "bowed" outward (*white arrows*), and excessive air (*blacker*) behind the sternum. Note, too, that the overall depth of the chest from the sternum to the spine is much greater in the overinflated chest. This is referred to as an *increased AP* (anteroposterior) *diameter.*

the plate where the bacteria are grown (Figure 3.12). If the antibiotic kills the bacteria, there will be a clear area around the disc, where the bacteria have not been able to grow (this clear area is called the *zone of inhibition*). If the bacteria are not killed by the antibiotic, they continue to grow right up to the disc, leaving no clear zone. Sometimes there will be a very small zone, sometimes a larger one. Most laboratories will define the response to the antibiotic based on the size of the clear zone. For example, when the antibiotic gentamicin is used in cultures of *Pseudomonas* organisms, the bacteria are proclaimed *sensitive* to the antibiotic if the clear area is 15 mm or larger; if the clear area is 13 to 14

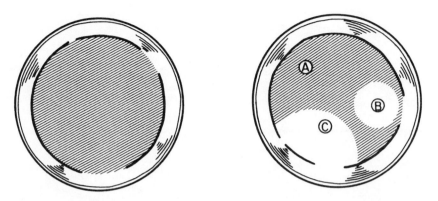

FIGURE 3.12. Culture and sensitivity testing, showing clear zones around the antibiotic discs. The larger the clear space around the disc, the more potent the antibiotic has been in preventing the bacteria from growing.

mm, it is considered *intermediate*, and if it is 12 mm or less, the bacteria are said to be *resistant* to the effects of the antibiotic. "Resistance" is thus a relative term, because the presence of even a very small clear space indicates that some bacteria have been killed. This also means that the laboratory might report a culture back as showing the bacteria to be "resistant" to a particular antibiotic, and your doctor might decide to use it anyway. Frequently in this kind of situation, the antibiotic has its desired effect despite the laboratory report. Many laboratories use an automated system of *microbroth dilution* for measuring antibiotic *sensitivity* or *susceptibility* to the various antibiotics. In this system, bacteria are placed in a series of test tubes, each containing progressively greater amounts (concentrations) of the antibiotic being tested, and the results are reported as which dilution of the antibiotic kills all the bacteria. Although less labor-intensive, microbroth dilution is probably not quite as accurate as the old Kirby–Bauer disc method.

SUMMARY

The respiratory system accounts for over 95% of the illness and deaths from CF, and therefore keeping it healthy is the most important thing that can be done for anyone with CF. Fortunately, there is much that can be done toward this end, and the tremendous improvement in life expectancy of patients with CF can be attributed largely to better prevention and treatment of lung problems. Most of the problems that develop in the lung are the result of bronchial blockage caused by thick mucus and infection that follows the blockage. Physical means, such as postural drainage and percussion treatments, and medications, including bronchodilators, help prevent and reverse bronchial obstruction. Antibiotics, given by mouth, aerosol, or IV injection, are very successful in treating bronchial infection.

4

The Gastrointestinal Tract

THE BASICS

1. Most people with cystic fibrosis (CF) need to take pancreatic enzymes with their meals and snacks to help digest their food.
2. People who skip their enzymes (or whose enzymes are not working right) have abdominal pain and frequent, large, smelly, loose bowel movements, and have trouble gaining weight.
3. With help from the CF center, everyone can learn how much enzyme to use.
4. Some patients with CF have intestinal blockage that needs to be treated promptly. The signs of this problem are "stomachaches" and fewer bowel movements than normal. If your child has no bowel movement for 24 hours, call the CF center right away.
5. Some babies and children with CF have gastroesophageal reflux (acid moving backward from the stomach into the esophagus), which can be treated with medicines and some diet changes.
6. To minimize reflux, put your baby to sleep on its stomach.
7. A few patients with CF (fewer than 5%) have serious liver problems.

THE NORMAL GASTROINTESTINAL TRACT

The gastrointestinal tract is made up of the organs that digest food (Figure 4.1). One way to understand how the gastrointestinal tract normally works in people without cystic fibrosis (CF) is to think about what happens to the parts of a meal when they are eaten. For this purpose we can use a (not completely well-rounded) meal consisting of meat, potato with butter, a glass of whole milk, and a dessert of candy. Each of these foods has a mix of nutrients: *protein*, *fat*, and *carbohydrate*. For this discussion, however, the meat will represent its main component, protein; the potato, starch (a carbohydrate with complex branching chains of molecules); the butter, fat; and the candy, sucrose (a carbohydrate that is simpler than starch). The milk contains another simple carbohydrate, lactose, as well as fat and protein.

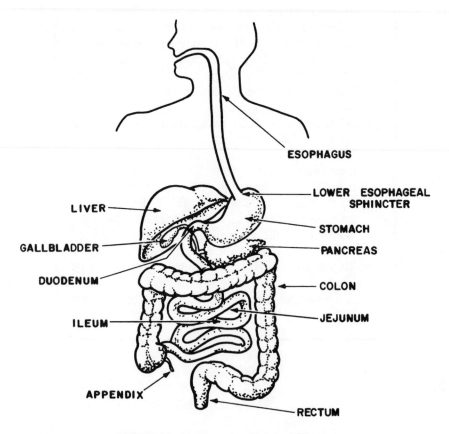

FIGURE 4.1. Anatomy of gastrointestinal tract.

None of this food would stay in the body if it were not broken down into small particles that can be absorbed into the bloodstream. This process of breaking down food is called *digestion*. When a person eats such a meal, digestion begins immediately in the **mouth**. Saliva contains digestive enzymes called *amylase* and *lipase*, and when these are mixed with the food during chewing, the amylase starts to break down the starch of the potato, and the lipase starts to break down the fat of the butter and milk. You will notice that most of the enzymes that break down food end in "-ase" or "-sin."

The *esophagus* is not actively involved in the process of digestion. It is a tube that moves the chewed food from the mouth to the stomach. It does have an important role, however, because it must move food down without air getting in, and it must let air or food come up when the need arises to belch or vomit. It is the esophagus that keeps food and liquid in the stomach, even when a person is upside down.

The chewed-up meat, potato, butter, milk, and candy have now passed through the esophagus into the *stomach*. Here, the protein in the meat and milk is acted upon by the enzyme *pepsin*, which is secreted by the stomach. The stomach makes a lot of acid, and the acid also helps begin the process of digestion.

When the food has been ground up by the stomach into small particles, the partly digested food is released slowly into the *duodenum*, the first part of the *small intestine*. Several inches beyond the stomach, in the duodenum, is a tiny opening through which juices from the *liver* and *pancreas* flow into the duodenum. These juices contain large amounts of important digestive enzymes made by the pancreas and bile salts (also called bile acids) made by the liver. Among the pancreatic enzymes are *proteases*, which digest proteins. *Trypsin, chymotrypsin,* and *elastase* are protein-digesting enzymes that continue the digestion of the protein from the meat and milk after it has passed from the stomach. Two other important pancreatic enzymes are *amylase*, which, like salivary amylase, continues to break down the potato's starch, and *lipase*, which digests nearly all the fat in the butter and milk. Lipase is a particularly important enzyme because it is the major fat-digesting enzyme in the digestive tract; it is also very fragile and is destroyed when in the presence of too much acid. Lipase also has other requirements to function well: Bile salts, made by the liver, and colipase, made by the pancreas, are both needed in the duodenum for lipase to work well.

The products of all of this digestion of protein and fat and starch are absorbed by the tiny cells of the wall of the small intestine as the muscles of the intestine squeeze the food slowly along toward the *large intestine* (also called the *colon*). There are enzymes attached to the cells of the wall of the small intestine that break down simple carbohydrates such as the sucrose of the candy and the lactose of the milk, just before they are absorbed by the intestinal cells. Other enzymes on these cells complete the digestion of starch and protein that was begun by the enzymes from the pancreas. Once the food has been broken down into these tiny particles and taken into the intestinal cells, it passes into the bloodstream and is carried to the various parts of the body where it is needed.

In a person whose gastrointestinal tract is working properly, nearly all of the nutritious food that is eaten is digested by the pancreatic enzymes and absorbed by the intestinal cells into the bloodstream. Very little of the food gets to the colon. That person's bowel movements contain nondigestible food products like fiber from the food, some water to keep the movement soft, and quite a lot of the bacteria that normally live in the large intestine. Very little of the carbohydrate and protein, and less than 7% of the fat, is wasted.

THE GASTROINTESTINAL TRACT IN CYSTIC FIBROSIS

The remainder of this chapter is devoted to the problems that occur in the gastrointestinal tract in patients with CF, with each problem being reviewed under the affected organ. Table 4.1 lists the problems and the frequency with which they occur.

Pancreas

Pancreatic Insufficiency

Abnormal mucus blocks the tiny tubes in the pancreas of people with CF, much as it does in the lungs. This means that the pancreatic digestive enzymes are not secreted into the intestine as they should be. (Remember that these enzymes are lipase, which digests fat; amylase, which digests starch; and the proteases, including trypsin, chymotrypsin, and others, which digest proteins.) Pancreatic insufficiency refers to the inability of the pancreas to secrete enough digestive enzymes for normal digestion and absorption. This does not happen until nearly all (90%) of the normal enzyme activity is lost; therefore, the pan-

TABLE 4.1. *Incidence of Gastrointestinal Conditions in Cystic Fibrosis*

Organ	Condition	Patients with Cystic Fibrosis with Condition, %
Pancreas	Pancreatic insufficiency	85–90[a]
	Pancreatitis	1
	Diabetes	1–5[b]
Liver and gallbladder	Cirrhosis	1–4
	Gallstones	10
Esophagus and stomach	Gastroesophageal reflux	10–20
	Ulcers	1–10
Intestines	Meconium ileus	10
	Meconium peritonitis	1
	Distal intestinal obstruction syndrome	10–30
	Rectal prolapse	10–20
	Intussusception	1

[a]At birth, only about 50% are pancreatic-insufficient.
[b]Diabetes is extremely uncommon before the age of 10 years; thereafter, it occurs in about 10% of patients until age 20 years, and in another 10% to 20% from 20 to 30 years.

creatic secretion must be quite low for pancreatic insufficiency to occur. In fact, most people with CF have extensive damage to their pancreas, so that it is largely replaced by scar tissue and fat, and they need to take enzymes by mouth with their meals. Until recently, it was thought that pancreatic insufficiency was present from birth. We now know that nearly 50% of infants with CF have pancreatic *sufficiency*, that is, they retain enough functioning pancreatic tissue for the digestion and absorption of their food, without needing enzyme supplements. In the first months and years of life, most of these *pancreatic-sufficient* infants lose pancreatic function, so that by age 8 or 9 years, 85% to 90% of patients with CF will have pancreatic insufficiency and will need to take enzymes with meals to digest their food. Somewhere between 10% and 15% of patients with CF remain pancreatic-sufficient all their lives. This one characteristic—whether people will be pancreatic-sufficient or pancreatic-insufficient—seems to be determined in large part by which particular CF gene mutations they have (see Chapter 11, *Genetics*, for more details).

Before effective treatment was available, most children with CF died in infancy, in part from starvation (malnutrition) due to their pancreatic insufficiency.

The intestinal cells have a "backup" group of enzymes that do fairly well at digesting starch and protein when the pancreas is not working properly. In this case, however, the digestion and absorption of starch is not complete, and the remaining starch may cause gas when it gets to the large intestine (colon). The digestion of protein is also not complete, so that some patients, especially infants, may have low levels of protein in the blood. If protein levels are too low, fluid may leak out of the blood vessels and cause puffy skin (*edema*).

The intestinal cells do not have a backup means to digest fat, and the effectiveness of the lipase produced by the salivary glands is limited. Therefore, most patients with CF do not digest and absorb fat well, and fat is passed out of the body in the bowel movements. Fat makes the bowel movements large, greasy, and more smelly than normal. Furthermore, all of the fat that comes out in the bowel movements is lost to the body. A given amount of fat has more calories than any other kind of food; so losing an ounce of fat means losing more than twice as many calories as would be lost in an ounce of carbohydrate or protein. Loss of fat in the bowel movements thus leads to malnutrition and poor growth, despite a huge appetite. The "textbook picture" of a youngster with undiagnosed CF is someone who is scrawny, has a huge appetite, and has frequent, large, smelly, greasy stools. This person is scrawny because most of the nutrients in the food consumed go directly into the toilet; the apparently huge appetite is really a way of compensating for losing half of what is eaten in the bowel movements—it's as if you've been fed a half portion, so you eat another portion to make up for that. Fat malabsorption may also lead to the lack of special kinds of fatty nutrients that are essential to health—"essential fatty acids" and fat-soluble vitamins (vitamins A, D, E, and K). (A detailed discussion of vitamins and fatty acids is in Chapter 6, *Nutrition*.)

Diagnosis

There are several ways in which a physician can determine if someone has pancreatic insufficiency. One method is simply a review of the history of bowel movements: Frequent, greasy, smelly, large bowel movements usually indicate pancreatic insufficiency. Another method is a test that involves taking a small sample of stool (bowel movement), staining it with a dye that will make whatever fat there is in the stool an easily noticeable color, and examining it under the microscope. A large amount of fat in the sample indicates that fat was not digested and absorbed, which suggests pancreatic insufficiency. A more accurate stool test is the *72-hour fecal fat test*, which—as you've probably guessed—involves collecting all bowel movements for 3 whole days and nights in a large, sealable container (usually the laboratory supplies a paint can). At the same time the stool collection is going on, the family keeps a careful food diary, listing every bite of every food the patient eats over the 3 days. The dietitian can then calculate how many grams of fat were eaten, and the laboratory staff can see how many grams of fat came out in the stool. Most healthy people will absorb at least 93% of the fat they eat. Put another way, less than 7% of the dietary fat should appear in the stool. More than 7% fat excretion means there is *malabsorption* (not as much absorbed as normal), which suggests incomplete digestion, usually caused by insufficient pancreatic enzymes.

Pancreatic insufficiency can also be evaluated by analyzing the amount of trypsin and chymotrypsin in the stools. Absent enzymes, or very low levels of enzymes, suggest that the pancreas has not released the enzymes. However, this test can be misleading, because some of the bacteria that live in the intestines can produce trypsin, whereas others can destroy it. A newer test measuring *stool elastase* seems to be much more accurate.

A final laboratory test for pancreatic insufficiency is more invasive than those just discussed. This test involves passing a tube through the nose, esophagus, and stomach into the duodenum, and collecting fluid directly from the point at which the pancreas empties its enzymes. The fluid can then be analyzed directly for enzyme content.

The test that is probably used more than any other is called a "therapeutic trial"; it is also called "trial and error," although physicians prefer the first term. In this test, enzymes are administered to the patient, and the physician observes what happens—particularly what happens to the patient's stools, appetite, and growth. Since enzymes in small doses are not harmful, and are not very expensive, this can be a good, sensible test. It may not always give the most accurate information in the fastest time, however.

One further test that is being used primarily as a newborn screening test for CF also relates to pancreatic function. This blood test is performed on the first or second day of life. A dried spot of blood is analyzed for *immunoreactive trypsinogen* (IRT), a substance that is found in higher quantities in the blood of newborns with CF than in those without CF. It is not known why this is so, but it may be that the trypsin, which can't get out of the pancreas into the duodenum, "backs up" into the bloodstream. One problem with this explanation is that even most CF babies with pancreatic sufficiency have an abnormal IRT. (Perhaps these pancreatic-sufficient babies have *some* pancreatic blockage—not total, and enough trypsin and other enzymes get into the duodenum to bring about normal digestion and absorption—but enough blockage that some trypsin backs up into the bloodstream and is detected by the IRT.) The test is not perfect for identifying CF, since there are many *false positives* (babies who don't have CF, but who test abnormal for IRT). Nevertheless, the test is being used in many hospitals (and even some statewide programs) in the United States and in several countries around the world. It is discussed a bit more in Chapter 2, *Making the Diagnosis.*

Treatment

Treatment of pancreatic insufficiency is simple and the results are dramatic now that pancreatic enzyme replacement is possible using powder or capsules (that contain microspheres or microtablets) taken with meals. Although it may seem complicated when families are first introduced to enzymes, virtually everyone who has CF or who has a child with CF soon becomes an expert at using enzymes. These enzymes are often *enteric-coated*, meaning that they are protected from the stomach acid by a coating that dissolves only when it is in a nonacidic surrounding. These enzymes pass through the stomach and begin to dissolve in the duodenum, which is a nonacidic environment (see Chapter 6, *Nutrition*, and Appendix B, *Medications*). Since the raw enzymes (especially lipase) are easily inactivated by acid, the introduction of enteric-coated enzyme preparations was revolutionary and made a huge difference in the effectiveness of this very important part of CF treatment. The quantity of enzymes to be taken is determined by evaluating such factors as bowel movements, appetite, and weight gain (and is discussed further in Chapter 6, *Nutrition*, and in Appendix B, *Medications*). On rare occasions, more formal tests, such as the 72-hour fecal fat test discussed previously, may be needed.

The amount of enzyme taken must be adjusted properly because too much enzyme can occasionally cause problems. Usually, taking too much enzyme has no medical consequences, and no change in bowel habits, appetite, or growth will result. The only consequences will be financial ones (paying for more enzymes than you need). On occasion, though, too much enzyme can cause one of two medical problems; one usually not serious, the other quite serious. A few patients who take too much enzyme will have a change in their bowel habits, most commonly with their stools becoming a bit looser than normal, and less commonly with patients becoming constipated. These problems are most often just a nuisance, and resolve quickly with lowering the enzyme dose. In the 1990s, with the availability of super–high-dose enzyme preparations, a new, serious, but rare, problem, called *fibrosing colonopathy*, was recognized: Some patients taking very high doses of enzymes had scarring of their large intestine, causing abdominal pain, often with bloody diarrhea, and many have needed surgery to correct the problem. This problem has never been seen except in those patients taking extremely high doses of enzymes and has become extremely rare since enzyme manufacture changed in the late 1990s. The usual enzyme dosages, and those that have been associated with fibrosing colonopathy, are discussed in Chapter 6, *Nutrition*. ("Fibrosing colonopathy" comes from "-opathy," meaning "disease" and "fibrosis," which means scar formation; thus, colon disease with scar formation.)

Since the CF pancreas also does not produce the bicarbonate-rich acid-neutralizing juice found in the normal pancreas, stomach acid is not always neutralized when it passes into the duodenum. This means the duodenum may be more acidic than normal, and enteric-coated enzymes may not be properly activated (the coating may not dissolve). Therefore, some children with CF need treatment with antacids (medicines that neutralize acid) or medicines that decrease the stomach's production of acid, like cimetidine, ranitidine, or omeprazole (see Appendix B, *Medications*) to make their enzymes work. Infants who are given the enzymes as non–enteric-coated granules or powder may develop an irritation around the mouth or buttocks, and mothers who are breast-feeding these infants may develop nipple irritation. For all these reasons, the enteric-coated enzymes are usually much better than the non–enteric-coated enzymes, especially in infants. (See Appendix B, *Medications*, for more details about taking enzymes.)

Pancreatitis

Pancreatitis is an inflammation of the pancreas that causes severe abdominal pain and, usually, vomiting. It occurs in people without CF, sometimes due to gallstones blocking secretion of the pancreas; due to drinking alcohol, as a side effect of medications; or due to other, less common, reasons. Pancreatitis is uncommon among patients with CF, probably in part because most patients with CF do not have enough intact pancreatic tissue to become inflamed. In fact, patients with CF and pancreatic insufficiency virtually **never** develop pancreatitis. Among the few patients with CF with pancreatic sufficiency, a few (about 10%) will get pancreatitis. Pancreatitis is diagnosed with blood and urine tests and radiologic tests. Eating calls on the pancreas to work, and this worsens inflammation. Therefore, the treatment of pancreatitis usually involves a stay in the hospital, during which time no food is given by mouth, and nutrition is given intravenously. Taking pancreatic enzymes may also help resolve this problem. Although the problem is rare, it often recurs in those unfortunate enough to have it. Since fat and protein are the main signals for the pancreas to secrete, a low-fat, low-protein diet may be recommended until the pancreatic inflammation has resolved.

Diabetes

In addition to producing digestive enzymes and acid-neutralizing juices, the pancreas produces hormones, especially *insulin*. Insulin is needed by the body to move glucose, the body's main simple carbohydrate used for energy, from the blood into the body's cells. When insulin is not produced as it is needed, *diabetes* results, with elevated blood glucose (blood sugar) levels.

Diabetes involves many complicated processes in the body. The high level of blood glucose causes glucose to be lost in the urine, and this glucose takes water with it that is needed by the body. The loss of glucose and water from the body produces other changes that can make people with diabetes malnourished, dehydrated, and quite ill. Sugar in the urine pulls extra water with it, so people with diabetes lose water in addition to sugar and calories. They urinate a lot, drink a lot, and may lose weight and feel "dragged out."

Nearly one half of all people with CF have some limitation of the ability of their pancreas to produce insulin, which is detectable with special tests. However, most patients produce enough insulin to prevent diabetes. Almost no patient with CF under the age of 10 years has diabetes, whereas between the ages of 10 and 20 years, approximately 10% of patients with CF develop it. From the ages of 20 to 30 years, another 10% to 20% develop it, and so forth, with an additional 10% to 20% developing diabetes with every additional decade. Stresses like pregnancy, worsened lung infection, or medications—most notably, steroids, which are sometimes used to control CF lung disease—can bring on CF diabetes. Diabetes that appears during these stresses often goes away when the stress is removed. The diabetes in patients with CF is often called CFRD (*CF-related diabetes*). CFRD tends to be milder than diabetes in other children, and is less apt to produce serious illness. The treatment for diabetes involves taking insulin by injection every day, in some cases several times a day, and cutting down on the amount of "simple sugars" (candy, soda pop, etc.) in the diet. Studies are being conducted to see if an oral medication can help to reduce sugar levels safely and prevent the need for insulin shots.

Diagnosing Diabetes

In some patients, the diagnosis of diabetes is straightforward: Someone with CF has lost weight, is very thirsty, and is urinating frequently (gets up two or three times at night to drink and pee). In others, the diagnosis requires blood tests: a "random" blood glucose sugar level (that is, a blood sample drawn at any time) above 200 mg/dL; a "fasting" blood glucose (taken after no food or drink for the previous 8 hours) greater than 126 mg/dL, or 2-hour value of greater than 200 mg/dL in an *oral glucose tolerance test,* abbreviated OGTT. This is an excellent test for detecting even unsuspected diabetes, and is recommended for patients 16 years and older. In this test, the patient has blood glucose levels measured before and 2 hours after drinking a special sweetened fluid. The normal response is for the glucose level to rise after the sweet drink, and then fall back to normal. In someone with a tendency toward diabetes, the glucose level will still be elevated 2 hours later. One final test that some centers use is the *hemoglobin A_{1c}* (HgA_{1c}), sometimes also called *glycosylated hemoglobin*. This test can give a rough estimate of whether glucose levels have been elevated over the previous weeks or months. In most labs, HgA_{1c} over 6 suggests diabetes.

There is conflicting information about the influence of diabetes on the overall health of people with CF, with some studies suggesting that patients with CF with diabetes die earlier than those without diabetes. Other studies have shown no difference in survival between patients with CF with diabetes and patients with CF without diabetes. Some CF physicians consider the diagnosis of CF to be "good news disguised as bad." The reason for this is that studies from Scandinavia showed that patients with CF who started insulin shots returned their body weight to what it had been several *years* before diabetes was suspected, and even improved their lung function. So, of course it's likely to sound like bad news if you hear you have yet another problem, but in this case, it's a problem for which there is good treatment, and treatment that might even help overall health.

Intestines

Meconium Ileus

Meconium is a baby's first bowel movement, formed in the intestine while the baby is still in the mother's womb. Since the baby has had nothing to eat, this bowel movement is formed from bits of mucus and intestinal cells shed into the intestines before birth. It is usually darker and stickier than the infant's stools will be once he or she starts taking milk.

In infants with CF, the meconium is much thicker and stickier than usual, probably because of the abnormal sticky mucus that patients with CF seem to make throughout the body, almost certainly related to the basic defect (see Chapter 1, *The Basic Defect*). In about 10% of babies with CF, this meconium is so thick that it clogs in the ileum [the third part of the small intestine, right near the appendix (Figure 4.1)] and blocks the intestines. This condition is called *meconium ileus*. This prevents the baby from having a bowel movement, and therefore causes the abdomen to swell—usually within the first 2 days after birth. In such babies, meconium ileus is usually the first clue that they have CF. Sometimes the intestines get so filled because of the blockage that a hole is broken in the intestinal wall, and meconium escapes into the abdomen. This is called *meconium peritonitis*, and can make the baby quite sick. It occurs in about 10% of infants with meconium ileus, meaning approximately 1% of all infants with CF.

Treatment for meconium ileus can be given with special radiologic procedures and enemas, but sometimes surgery is required. The radiologic procedure and enema, called a *Gastrografin enema*, involves putting Gastrografin, or a similar product, into the rectum, and letting it run back through the colon. Gastrografin is a liquid with three characteristics that make it ideal to use in this situation: (a) it is very slippery and can get by just about any obstruction; (b) it is very concentrated and acts like a dry sponge, pulling fluid into the intestines and watering down the thick meconium; and (c) it appears on a radiograph (x-ray film) so the progress of the whole procedure can be followed. When this procedure is carried out by radiologists experienced in its use in infants (ideally with the cooperation of surgeons and CF specialists), it is safe and very effective. However, in some infants, these enemas will not relieve the obstruction and surgery becomes necessary. All infants with meconium peritonitis require surgery. When the surgery is performed by surgeons with experience in infants, it is usually successful. Babies who have had surgery have a slightly higher likelihood of developing intestinal obstruction later in life because after abdominal surgery in *anyone* (infants or older people; CF or non-CF), scars (adhesions) may form and block the intestines.

Meconium ileus is a serious problem, but most infants who have it do very well after it is treated. If they make it through the difficult first few weeks, their outlook is similar to that for other CF babies who have not had meconium ileus. Meconium ileus occurs almost exclusively in infants with CF; therefore, a baby with meconium ileus should be diagnosed immediately, and general CF care should begin right away. A sweat test should be performed, despite a commonly held misconception that babies do not sweat enough for a valid sweat test. In fact, most babies do give plenty of sweat for analysis and diagnosis. In those few infants who do not produce enough sweat, the baby should be treated *as though he or she has CF* until a definite diagnosis can be made, perhaps with genetic testing, perhaps with a repeated sweat test (see the *Introduction* and Chapter 11, *Genetics*, for more discussion of tests used to diagnose CF). There seems to be an increased risk of meconium ileus in patients carrying the 621+ G→T mutation and in children born into families with prior children with meconium ileus.

Distal Intestinal Obstruction Syndrome

Distal intestinal obstruction syndrome (DIOS) involves blockage of the intestines that is similar to meconium ileus, but occurs after infancy. Because of its similarity to meconium ileus, the problem used to be called "meconium ileus equivalent," even though intestinal contents are not referred to as "meconium" in anyone older than a newborn. The intestinal contents usually block the same area of the ileum (just before the colon) as in meconium ileus, but sometimes the blockage occurs farther along, in the colon.

DIOS may be brought on by too few enzymes (since that will make the stools very large and bulky), by dehydration (for example by not drinking enough fluid during exercise in hot weather), or by dietary changes. It is somewhat more common in children who have had meconium ileus as newborns, especially if they had surgery. In rare cases, it may be caused by an excess of enzymes. In many cases, it is not known what caused the blockage, other than the thickening of the intestinal mucus.

Crampy stomachaches and constipation are the symptoms produced by DIOS. Often, doctors can feel the blockage when they examine the patient's abdomen. It can also be seen on radiographs. If a person with CF has severe abdominal pain and no bowel movements, it is most likely due to this problem. No bowel movements for 24 hours should prompt an urgent call to the CF center.

Treatment for this complication of CF may involve continuing to take enzymes, taking stool softeners or special laxative preparations, and having special radiographic examinations and enemas. Although it rarely requires surgery, it must be attended to promptly so that more serious problems, such as perforation or leaking of the bowels, do not occur.

Intussusception

Intussusception is a very rare problem that occurs when part of the intestine is pulled along inside another part of the intestine in much the same way that a telescope collapses in on itself (Figure 4.2). Intussusception can be a complication of DIOS, and the part of the intestine that is pulled along is usually the end of the ileum, which is pulled into the colon. What probably causes this action is that sticky stool and mucus, which adhere to the inside of the intestines, are pulled along by the powerful waves that pull the food along, drawing the intes-

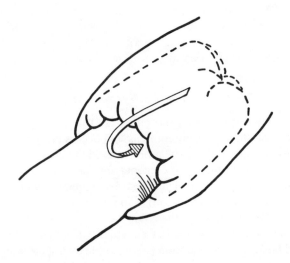

FIGURE 4.2. Intussusception. This condition occurs when the intestine slides within itself, like a telescope.

tine with them. This "telescoping" may cause the blood vessels that normally nourish the intestines to be blocked off, which may damage the intestine, causing bleeding or even destruction of that part of the bowel. Intussusception, like DIOS, causes abdominal pain (which may be intermittent or constant), and may cause vomiting or a decreased number of bowel movements. Intussusception may be treated by barium enema radiograph or may require surgery, but patients with this problem tend to do well if promptly treated.

Fibrosing Colonopathy

Fibrosing colonopathy is very unusual problem that affected a few patients with CF, especially in the 1990s, and was seen only among the patients taking very large doses of pancreatic enzymes with each meal. People who developed the problem had abdominal pain and some had bloody diarrhea. It is a serious problem that may require surgery. It has practically disappeared in the 2000s. It is discussed at greater length in Chapter 6, *Nutrition*.

Rectum

Rectal Prolapse

Rectal prolapse is similar to intussusception, involving the same "telescoping" action. In this case, the rectum is pulled along through, and right out of, the anus, to a point where it becomes visible (Figure 4.3). This usually happens during a bowel movement. Rectal prolapse may occur repeatedly in a young child, before the diagnosis of CF is made. It is fairly common, occurring in nearly 20% of patients with CF. Although it is frightening for a parent to see, it is seldom dangerous or painful.

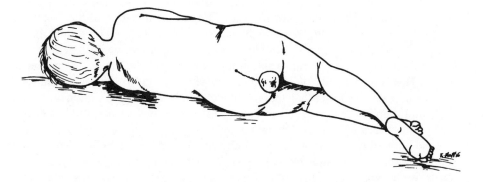

FIGURE 4.3. Rectal prolapse. This condition is similar to intussusception in that the bowel turns partly inside out. In rectal prolapse, the last part of the bowel (the rectum) turns inside out, and protrudes from the anus.

Rectal prolapse may be the first CF-related problem to appear before CF is diagnosed in a child. Several factors related to undiagnosed CF can cause rectal prolapse. Malnutrition affects the structures that usually support the rectum, and coughing and straining during sticky, bulky bowel movements increase the pressure on the rectum, pushing it out. Treatment of each episode of prolapse usually consists simply of pushing the rectum gently back into place by hand. If it is difficult to restore it to its normal position, a doctor's help should be obtained immediately. The prolapse usually stops occurring when treatment of the CF (especially with enzymes) improves the bowel movements, reduces coughing, and increases overall nutrition. Rectal prolapse rarely requires surgery. Since rectal prolapse is very uncommon in developed countries except in youngsters with CF (and a very few with severe constipation or diarrhea), anyone with rectal prolapse should be tested for CF.

Esophagus

Gastroesophageal Reflux

Gastroesophageal reflux occurs when the stomach contents (acid and partially digested food) come back up into the esophagus ("gastro" refers to the stomach; and "reflux" indicates a fluid going backward from the way it's supposed to go). A certain amount of this is normal, and we are usually unaware that it is happening. However, when this occurs often, or when the acid from the stomach remains in the esophagus for very long, the mucous membranes of the esophagus become irritated and inflamed. *Esophagitis* (inflammation of the esophagus) then results, producing the feeling called "heartburn," which has nothing to do with the heart. In addition to the discomfort this causes, on rare occasions the damage can be severe enough to cause bleeding or a narrowed area of scar tissue (*stricture*) within the esophagus, which can make swallowing very difficult.

Gastroesophageal reflux—often abbreviated to "acid reflux" or just "reflux"—can lead to other problems in addition to the irritation of the esophagus itself. One problem occurs when the refluxed material comes up farther than the esophagus and is actually vomited. Besides being messy, vomiting entails a loss of food and crucial nutrients and, if it occurs frequently, can lead to malnutrition. This is a particular problem in babies who have reflux, because a baby's esophagus is much shorter than that of older children. Although a certain amount of "spitting up" is quite normal in babies, too much may be harmful, such as when it interferes with normal weight gain.

In addition to the irritation of the esophagus and the loss of calories, gastroesophageal reflux can cause pulmonary (lung or breathing) problems. This may occur two different ways: (a) refluxed material may reach the back of the throat and actually be breathed (*aspirated*) into the lungs. There are normally good protections that keep refluxed material from getting into the lungs, so most breathing problems caused by reflux occur in the second way; (b) when nerves in the esophagus are irritated by stomach acid, they can send a signal to the bronchial tubes to get narrower, making the bronchial wall muscles squeeze down. [In certain instances, this reaction is actually a protective mechanism (see Chapter 3, *The Respiratory System*).]This reaction of the bronchi causes breathing difficulties that are similar to those of asthma, and may make the breathing problems of CF worse.

Acid reflux is somewhat more common in people with CF, for several reasons. Some medications and treatments have a side effect of relaxing the muscle at the bottom of the esophagus (lower esophageal sphincter) (Figure 4.1). If that sphincter relaxes too much, food is more likely to pass backward through it from the stomach into the esophagus. People with CF spend more time upside down (for treatments) than other people. If the muscle at the bottom of the esophagus relaxes when you are upright, gas escapes, and we call that a burp, but if it happens when you are upside down, the stomach contents escape into the esophagus. The esophagus enters the stomach from above, which is obvious from the diagram in Figure 4.1. What is not as obvious is that it goes into the *back* part of the top of the stomach. This means that lying on your belly is similar to standing up: What's in your stomach will fall to the front (away from the opening to the esophagus), and if the muscle at the bottom of the esophagus relaxes, it produces a burp; but if you lie on your back, the fluid in the stomach is right at the esophageal opening, just waiting for it to relax so it can go back into the esophagus. (Okay, so it's not really *waiting* for this to happen, of course, but it might as well be. Studies have shown clearly that babies have much less reflux when they sleep on their bellies than when they sleep on their backs.) Coughing, which is helpful in clearing lung mucus, also tightens the abdominal muscles and may put pressure on the stomach that forces material up into the esophagus. People with CF may produce more stomach acid than normal, and this may also make reflux worse.

Treatment for reflux is divided into three categories: simple measures, medications, and surgery. The simple measures include body position and meal characteristics. Head-down positions and lying on the back or slouching while sitting make reflux worse. Infant seats and swings, which put babies in a partly back-lying and partly slouching position, can cause infants to have more reflux than when they are lying face down. Sitting or standing straight up or lying face down makes reflux less likely to occur. Babies with CF should be put to sleep on their stomachs, unless they are very unhappy that way, despite recent recommendations to put babies to sleep on their backs. Older children with CF should eat meals at least 2 hours before bedtime, and they should avoid acid foods (tomatoes, soft drinks, fruit juices) and spicy foods. Caffeine (as in tea, Coke, Mountain Dew) may relax the lower esophageal sphincter and make reflux worse. Tight jeans may increase pressure on the belly and push stomach contents into the esophagus. Thickening infants' formula with 1 tbsp of dry rice cereal for each ounce of formula helps decrease spitting up and adds calories to the formula. Smoking (or being around smoke) can make reflux worse, so children with

CF and reflux should avoid smoke exposure. (Of course, the smoke has an even worse effect on the lungs themselves, so there are several reasons to avoid being around smoke.)

The first-line medications to treat reflux are those drugs that decrease the stomach's acid production. There are two main classes of these drugs, namely "histamine 2 (H_2) blockers" and "proton pump inhibitors." The most commonly used H_2 blockers are cimetidine (Tagamet), ranitidine hydrochloride (Zantac), and famotidine (Pepcid). Among the proton pump inhibitors are omerprazole (Prilosec), lansoprazole (Prevacid), pantoprazole sodium (Protonix), and esomeprazole (Nexium). Liquid antacids (Maalox, Mylanta, etc.), which do not stop the production of acid, but work to neutralize the acid that has been produced, can be helpful in some cases, and are often used in a "therapeutic trial." If a quick swig of Maalox makes the pain go away, the pain was probably caused by excess stomach acid.

One other medication that some physicians (and patients) have found helpful in decreasing reflux is the antibiotic erythromycin. Given in much lower doses than those used to kill bacteria, erythromycin helps speed up stomach emptying. An empty stomach has less fluid to reflux.

If the simple measures and medications do not produce enough relief from the reflux, a surgical procedure called a *fundoplication* (or a Nissen fundoplication) can be performed. This involves wrapping the upper part (the *fundus*) of the stomach around the bottom of the esophagus to strengthen the muscle at the bottom of the esophagus. When performed by a surgeon experienced in children's problems, this procedure is nearly always successful in treating reflux. It has also recently been done using a *laparoscope,* without as large an abdominal incision as previously required (a *laparoscopic fundoplication*), which helps make the procedure and recovery simpler for the patient.

Stomach

Increased Acid

There may be an increase in the amount of acid the stomach makes in CF. Although this does not seem to make ulcers common in people with CF, it may add to the problem of gastroesophageal reflux and cause pancreatic enzymes to be less effective. These possibilities have been discussed in other sections.

Liver

Fatty Liver

The livers of people with CF often become enlarged because the liver cells get packed with fat. This also happens in malnourished people without CF and it may be due to the malnutrition itself. (It is not known why malnutrition, which makes the rest of the body lose fat, makes the liver gain fat.) Fatty liver may happen at any age, and may improve as nutrition improves. By itself, it probably does not cause any problems.

Blocked Bile Ducts

In addition to blocking the small tubes in the lungs and in the pancreas, abnormally sticky mucus can block the bile ducts. The bile ducts are the small tubes in the liver that take the bile, including the bile salts needed for digestion, to the pancreatic duct and then to the duodenum. Thus, when the bile ducts are blocked, the digestion of fat may become more difficult, because fat digestion is more efficient if bile salts reach the intestine.

When the bile ducts become blocked in babies, the yellow bile cannot get out of the liver and backs up into the blood, where it is carried to the skin, causing a temporary yellow discoloration of the skin called *jaundice*. Jaundice in infants with CF is much more common in those who have meconium ileus (blockage of the intestines, which was discussed in an earlier section). In older children, the blocked ducts are less likely to cause jaundice, but they may cause scarring in the liver (*biliary fibrosis*), which may often be present without producing any signs or problems. If this scarring becomes severe, it is called *biliary cirrhosis* and can cause serious problems. This problem is quite uncommon, occurring in only 1% to 4% of people with CF.

The complex problems caused by cirrhosis of the liver include fluid (*ascites*) building up in the abdomen, and life-threatening bleeding from large veins (*varices*) that form in the esophagus and other areas of the gastrointestinal tract. A third problem resulting from cirrhosis is called "hypersplenism": The spleen, an organ in the left side of the abdomen (whose usual job is to filter old and damaged blood cells out of the circulation) swells. As it enlarges it traps many more blood cells flowing through it than normal, and it traps not just the old, damaged cells, it also traps cells that are still healthy and needed. If it traps blood-clotting cells called *platelets*, it may cause bleeding problems; if it traps the red blood cells, *anemia* may result; if it traps white blood cells, it can decrease the overall number of these infection-fighting cells. An enlarged spleen can rupture, causing rapid blood loss, so patients with large spleens are usually advised not to participate in contact sports.

If cirrhosis advances, it may interfere with the proper functioning of the liver, and certain blood tests of liver function may become abnormal. Many CF centers monitor these blood tests periodically (annually, for example). Patients with abnormal liver tests usually need to take extra vitamins (especially vitamins A, D, E, and K). The liver problems of CF may be quite stable for many years, without interfering with patients' overall health or feeling of well-being. In a very small percentage (1% to 2% of all patients), the liver may fail to work at all. Since the liver is essential to life, liver failure can cause death or prompt the need for liver transplant (see Chapter 8, *Transplantation*, for more details about liver transplantation).

There is no definite way at present to interrupt the scarring caused by the duct blockage in the liver, any more than in the pancreas. However, there is a relatively new medicine, called ursodeoxycholic acid ("urso"; Actigal) that is showing some promise. Urso (which means "bear") is a bile salt found in bears. Whether urso or other newer medications prove to be helpful in reducing or delaying the liver scarring itself, there are effective treatments for some of the problems caused by the liver scarring. If hypersplenism causes dangerously low levels of a particular type of blood cells, they can be replenished by transfusion, but this is rarely needed. If varices form and bleed, they can be treated by *sclerotherapy* or *variceal banding*. In sclerotherapy, a physician, usually a gastroenterologist, passes a flexible, lighted tube (an *esophagoscope*, or *endoscope*) down the throat and into the esophagus, and injects a chemical into these large vessels in order to make them scar until closed. Sclerotherapy is usually repeated at intervals ranging from weeks to many months, and is quite effective in treating varices. Variceal banding is similar, in that it is also performed by a gastroenterologist, operating with an endoscope in the esophagus, but instead of injecting a chemical into the swollen veins, the gastroenterologist slips a rubber band around the veins and pulls it tight to close those vessels.

Another method used to treat varices is a surgical technique that directs the blood flow away from the varices; this is called a *shunt* or *portosystemic shunt*. These shunts are major surgical procedures and make subsequent liver transplantation extremely difficult or impossible. A newer procedure called TIPS (for transjugular intrahepatic portosystemic shunt) can be performed by specially trained radiologists. This method can relieve some of the pressure that causes hypersplenism and esophageal varices, and it does not make it more difficult to do a liver transplantation later. In an even newer surgical approach to varices, a very few patients have had a *partial splenectomy* (removal of part of the spleen), with decreased varices and correction of the hypersplenism, with blood counts returning to normal. A liver transplantation might still be possible after a partial splenectomy.

Ascites, the collection of fluid in the abdomen, can be treated by changes in the amount of salt and water a person eats and by drugs (diuretics) that increase urination. There are other treatments for the complexities of liver failure, which your doctor can discuss with you if they are ever needed.

Liver transplantation can be performed for someone whose liver function has failed, or whose problems from esophageal varices cannot be controlled. Dozens of liver transplantations have been performed successfully in patients with CF. Any transplantation procedure is an extremely serious undertaking, often with unpredictable consequences, and should not be done if the risks are not fully understood by patient and family. Liver transplantation is discussed at greater length in Chapter 8, *Transplantation*.

Gallbladder

The gallbladder is a pouch attached to the bile ducts just outside the liver. It collects the bile made by the liver and releases it into the intestine at the time of a meal, when it is needed. The gallbladder and the tube that connects it to the liver are abnormal in one third of all people with CF, but this does not usually cause any problems. Approximately 10% of all patients with CF may have gallstones. If the gallstones cause pain, which they sometimes do, they are treated by surgery to remove the gallbladder and the stones.

Abdominal Pain

"Stomachaches" are a common problem for people with CF, and there are many possible causes. Several of the complications listed in Table 2.1 cause abdominal pain. DIOS may be the most commonly diagnosed cause of stomachaches, but reflux disease, gallstones, ulcers, pancreatitis (almost exclusively in those patients who do not need to take enzymes), and intussusception, all of which occur more often in patients with CF than in other people, are also major causes of abdominal problems. For patients who take enzyme supplements, it is important to take them regularly, because skipping enzymes is almost guaranteed to result in discomfort. In recent years, with insurance companies insisting on generic medications, many patients have had generic enzymes substituted for their usual brand (sometimes without their knowing it), a change that has resulted in abdominal pain, as the generic enzymes available through the 1990s and early 2000s have not been nearly as effective as the brand-name enzymes. Other sources of abdominal pain include excessive coughing, which can cause the abdominal muscles to become sore, and medications, some of which cause abdominal pain as well. People with CF can have the same abdominal problems as everyone else, including constipation, gastroenteritis (this is an intestinal infection, often inaccurately called a "stomach flu," and is frequently accompanied by nausea, vomiting, and/or diarrhea), urinary tract infection, and appendicitis. Lactose intolerance (the inability to digest the main carbohydrate in milk) is a common cause of abdominal pain in children with or without CF. In young women, gynecologic problems can be responsible for abdominal pain, and a rare cause of apparent abdominal pain in boys is *testicular torsion* (a twisted testicle). Finally, psychological stress can be a cause of stomach problems in some people.

Lippincott Williams & Wilkins
530 Walnut Street
Philadelphia, PA 19106 USA
LWW.com

Cystic Fibrosis: A Guide for Patient and Family
Third Edition
David M. Orenstein

NOTICE TO READERS

ERRATUM

Treatment of the lungs:

Important recent studies suggest that use of head-down positions for airway clearance treatments (as part of "postural drainage") for infants increases the likelihood of gastroesophageal reflux (see Chapter 4), and may even make lung disease worse, without improving airway clearance.

Airway clearance remains a mainstay of cystic fibrosis care, but most experts now recommend avoiding the head down positions during these treatments, especially for infants.

Appendix C (Airway Clearance Techniques) includes drawings of all the positions (including head down) that were formerly used, but I recommend NOT using the positions illustrated where the infant's head is below his or her chest.

Lippincott Williams & Wilkins
530 Walnut Street
Philadelphia, PA 19106 USA
LWW.com

Cystic Fibrosis: A Guide for Patient and Family
Third Edition
David M. Orenstein

NOTICE TO READERS

ERRATUM

Treatment of the lungs:

Important recent studies suggest that use of head-down positions for airway clearance treatments (as part of "postural drainage") for infants increases the likelihood of gastroesophageal reflux (see Chapter 4), and may even make lung disease worse, without improving airway clearance.

Airway clearance remains a mainstay of cystic fibrosis care, but most experts now recommend avoiding the head down positions during these treatments, especially for infants.

Appendix C (Airway Clearance Techniques) includes drawings of all the positions (including head down) that were formerly used, but I recommend NOT using the positions illustrated where the infant's head is below his or her chest.

5

Other Systems

THE BASICS

1. Sweat glands make sweat that is very salty in people with cystic fibrosis (CF). This gives us the sweat test; and occasionally patients, especially babies, lose excess salt in hot weather.
2. Thick mucus in the reproductive system means that most men with CF are sterile (although their sex life is completely normal), and women have a harder time getting pregnant than other women.
3. Both boys and girls may go through puberty later than their classmates, but most will develop normally, a year or two later.

SWEAT GLANDS

Normal Sweat Glands

Sweat begins in the coil of the sweat gland, below the surface of the skin (Figure 5.1) as a fluid that is chemically very similar to blood. As it makes its way toward the skin, sodium—with its positive electrical charge—is pumped out of the duct, and eventually back to the bloodstream. Whenever a positive charge leaves any tube or duct in the body, a negative charge accompanies it in order to maintain the same total electrical charge. In the case of the sweat, it is chloride and its negative charge that are carried out of the sweat fluid to follow the positive charge of sodium. By the time the fluid reaches the skin surface as sweat, it still has some salt, but the sodium and chloride contents are very low compared with those in the blood. This helps the body conserve sodium and chloride, especially in hot weather or when someone is exercising heavily.

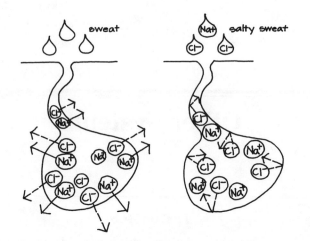

FIGURE 5.1. Sweat abnormality. In the normal (*left*) and cystic fibrosis (*right*) sweat gland, fluid begins in the base of the duct with a salt (sodium chloride) content close to that of blood. Then, in the normal sweat gland, as the fluid moves up the gland toward the skin, sodium (*Na⁺*)—with its positive charge—leaves the gland, and chloride (*Cl⁻*)—with its negative charge—follows, in order to keep electrical neutrality (same number of positives and negatives in all body compartments). But, in the cystic fibrosis sweat gland, because of the missing or blocked CFTR (cystic fibrosis transmembrane conductance regulator) (see Chapter 1, *The Basic Defect*), chloride cannot leave. Since chloride can't leave, it holds the sodium back too, and the fluid that emerges from the skin as sweat has a much higher concentration of sodium and chloride than normal.

Sweat Glands in Cystic Fibrosis

It has been known for many years that people with cystic fibrosis (CF) have an extremely high salt content in their sweat. You've seen in Chapter 1, *The Basic Defect*, that CF cells set up a roadblock to chloride trying to pass through their membranes. This block in the cells of the sweat duct means that chloride is stranded within the duct fluid. Because the negatively charged chloride can't leave, it holds sodium and its positive charge back as well. This means the fluid that emerges from the skin surface as sweat has abnormally large concentrations of sodium and chloride (salt).

The sweat abnormality is important for two reasons: (a) it allows the diagnosis of CF to be made, through the sweat test, and (b) it means that some patients, especially babies, may become sick by losing more salt than they take in during the summer (see the section *Salt Loss* below).

Over 99% of people with CF have abnormal sweat. They sweat the same *amount* of sweat, but there is an excess of salt (sodium and chloride) in their sweat. People without CF have less than 40 milliequivalents per liter (mEq/L) of chloride in their sweat (and a similar concentration of sodium), whereas people with CF have more than 60 mEq/L (and usually more than 80 mEq/L). This means that an analysis of the sweat can tell physicians whether someone has CF or not. Once the result of a test is positive, it will always be positive (meaning that if someone has CF, he or she will always have it). Also, a "positive test" is positive. Period. There are no differences between someone whose sweat chloride concentration is 83 mEq/L and someone whose concentration is 115 mEq/L. Both have CF. The higher number does not mean a worse case of CF. There are a few very uncommon CF mutations that cause CF with normal sweat chloride (and sodium) levels (see Chapter 11, *Genetics*, Table 11.4).

The Sweat Test

Much of the following information can also be found in Chapter 2, *Making the Diagnosis*.

Informal sweat testing has been done for centuries. There was a folk belief in Europe in the Middle Ages that "a child who tastes salty from a kiss on the brow . . . is hexed, and soon must die." Modern-day parents of children with CF frequently notice that their babies taste salty when they kiss them and that their older children have salt crystals on their faces and in their hair when they are active in the summertime. However, not everyone's taste buds are sensitive enough to distinguish between CF sweat and non-CF sweat. Fortunately, although a positive result of a sweat test means a child has CF, it is no longer true that he or she "soon must die." (Nor do we believe that he or she is "hexed"!)

Since the 1950s, a more accurate method of sweat testing has been available. The *Gibson–Cooke* method is a sweat test that is highly accurate. When sweat testing is done by any almost other method, mistakes frequently arise, resulting in *false positives* (children who *do not have CF* but whose tests indicate that they *do* have it) and in *false negatives* (children who *do* have CF but whose tests indicate that they *do not* have it). The correct method is the Gibson–Cooke method of sweat testing by *pilocarpine iontophoresis with quantitative analysis of sodium and/or chloride*. Here's what all that means:

The Gibson–Cooke method uses the chemical *pilocarpine* to stimulate the sweat glands to produce sweat. Pilocarpine reaches the working part of the sweat gland by first being placed on the skin and then directed into the sweat gland by a small electrical current; this process is called *iontophoresis*. The sweat is then collected on a cloth or paper pad or in a tiny coiled tube. It is then weighed carefully, and the sodium and/or chloride concentrations are measured very precisely (*quantitatively*).

To perform the test and collect the sweat takes 30 to 60 minutes. The laboratory analysis takes another 30 minutes or so. Therefore, it's usually several hours between the time someone comes into the laboratory and the time the results are ready.

The first step in the test is that the forearm (or occasionally, in a small baby, the lower leg, or even the back) is washed off, to remove any salt that might be on the skin. Then some pilocarpine is placed on the skin. Pilocarpine is colorless, odorless, and looks and feels like water. Two flat metal electrodes are placed on the skin and connected to a small box that sends a slight electrical current (approximately 2 to 5 mA) into the skin, driving the pilocarpine into the vicinity of the sweat gland, where it can "turn on" the sweat gland. The electrical current is usually not felt at all, but some people feel a mild tingling, and a few may even feel a harsher tingling or burning. It should not burn, and if it does, you should tell the technician, so that the current can be turned down.

After about 5 minutes with the electrodes in place, they are removed, the arm (or leg or back) is again wiped off, and that piece of absorbent material (gauze or filter paper) or coiled tube is placed on the skin. The technician then wraps the arm, covering the gauze with a dressing that is airtight and watertight, so that no sweat will evaporate or leak out. During the next 30 to 60 minutes, the dressing is left in place while the "revved up" sweat glands are making sweat. The technician then removes the dressing with tweezers or forceps, taking care not to touch the gauze or filter paper with his or her fingers, puts the paper (now soaked with sweat) or tube (now filled with sweat) into a bottle, and takes it to the laboratory. In the laboratory, the technician weighs the bottle to see how much sweat there is, rinses the sweat out of the paper or gauze or squirts it out of the coiled tubing into a container, and then puts it through the chemical analyzers to find out precisely how much sodium and/or chloride is in the sweat. Some laboratories measure the chloride, some measure the sodium, and some measure both. As long as the sweat is obtained by this method, it doesn't matter which part of the salt is measured.

When the test is performed by this method, *by a laboratory experienced in performing this test*, the result should enable the physician to make a definite and accurate diagnosis.

One other method of sweat testing is also acceptable, one that is not very widely used: the *Macroduct Sweat Collection System* (Wescor, Logan, UT), whose use is mostly confined to a "screening" test in doctors' offices or hospitals that are not near a CF center. Positive tests from this method should then be confirmed with a test by the Gibson–Cooke method.

Problems with Sweat Testing

In an experienced laboratory, not getting enough sweat is the only major problem that interferes with obtaining a reliable result. Most laboratory experts say that they must have 100 mg of sweat in order to do an accurate analysis. Some people, especially some very young babies (under 1 month old) may not make enough sweat to analyze. There is a common (incorrect) belief that sweat testing cannot be done in very young babies. However, it *can* be done, and *should* be done in any baby for whom the possibility of CF has been raised. If enough sweat is collected—as it will be for most babies—the results will be valid, even within the first weeks of life, and even in a premature infant.

Adults have higher sweat sodium and chloride levels than children, but even in adults, a sweat chloride concentration greater than 60 mEq/L is abnormal.

There are a very few conditions that give elevated sweat chloride or sodium levels, and these are usually readily distinguished from CF. Similarly, there are very few people with CF whose sweat sodium and chloride concentrations are below 60 mEq/L. Finally, there are very few people whose sweat sodium and chloride concentrations are between 40 and 60 mEq/L. These few people are said to have test results in "the gray zone," or the "intermediate range," meaning neither definitely positive nor definitely negative. Some uncommon CF mutations have been found to cause CF with intermediate range, or even normal, sweat chloride and sodium levels. Tests in this range are discussed in Chapter 2, *Making the Diagnosis,* and the various mutations are discussed in Chapter 11, *Genetics.*

That a hospital or laboratory says they can perform a sweat test is not adequate assurance that they can do it correctly. *Nearly one half of all patients who come to CF centers having had sweat tests done in outlying hospitals have received incorrect results from these tests.*

Salt Loss

In addition to making the sweat test possible, the sweat abnormality can also affect the health of some people with CF. For each drop of sweat made, considerably more sodium and chloride are lost from the body than would be lost in someone without CF. In most children and adults with CF, the body is able to regulate the amount of salt in the bloodstream amazingly well. When more salt is lost, people want and take in more salt, and the kidneys reduce the amount of salt lost through the urine. Under most circumstances, even including active exercise in hot weather, if adequate salt is available, children and adults with CF will take in the proper amounts after they've stopped exercising. Pretzels and other salty snacks may be available for toddlers, whereas older children and adults can have access to the saltshaker, and no further supplements are needed. Salt tablets are not needed.

Infants with CF may lose too much salt in their sweat, and are not able to let their parents know that they feel like having a pickle or pretzel or other salty food. Each year, especially during summer months, some infants with CF become ill because of having lost too much salt. They become lethargic, their appetite falls off, and they seem sickly. If this happens, they may require hospitalization and intravenous fluids containing replacement sodium and chloride. In order to prevent this problem, it's advisable for infants to be given a tiny bit of salt in their bottles during hot summer months. An amount as small as ⅛ tsp, once or twice a day, is probably adequate. Because too much salt can cause problems, it's best to provide moderate, regular supplements.

Some older children and adults who are very active during hot weather will need to be careful about replacing lost fluid and salt. The only immediate danger for a teenager under extreme exertion, such as marathon running or a long, tough football practice in full uniform in hot weather, is fluid loss. Athletes should drink more water or—especially good—a sports drink like Gatorade than they feel they need, since thirst is not as sensitive a guide as is the taste for salt. Neither of these tastes is great *during* exercise. All children underestimate their need for fluid when they exercise in the heat, and young people with CF underestimate their fluid needs even more than other children. Salt replacement does not need to be immediate, and will be accurately guided by taste.

BONE AND JOINT PROBLEMS

People with CF who have absolutely no lung problems will not have any skeletal problems that can be attributed to CF. However, almost everyone with CF who has even the slightest degree of lung involvement (and that means almost everyone with CF) will have a condition called *digital clubbing*. This is an unfortunate name for this condition, since it sounds rather grotesque, and while in its most extreme form it can be very noticeable, in most cases it affects only slightly the shape of the fingers and toes. As shown in Figure 5.2, two features distinguish clubbed fingers from nonclubbed fingers. The first is the angle at which the base of the nail meets the finger. This angle becomes progressively flatter as clubbing increases. The second characteristic of a clubbed finger is that the thickness of the tip of the finger, the part beyond the last joint, when measured from the base of the nail to the bottom of the finger pad, becomes thicker than the finger at the joint itself.

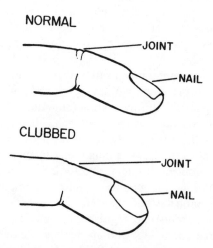

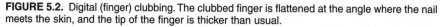

FIGURE 5.2. Digital (finger) clubbing. The clubbed finger is flattened at the angle where the nail meets the skin, and the tip of the finger is thicker than usual.

The cause of digital clubbing is not known. In general, as lung disease worsens, so does clubbing. However, many people with fairly mild lung disease may also have pronounced clubbing. Therefore, clubbing itself does not precisely reflect the degree of lung involvement.

There are other conditions aside from CF that are associated with clubbing, including some forms of liver disease, inflammatory bowel disease, and heart diseases in which the blood oxygen level is too low. Clubbing is a very helpful diagnostic clue when a child with lung problems is being evaluated, since clubbing is found in most patients with CF over the age of 2 or 3 years and is very rare in children who do not have CF. Any child with chronic or recurrent respiratory problems and digital clubbing should be tested for CF.

Another complication of CF that may affect the skeletal system is one that causes bone or joint pain in the legs, particularly the knees. This problem is called *hypertrophic pulmonary osteoarthropathy* (HPOA). The name indicates that it is seen in people with pulmonary problems, and refers to "something wrong with" (-*opathy*) the bones (*osteo*) and/or joints (*arthro*). The term "hypertrophic" refers to radiographic findings in this condition, which include an elevation of the *periosteum* (the membrane covering the bone). This periosteal elevation makes it appear as though there is extra (*hyper*) growth (-*trophy*). The condition can be painful. It is not very common, and occurs mostly in people with severe lung disease. It usually improves as the lungs improve with treatment, but specific treatment for the bone/joint problem (see below) can also be helpful.

Finally, there is an uncommon and poorly understood arthritis—most commonly of the ankle or knee—that some people with CF get. The joint is tender, and may have a skin rash associated with it. It usually gets better with antiinflammatory treatment, like aspirin or ibuprofen.

Treating Bone and Joint Problems

The degree of digital clubbing roughly corresponds with the degree of lung involvement, so treating the lungs may indirectly lessen the amount of clubbing. There is no treatment for clubbing aside from treatment of the lungs. Fortunately, a specific treatment is not required for clubbing, since it is not a painful condition. The only problem with clubbing is the embarrassment it can cause some people in adjusting to having fingers that look different from normal.

Osteoarthropathy may cause some physical discomfort, and people often will not mention it to their CF physicians, being unaware that leg or knee pain could be related to CF. As with clubbing, osteoarthropathy improves when the lungs improve. Regardless of the condition of the lungs, the discomfort of osteoarthropathy responds very well to aspirin, ibuprofen, and other similar antiinflammatory drugs (see Appendix B, *Medications*).

REPRODUCTIVE SYSTEM IN CYSTIC FIBROSIS

Although the reproductive systems of people with CF are normal, the thick mucus found in so many other places in the body also affects this system. (The reproductive system is discussed at greater length in Chapter 14, *Cystic Fibrosis and Adulthood*.)

The Male Reproductive System in Cystic Fibrosis

In boys and men with CF, the reproductive system is completely normal, with one exception. In 98% of boys and men with CF, the *vas deferens* is incompletely formed or totally blocked. The *vas deferens* is the tube that carries sperm from the testicles to the penis. This is the tube that is cut and tied when a man has a vasectomy. Sperm is formed normally in the testicles, but because of the blockage, it cannot be released. Men with CF have completely normal sex lives, but the 98% of men with CF who have this blockage are sterile. (It is very much as though everything had been normal, and they had gotten a vasectomy.) A small proportion of men with CF (about 2%) are not sterile, and some have fathered children.

It is possible to test whether a teenager or adult with CF is one of the 98% who are sterile or one of the 2% who are not. The patient simply gives a semen specimen to the laboratory, where it is analyzed for sperm.

The Female Reproductive System in Cystic Fibrosis

In women with CF, the problems related to the reproductive system are subtler than those in men. The main problem is that the mucus lining the cervix (the opening to the uterus, or womb) is thick, just like mucus elsewhere. As a result, it is harder for women with CF to get pregnant than it is for women without CF. It certainly is possible though; several hundred women with CF have gotten pregnant, and many of these women have delivered babies.

Women whose lungs are in excellent shape when they get pregnant usually do well with the pregnancy. Women whose lungs are at all involved with CF lung disease may have a very hard time with the pregnancy. There are many women with CF who have been in fairly good health before they became pregnant, but whose health deteriorated during the pregnancy.

DELAYED PHYSICAL DEVELOPMENT

Both boys and girls with CF may go through puberty 1 to 2 years later than their classmates. This occurs as an indirect result of CF and is likely to be a direct result of poor nutrition or of chronic lung infection. Delayed development can be a problem in any chronic illness, for energy expended to fight the illness depletes the body's energy reserve for growth. This can be difficult emotionally for young people, too, if all their friends are shooting up in height, filling out, and growing into physical adulthood, and they are left behind, with the body of a small child. It may soften the blow somewhat if they know that most young people with CF eventually go through puberty, although it may be a year or two behind their friends. The treatment for this problem is directed at the underlying causes and in CF, that means treating the lungs and improving the nutrition.

6

Nutrition

THE BASICS

1. Nutrition is important for people with cystic fibro-
    sis (CF) for growth and overall health, including the
    health of their lungs.
2. Good nutrition for patients with CF has three parts:
    a. High-calorie diet
    b. Pancreatic enzymes with every meal and snacks
        containing fat and protein.
    c. Vitamins
3. If someone can't gain weight on a regular diet, oral
    high-calorie supplements may help; if not, tube feed-
    ings may be helpful for weight gain.

THE IMPORTANCE OF NUTRITION IN CYSTIC FIBROSIS

Malnourished people do not grow well, and often they do not feel well. Malnutrition damages the immune system, which is the body's defense against infection and, in someone with cystic fibrosis (CF), may contribute to the pulmonary
disease and hasten death. Patients with CF who are better nourished grow better,
have better pulmonary function, and live longer than patients with poor nutrition.

MONITORING GROWTH AND NUTRITION

In an adult, generalized malnutrition shows up first as weight loss. In children,
who should grow and gain weight steadily, a slowing down of weight gain may
be the first sign of malnutrition. This is most easily detected by plotting a child's
weight on a growth chart (Figure 6.1), which compares an individual's growth to

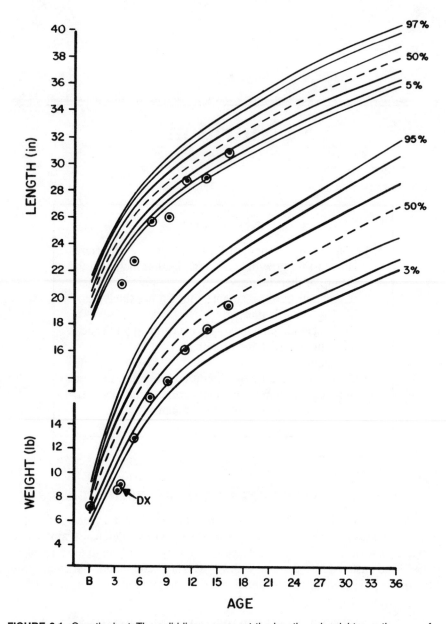

FIGURE 6.1. Growth chart. The solid lines represent the length and weight growth curves for normal children at various ages (in months). The *"3%"* line refers to the length and weight of healthy children in the lowest 3% for their age; that is, 3% of healthy children will have a weight that falls on or below the 3% line, whereas 97% will be heavier. The *"50%"* dotted lines represent the 50th percentile, or the average length and weight for healthy children. The circles represent the specific measurements for one youngster with CF. This child's weight was near average at birth and fell below the third percentile by the time of diagnosis (*Dx*). Treatment began after diagnosis, and the child's weight reached just below the average for age by 18 months.

that of other children of the same age and sex. If the child's growth does not keep up with the curves, malnutrition may be the cause. This growth curve should not be used as a "grade" where you strive to attain a high number, but as a form of tracking a child's growth over time. The growth curve shows the child's individual growth pattern over the years and is an indication of how the child is doing nutritionally. In 2000, new growth charts were distributed to health professionals by the Centers for Disease Control and Prevention, with updated normal values, and percentile lines representing the third, tenth, 25th, 50th, 75th, 90th, and 97th percentiles. The revised growth charts also include the standard measurements for height and weight, and in addition, a chart for body mass index (BMI), which looks at *weight in relation to height*. The BMI can be used to identify individuals who are under- or overweight better than just the weight alone.

When malnutrition affects growth, it usually affects weight first. When weight has been severely affected, the poor nutrition can affect height in a similar fashion, and a child may begin to show signs of falling behind in on the height curves (that is, he or she may not grow tall as fast as a healthy child of the same age). Finally, if severe malnutrition affects a very young child at a time when the brain is actively growing (up to about 36 months old), the head circumference may grow more slowly than normal. Weight, height, and head circumference should be plotted regularly for babies and weight, height, and BMI for all children and adolescents to identify evidence of malnutrition.

Another method of assessing a person's nutritional state is called anthropometrics ("measuring people"). Measurements are taken, such as skinfold thickness, which gives an estimate as to how much fat is stored in the body, and mid arm circumference, which gives an estimate of the amount of muscle protein. It is important to have both fat and muscle protein. When someone is not eating well, fat stores can be broken down to be used for energy, sparing the muscle protein, so that the person does not become too weak. When the fat stores run out, the body is forced to use protein for energy, and muscle wasting takes place. Low muscle mass may also result from lack of use (not enough exercising). By comparing annual measurements of muscle and fat mass, the dietitian and physician can determine the adequacy of the fat and muscle mass. Diet and exercise recommendations can be made when these measurements need improvement.

Many aspects of a person's nutritional state can also be measured by blood tests such as albumin, total protein, glucose, liver function tests, fat-soluble vitamins, and hemoglobin/hematocrit levels.

CAUSES OF MALNUTRITION IN CYSTIC FIBROSIS

At one time, it was assumed that the malnutrition that affects so many children and adults with CF was entirely due to the poor digestion of food, which, in turn, was due to the lack of pancreatic enzymes and bile salts, as was discussed in Chapter 4, *The Gastrointestinal Tract*. Although enzyme deficiency is a major cause of malnutrition in CF, there are additional factors contributing to malnutrition: (a) enzyme supplements do not work perfectly; (b) people with CF may not take in enough calories, even for someone with normal needs; and (c) there are increased caloric needs in CF.

Enzyme Deficiency

Although oral enzyme supplements help a great deal, they do not work perfectly. The digestion of most patients with CF is not complete, even with enzymes, and some degree of malabsorption of foods still occurs. (Remember that digestion is the process of breaking down food into particles tiny enough for them to be absorbed into the bloodstream from the intestines; enzymes are needed for digestion; digestion is needed for absorption; and absorption of food is needed for growth and energy.) The imperfection of oral enzyme supplements is due to the difficulty of mimicking perfectly the body's finely tuned system for trickling the pancreatic enzymes into the duodenum just as the food arrives from the stomach. When pancreatic enzyme capsules are swallowed with the meals, they may not arrive in the duodenum at the precise time to meet up with the food. The oral enzyme supplements can also be inactivated in the stomach by the stomach acids. We do not usually supplement bile salts (similar to those naturally produced in the gallbladder), and the possible lack of bile salts may prevent the oral enzymes from acting optimally. Finally, with CF, the secretion of bicarbonate from the pancreas is also limited, causing incomplete neutralization of stomach acid, which may prevent the enteric coating on the oral enzymes from dissolving. All of these factors may contribute to malabsorption and poor nutrition, even in patients who take all of their enzymes as prescribed. Not taking the prescribed enzymes can also be a problem, and it is not unheard of for patients with CF to "forget" to take enzymes because of not wanting their classmates to see them.

In addition to interfering with good nutrition, malabsorption of food can also cause bothersome side effects. Some signs of malabsorption include the following:

• Gas and bloating
• Stomach cramps
• Frequent stools
• Greasy or floating stools
• Larger and looser, bulky stools
• Bad-smelling stools
• Lighter brown or yellow stools

Often, malabsorption can cause the child's appetite to become bigger to make up for the food he or she is not absorbing. In fact, the "textbook picture" of a baby or child with untreated CF is someone with a voracious (huge) appetite, but poor weight gain. If you see a large increase in your child's appetite, you should watch for the other signs of malabsorption listed above. If you suspect malabsorption, discuss with the CF team how to adjust the oral enzyme supplements.

Intestinal infections can cause diarrhea with an increase in the number of stools that become watery instead of bulky. Diarrhea is different from malabsorption in that it is not treated by adjusting oral enzymes. To treat diarrhea that persists for more than 1 day, contact your doctor.

Inadequate Caloric Intake

It is commonly believed that people with CF have a large appetite, and some do. But, many children, teenagers, and adults with CF actually eat less food than their friends do. Malnutrition itself may decrease a person's appetite (this is called the "anorexia of malnutrition"). Feeling sick and coughing a lot can also decrease a person's appetite. In the past, patients with CF were prescribed a low-fat diet, because it resulted in less fat in the stools. Having less fat in the diet meant less fat in the stools; unfortunately, it also meant fewer calories for the body to use for growth. The low-fat diet attempted to make up for the lost fat calories by increasing calories from carbohydrates. However, an ounce of fat has more than twice as many calories as an ounce of carbohydrate; so, if you are on a low-fat diet, you have to eat a lot more to get the same number of calories for growth. On low-fat diets, many people with CF were unable to eat enough calories and became malnourished. With the right amount of oral enzymes, even a high-fat diet can be digested and absorbed, giving more calories with less food. A low-fat diet is no longer recommended except under very special circumstances. Instead, a high-fat, high-protein diet is recommended for all patients with CF unless otherwise instructed. Even so, it simply may be impossible for some patients with CF—try though they will—to eat enough to supply their needs. In this case, it still is possible to reestablish good growth, with one or more of the available additions to a well-rounded diet (see later, after the section on enzymes).

Increased Caloric Demands

The third main reason for malnutrition in CF is an increased use of calories. Coughing, breathing hard, and fighting an infection all require additional calories. If you are using more calories in these ways all day, the need for extra calories accumulates. It may be difficult for the person with CF to keep up with this high calorie demand. The caloric intake required to maintain good growth in someone with CF is usually 30% to 50% *more* than that required for a person of the same age and sex without CF.

SPECIAL DEFICIENCIES IN CYSTIC FIBROSIS

Hypoalbuminemia (Low Blood Albumin Levels)

Albumin is the main body protein in blood. One of its primary roles in the blood is to keep water in the arteries and veins. If there is not enough albumin in the blood (hypoalbuminemia), water leaks out into the skin and other organs and produces skin puffiness called edema. Hypoalbuminemia and edema may occur in infants with CF before they are diagnosed, and may be the clue that leads to the diagnosis of CF. A few decades ago, it seemed to be a bigger problem among undiagnosed infants fed with soy-milk formula, perhaps because the protein in soy formulas was missing an essential amino acid. Modern-day soy formulas are now fortified with this missing product, but most CF physicians still shy away from soy formulas. Hypoalbuminemia is treated by giving pancreatic enzymes and plenty of protein in the diet.

Essential Fatty Acid Deficiency

Fatty acids are the parts of the fat (triglyceride) molecule. Essential fatty acids are fatty acids the body needs that it cannot make from other nutrients; therefore, they have to come from the diet. Two essential fatty acids, linoleic acid and α-linolenic acid, are found in breast milk, fresh-water fish, and vegetable oils such as canola and safflower. Linoleic acid is further metabolized (processed) in the body to arachidonic acid; α-linolenic acid is metabolized to d ocosohexaenoic acid (DHA). DHA has gotten a lot of publicity recently, with speculation that abnormal fatty acid metabolism is a primary problem in CF and that DHA supplements can be helpful. More research needs to be done in this area before we can recommend jumping on the DHA bandwagon. All of the essential fatty acids are used for a number of complex and necessary functions, including the manufacture of cell membranes. They also appear to be needed for optimal lung function. The difficulties in fat digestion and absorption in untreated CF patients can show up early in life as deficiencies of these essential fatty acids, since the body's need for them cannot be met by making them out of other nutrients. In addition, the essential fatty acids that do get absorbed may get used for other caloric needs: For example, they may get "burned up" to supply energy for breathing. With infants being diagnosed and started on enzymes at a younger age, fewer infants have this problem now than in the past.

Iron Deficiency

Iron is concentrated in the blood, but some is present in every living cell of the body. Iron's main function is to carry oxygen and carbon dioxide from one body tissue to another via the blood. Most iron is present in the hemoglobin molecule of the red blood cell. Any more than very mild iron deficiency will lead to low hemoglobin levels and anemia (low red blood cell concentration). Symptoms of iron deficiency include fatigue, decreased resistance to infection, and soreness in the mouth. To screen for iron deficiency, hemoglobin levels are measured.

Good dietary sources of iron are fortified cereals, meats, dried fruits, and deep-green vegetables. Iron in meat, poultry, and fish is absorbed better than the iron from vegetables. Iron-deficiency anemia is the most common nutritional deficiency in children in North America, affecting almost 40% of young children. It is most common after 1 year of age (between 12 and 36 months) when children stop taking breast milk or iron-fortified formulas and begin taking whole milk, which is low in iron. It also occurs in adolescent males, and females from adolescence through adulthood. Iron deficiency may occur from inadequate iron intake, impaired absorption, or blood loss. It is important during times of higher iron needs to encourage the intake of iron-rich food sources, or to supplement the diet with a multivitamin with iron. These times of high iron needs include times of blood loss, either through healthy causes (especially menstruation), bleeding from injury or disease, or times of multiple blood tests.

If anemia is detected, an oral iron supplement will be prescribed. When taking iron supplements, it is important to remember to take them without pancreatic enzymes, because (unlike the case for fat or protein, where enzymes help absorption) the enzymes interfere with the iron absorption. To improve iron absorption, take the oral iron supplements with a beverage that contains vitamin C (orange or grapefruit juice).

Fat-soluble Vitamins (Vitamins A, D, E, and K)

Vitamins A, D, E, and K require fat to be absorbed and, since patients with CF have trouble digesting and absorbing fat, the bloodstream levels of these vitamins are often low in patients with CF. As part of their daily medical therapy, patients with CF are put on a "standard CF dose" of vitamins, based on age. This dose is higher than that recommended for people without CF. It is important that the vitamins prescribed are taken daily to prevent deficiency of those vitamins. To make vitamins easier to absorb, they should be taken with meals when oral enzymes and food are supplied. A physical examination and blood tests can then tell if more vitamins are required. If a vitamin level is low, this could be from not taking the prescribed dose daily, or not taking the dose with enzymes. Whatever the reason for the low vitamin level, extra vitamins may be prescribed to help improve the blood levels.

There are vitamin supplements especially made to meet the fat-soluble vitamin needs of patients with CF, and for some patients this may be more convenient. Some of these CF vitamin preparations include ADEK (Axcan Scandipharm, Birmingham, AL), Vitamax (Ambix Labs, East Rutherford, NJ), and Source ABDEK (SourceCF, Huntsville, AL).

Some people may want to take more vitamins and minerals than have been prescribed, thinking that more may be better. Actually, the body uses only a certain amount of each vitamin and mineral, and a large excess cannot be used. For some vitamins (water-soluble vitamins), the extra amount just ends up in the urine. (Some public health experts who laugh at Americans' overzealous use of vitamins say that "Americans have the most nutritious urine in the world!") The fat-soluble vitamins are not excreted in the urine, and taking an excessive amount can be dangerous.

"Complementary" and "Alternative Medicine" Products

There are several "complementary" and "alternative medicine" or health food products available that make claims to cure or help CF. These products can be problematic for two reasons. First, these products are classified as nutritional supplements and are not regulated by the FDA (Food and Drug Administration) nearly as carefully as medicines or drugs. No proof of safety or effectiveness is required. Furthermore, there is no assurance of purity or potency in most of these products. If you want to try one of these products, first discuss it with your CF team. Some products could interfere with the CF medicines that you take daily, others might not help, and, some might actually be dangerous.

Vitamin A

Vitamin A is needed for fighting infections, preventing night blindness, and general growth and maintenance of the body. Retinol and carotene are two types of vitamin A. Vitamin A is found in animal products, particularly liver, egg yolks, and fortified milk. Carotene is found in dark-green, deep-yellow, and orange vegetables and fruits and is converted to active vitamin A in the body. Vitamin A is normally absorbed from the intestine and then stored in the liver to be used when it is needed. Two proteins made by the liver—prealbumin and retinol-binding protein—are needed to extract the vitamin A from the liver. Blood levels of vitamin A have been found to be below normal in some people with CF, even when supplemental enzymes and vitamins are given. The abnormal fat digestion is part of the problem with vitamin A in CF, but even when vitamin A is absorbed and stored in the liver, it will not be available to the body if there are low levels of prealbumin and retinol-binding protein (two forms of albumin). Zinc is a mineral that helps retinol-binding protein extract vitamin A from the liver, so it is important that patients receive zinc in their diet and multivitamins. Vitamin A levels can be decreased with acute illness, so levels measured during an illness may yield misleading low results.

A standard multivitamin preparation that contains 5,000 to 10,000 IU (international unit) of Vitamin A should be given daily to help prevent deficiency. Vitamin A is better absorbed when it is taken with a meal and enzymes. B-carotene is a precursor to vitamin A and functions as an antioxidant in fighting inflammation. It is uncertain whether a β-carotene deficiency exists in patients with CF, but this question (and others about β-carotene in CF) is being studied.

Vitamin D

Vitamin D is needed for growth of strong bones and teeth and for normal functioning of many other organs. It is important for the absorption of calcium and phosphorus from the diet into the bloodstream. Vitamin D has taken on added importance over recent years with our increasing awareness of problems with bone health in older patients with CF. Severe vitamin D deficiency causes a bone disease called rickets, in which the bones are abnormally soft. This problem is unusual in CF. More subtle vitamin D deficiency can contribute to problems that are much more common, especially in older patients and those who have received many steroid medications. These more common bone problems are *osteopenia* and *osteoporosis*. *Osteopenia* means a decreased bone mass or density; *osteoporosis* is osteopenia that is bad enough to reduce the bone strength so much that fractures are more likely. Vitamin D is found in fortified milk and dairy products. It is also made in the skin by the action of sunlight, but in areas of limited sunlight, in people who stay indoors, or who use sunscreen with sun-protection factors (SPF) of greater than 8, the exposure to the sunlight might not be enough to meet the vitamin D needs. Vitamin D from the diet or skin must be activated by the liver and kidneys, which means that people with liver disease or kidney disease are more susceptible to vitamin D deficiency. The Cystic Fibrosis Foundation recommends checking vitamin D levels annually to screen for deficiency. If deficiency does occur, the diet should be reviewed for adequate calcium and vitamin D intake and additional vitamin D may be needed to correct the low blood levels. Plenty of sunshine is also helpful to keep an adequate amount of vitamin D in the body, and weight-bearing exercise (like walking or jogging) is also important to maintain bone strength.

Vitamin E

Vitamin E is important for the functioning of a number of important body parts, especially nerves. Good sources of vitamin E are vegetable oil, wheat germ, dried beans and peas. Symptoms of vitamin E deficiency may include unsteadiness while walking. Vitamin E deficiency also causes an abnormal knee-jerk reflex, which the doctor checks by hitting the knee with the rubber reflex hammer.

Vitamin E deficiency can be detected by blood tests. Low vitamin E levels are common even with patients taking supplements and pancreatic enzymes. Standard multivitamin supplements do not contain the amount of vitamin E needed to maintain adequate levels, and a separate vitamin E supplement is recommended. It is important for patients with CF to take extra vitamin E daily. If blood tests indicate a deficiency, a higher dose of vitamin E can be prescribed. Water-soluble forms of vitamin E are more easily absorbed than the more expensive health food store preparations of vitamin E.

Vitamin K

Vitamin K is needed by the liver for making some of the clotting factors that stop bleeding. When the vitamin K level is low, the clotting times are prolonged. Vitamin K is also important for bone formation. Green leafy vegetables and cauliflower are good food sources of vitamin K, and it is also found in dairy products. In addition, bacteria that normally live in the intestines make vitamin K. People with CF may need extra vitamin K, though, because both dietary and intestinal sources of vitamin K may be less than normal: First, vitamin K may not be well absorbed by the patient with CF. A second problem that someone with CF might have is that antibiotics given to treat infection in the lungs may kill the bacteria in the intestines, cutting down on the number of intestinal bacteria available to make vitamin K. This means that some people with CF who take a lot of antibiotics may need additional vitamin K.

Low blood levels of vitamin K can lead to very serious bleeding. There are two blood tests for clotting factors to estimate vitamin K levels. These are the "PT" test (prothrombin time) and the "PTT" test (partial thromboplastin time). The PT becomes abnormal if levels of vitamin K are too low, and in more severe deficiencies, the PTT may also become abnormal. Vitamin K deficiency can be corrected by adding oral or injected vitamin K supplements. Since the liver is needed to make the clotting factors, even vitamin K given by injection may not provide enough if the liver is failing to work (as in severe cirrhosis, discussed in Chapter 4). In this case, the already-made clotting factors may be administered by giving a transfusion of "fresh-frozen plasma." The CF multivitamins contain some vitamin K but more research needs to be done to determine they contain enough. If you take an over-the-counter multivitamin, look for one containing vitamin K. Further studies need to be done to determine the optimal dose of vitamin K for patients with CF.

Hypomagnesemia (Low Blood Magnesium)

Magnesium, like calcium, phosphorus, sodium, and chloride, is one of the minerals the body needs. Good food sources of magnesium include whole grains, dark-green leafy vegetables, milk, soybeans, and molasses. Normally, magnesium is absorbed from the diet, and the kidneys get rid of any extra through the urine. When there is too little magnesium in the blood (hypomagnesemia), the signs include weakness, shakiness, and muscle cramps. In CF, there are a number of causes for hypomagnesemia. Maldigestion and malabsorption may prevent the magnesium from being absorbed from the intestine. Some antibiotics given for lung infections [especially the "aminoglycosides" (see Appendix B, *Medications*)—most of these end in "-micin" or "-mycin"] and diuretics given for heart or liver problems may cause too much magnesium to be lost in the urine. During a physical examination, hypomagnesemia can be checked for by assessing the knee-jerk reflex. If the knee-jerk reflexes are too brisk (the opposite of what happens with vitamin E deficiency), this could indicate low magnesium levels. The hands and face muscles can be evaluated for muscle spasms. Blood measurements of magnesium can confirm the diagnosis of hypomagnesemia. The treatment is by oral or intravenous (IV) magnesium supplements. Sometimes a large amount is needed to correct a deficiency.

Hypoelectrolytemia

The main chemicals in the bloodstream that carry an electrical charge, such as sodium, chloride, and potassium, are called *electrolytes*. People with CF lose a lot of salt in their sweat, and since salt consists of sodium and chloride, they may lose enough sodium and chloride to lower the blood levels of these electrolytes. This is especially likely to happen during exertion (exercise) in hot weather, or in infants whose diet is low in salt, and who can't tell us they feel like having something salty to eat.

Once CF is diagnosed, the problem can usually be prevented, and most CF experts advise adding extra salt to the diet. Infants receiving formula and plain baby foods that are low in salt should have a small amount of salt added to the formula (about ⅛ tsp per day should be about right). This small amount of salt should prevent any problems from developing and will avoid the serious problems that could be caused by giving too much salt at one time. During hot weather or times of increased sweating, this amount of salt may need to be increased. Older children need no special treatment, other than free access to salty foods or the saltshaker. Their taste will tell them how much salt they need. This is discussed more in Chapter 5, *Other Systems*.

NUTRITIONAL TREATMENT

Basic dietary treatment in CF consists of a well-rounded diet with plenty of fat, protein, and carbohydrates, taken with enough pancreatic enzymes to provide maximum absorption. Tables 6.1 and 6.2 contain guidelines and sugges-

---

TABLE 6.1. *Suggestions for Improving Your Child's Nutrition*

1. Plan a definite eating schedule with three well-balanced meals and at least two snacks daily. Try to have the meals around the same time each day.
2. Meals should last 20–30 min. Young children have short attention spans and usually lose interest in eating after spending this amount of time at the table.
3. If the child refuses to eat for more than 10 min, remove him or her from the table and offer nothing to eat until the next scheduled meal or snack.
4. Scheduled snacks are important, but all day snacking or "grazing" should be avoided. Grazing keeps the child full and he or she never really feels hungry.
5. Give a large, high-calorie snack at bedtime, unless the child has reflux (see Chapter 4).
6. Keep food offered simple. Children can be overwhelmed by too many foods at one meal.
7. Try to make foods attractive and appealing. Offer foods that the child can easily manage (cut-up meats, etc.).
8. Make the child's eating environment comfortable. Children should sit in sturdy chairs with their feet supported. The table and food should be easily reached.
9. Avoid distractions at meal time, such as television. Television provides too much stimulus and the child does not focus on eating.
10. Be sure the child is not filling up on fluids. Do not give any beverage 30–60 min before a meal.
11. Reward positive behavior with verbal praise. Sticker charts may work well with younger children.
12. Parents should set good examples by eating nutritious meals with their children. If you don't eat well, you can't expect your child to eat well.

TABLE 6.2. *Ways to Increase Calories*

1. Add margarine to the bread of sandwiches; grill sandwiches. Melt margarine on vegetables, waffles, and potatoes.
2. Add grated Parmesan cheese to spaghetti, casseroles, popcorn, and salads.
3. Melt cheese with scrambled eggs and casseroles and add to sandwiches. Order extra cheese on pizza.
4. Chopped nuts add lots of calories; add to cookie dough, breads, and pancakes. Buy breakfast cereals with nuts and dried fruit for higher calories per serving.
5. Drink whole milk instead of 2% or skim milk. Use whole-milk cheeses instead of skim-milk cheeses.
6. Add powdered nonfat dry milk to whole milk to increase the calories (¼ cup powder milk to 8 oz whole milk). Use the high-protein milk in cooking.
7. Use cheese sauce on vegetables, potatoes, pretzels, nachos, and french fries.
8. Use gravy on meats, potatoes, rice, noodles, and french fries.
9. Top hot chocolate, pudding, gelatin, and milkshakes with whipped topping.
10. Use extra eggs in pancake, waffle, or french toast batter.
11. Add a package of vanilla instant breakfast to instant pudding mix.
12. Choose glazed doughnuts instead of cake doughnuts (275 cal vs. 105 cal), or chocolate-covered sandwich cookies instead of vanilla wafers (90 cal vs. 10 cal).

tions for maintaining good nutritional intake. There is a whole section later in this chapter on how to use pancreatic enzymes.

NUTRITION THROUGH THE YEARS

For infants, either formula or breast milk is recommended. If formula is used, a milk-based formula fortified with iron is advised until 1 year of age. Since pancreatic enzymes are often given in baby fruit at a young age, it is fine for babies to start baby foods as early as 3 to 4 months of age. Remember, though, before going overboard with solids, ounce-for-ounce, formula usually has more calories than solid baby foods, so you want to avoid filling up with foods that are lower in calories than regular infant formula. If the infant needs to "catch up" on the weight curve, the dietitian can give you special recipes to concentrate formulas or breast milk for higher calories (Table 6.3 shows examples). Babies who are tiny and cannot put on weight before they are diagnosed often catch up on their growth curve and begin to look much healthier very soon after starting their oral enzymes and general CF care (Figure 6.1).

Toddlers and preschool-aged children with CF should use whole milk (3% fat). Continual snacking or "grazing" is discouraged because it makes it harder to time the oral enzymes accurately, and hard to make the diet nutritious. Three meals and two to three snacks a day work well for most children with CF.

Feeding problems are common in all children, with meals often becoming battlegrounds, and the problem can be worse in someone with CF—the parents know the importance of nutrition, and the child senses how important this is to the parent. Furthermore, it is one area of a child's life where he or she can exert a lot of control—you cannot force a child to eat if he or she truly does not want to. The parents' responsibility is to offer their children nutritious foods at meal-

TABLE 6.3. *Ways to Increase Calories for Infants*

1. If your baby seems thirsty, feed formula, rather than juice or water, since the formula has more calories and nutrition.
2. Regular infant formula has 20 cal per ounce. You can use several different kinds of supplements to increase that to 24 cal per ounce. Here are some examples *(DO NOT USE ANY OF THESE FORMULAS WITHOUT CHECKING FIRST WITH A CYSTIC FIBROSIS DIETITIAN OR PHYSICIAN—WHILE THESE ARE SAFE AND EFFECTIVE FOR MOST BABIES, SOME COULD BE HARMFUL FOR INDIVIDUAL BABIES):*
   a. Concentrated formula: The usual recipe for 8 oz of 20-cal-per-ounce formula is four scoops of powder and 8 oz of water. By using five scoops of powder and 8 oz of water, you can increase the calories to 24 cal per ounce.
   b. Polycose powder (a special sugar): add 4 tsp of Polycose powder to 8 oz of 20-cal formula to make 24 cal per ounce.
   c. Corn oil safflower oil is a very inexpensive way to add extra calories: add <fr3/4> tsp of corn oil to 8 oz of 20-cal formula to make 24 cal/oz formula.
3. MCT oil is more readily absorbed fat than corn or safflower oil, but is more expensive: add 1 tsp of MCT oil to 8 oz of 20-cal formula to give 24-cal formula.
4. Baby rice cereal: add 2 tbsp to 8 oz of 20-cal formula to give 24-cal formula.

MCT, medium-chain triglyceride.

times and snacks and encourage them to eat, but in the end, it is up to the child how much he or she will eat. Avoid force-feeding your child. By making the mealtime enjoyable, you can keep eating a pleasant part of CF care. A child may enjoy a picnic lunch outside, eating with a friend, or in another room of the house for a change. If you have a picky eater who is eating just a small amount of food, the goal is to make that small amount as high in calories as possible. Children at this age will start learning the importance of taking oral enzymes, and some will start swallowing the capsules.

School-aged children with CF will be learning to take more responsibility for their care as they start spending more time away from home. They will be responsible for deciding what foods to eat and when to take their enzymes. The frequent smelly stools caused by malabsorption can be embarrassing for school-aged children. They may find it hard to discuss their stools and symptoms, but it is important that they overcome this embarrassment so they can learn to take care of themselves. The wish that most children have to be the same as all their friends is difficult to fulfill with the CF diet and enzyme capsules required for each meal. The routine of taking enzymes needs to be continued no matter where they eat, at home or away. With sports and other physical activities, children with CF will need to use extra salt and drink more fluids than their friends.

Teenagers are in a category all their own (some people think they are actually from another planet, but we'd like to deny those rumors here and now). Teens are often on the run, and don't seem to have time to sit still for their regular meals; they often like fast food. They need to remember (and sometimes need reminding) that food is important, and taking enzymes with their meals is crucial. Well-balanced meals are important. However, heavy reliance on fast food is not necessarily all bad. The same thing that makes much fast food bad for most people—big portions, lots of calories, lots of fat—can actually be helpful for the busy teenager with CF, *IF* he or she remembers to take enough enzymes.

HOW TO USE PANCREATIC ENZYMES

See also Appendix B, *Medications*.

Remember from the previous discussion of how pancreatic enzymes work that, normally, these digestive chemicals are released from the pancreas into the duodenum (the part of the intestine right after the stomach) just as the food passes into the duodenum from the stomach. We try to duplicate this process by using oral pancreatic enzyme supplements. These enzymes should ideally mix with the food in the duodenum, just as happens in people without CF. This means several things. First, **enzymes need to be taken with meals (and with *each* meal)**: These are not a once-a-day or a three-times-a-day medication. If someone has two meals, the enzymes should be taken twice; if someone has three meals and two snacks, the enzymes need to be taken five times, directly with the food. Some physicians recommend taking the whole enzyme dose at the beginning of each meal, while others think it's better to take one half the enzymes at the beginning and the rest halfway through the meal. Once you take the oral enzymes, they are effective for about 45 minutes to 1 hour. This means that if you are a slow eater, or are eating over a long period of time, then the dose should be split, and some enzyme given later in the meal. If you finish eating, and have a snack 5 minutes later, no more enzymes are needed, but if you have a snack 1½ hours after your last enzyme capsule, you need to take more enzymes.

Enzymes come in two main types: enteric-coated (the most common) and non–enteric-coated. The enteric-coated enzymes come in capsules with little beads inside (these beads are called "microspheres" by some drug companies, and "microtablets" by others). These beads are a bit like an M&M: There's a thin coating, and the good stuff (in this case, the enzyme itself) is inside the coating. The coating protects the enzymes from stomach acid, since acid destroys the enzymes. The coating is designed to dissolve when it's in a nonacid environment, which is usually the case in the duodenum. So, it "melts in your duodenum, not in your stomach," like the M&M melts in your mouth and not in your hand. This works beautifully, because it means that when the system works as designed (most of the time), the coating dissolves, and the enzymes are released in the duodenum, exactly where the body's own pancreatic enzymes are designed to enter the intestine and mix with the food to begin digesting fat and protein. When enteric-coated enzymes were introduced in the 1970s, they provided a revolutionary change in the ability of CF patients to digest and absorb food. [The older, non–enteric-coated enzymes are still available and are useful in a few situations. These enzymes come as a powder, tablet, or capsule (with powder in it).]

The enzyme capsules can be swallowed whole (that's the most convenient way, once a child is old enough to swallow capsules), or opened up and the beads taken separately. The beads can be mixed with some soft food, such as apple-sauce. This is the most common way for babies to take the enzymes. Applesauce is a good food to mix the beads in, because applesauce is acid, and therefore the enzyme's coating will not dissolve while it's sitting in the food waiting to be eaten. The applesauce or other food should not be heated, because the heat will dissolve the coating. Even with cool applesauce, the beads should not be allowed to sit in the applesauce (or other food) for long: They should be mixed in just before the meal. If they sit too long and the coating does dissolve, the enzyme will start to digest the food, and may make it less tasty. It won't be dangerous, but it just won't be quite as attractive or effective. The beads can also be just placed on a baby's tongue, and rinsed right down with a bottle or breast-feeding. For older children and adults, beads can be taken alone, in their capsules, or mixed with most any foods, but it's important that they not be chewed, because that will break the protective coating, with two bad results: The patient will get a bitter taste (and possibly some lip or mouth irritation), and the enzymes will likely be destroyed by acid once they get to the stomach.

It's a good idea for anyone using enzymes to practice good mouth care and be sure that all the beads are out of the mouth at least by the end of the meal. For people (usually this is little people: babies) using the powdered enzymes, this is essential to prevent irritation from the raw enzyme. Breast-feeding mothers will need to clean their breasts carefully to avoid nipple irritation. In some babies, enzymes passing out with the stools can cause a burn to the buttocks if the dia-pers are not changed frequently or the bottom not cleaned thoroughly.

The enteric-coated enzymes come in many different strengths, based on how much fat-digesting enzyme (lipase) they contain. These different preparations (Table 6.4) are labeled by their strength with numbers representing how many thousand units of lipase are in each capsule: An MT4 is a capsule of microtablets containing 4,000 units of lipase, while an MT20 has 20,000 units. The high-dose capsules are convenient for people who need a lot of enzyme, since one MT20 is easier to swallow than five MT4s. But, it's harder to make small adjustments in dosage: If someone taking two MT4s needs a little more enzyme, it's easy to increase by one capsule per meal. If you take MT20s, and increase by one cap-sule, it's like increasing by five standard MT4 caps. The high-dose capsules also cost much more than the low-dose caps (although the cost is roughly the same unit-for-unit of lipase).

Who Needs Enzymes?

Most people with CF (85% to 90% of all patients with CF) need to take enzymes with their food in order to digest that food. As many as one half of all newborn babies with CF do *not* need to take enzymes, but most of these

TABLE 6.4. *Pancreatic Enzymes Comparison Guide*

Product	Manufacturer	Lipase[a]	Protease[b]	Amylase[c]	Special Features
Creon 5	Solvay[d]	5,000	18,750	16,600	Capsules, enteric-coated minimicrospheres
Creon 10	Solvay	10,000	37,500	33,200	Capsules, enteric-coated minimicrospheres
Creon 20	Solvay	20,000	75,000	66,400	Capsules, enteric-coated minimicrospheres
Pancrease	Ortho-McNeil[e]	4,500	25,000	20,000	Capsules, enteric-coated microtablets
Pancrease MT4	Ortho-McNeil	4,000	12,000	12,000	Capsules, enteric-coated microtablets
Pancrease MT10	Ortho-McNeil	10,000	30,000	30,000	Capsules, enteric-coated microtablets
Pancrease MT16	Ortho-McNeil	16,000	48,000	48,000	Capsules, enteric-coated microtablets
Pancrease MT20	Ortho-McNeil	20,000	44,000	56,000	Capsules, enteric-coated microtablets
Pancrecarb MS4	Digestive Care[f]	4,000	25,000	25,000	Capsules, enteric-coated, bicarbonate buffer, microspheres
Pancrecarb MS8	Digestive Care	8,000	45,000	40,000	Capsules, enteric-coated, bicarbonate buffer, microspheres
Ultrase	Axcan Scandipharm[g]	4,500	25,000	20,000	Capsules, enteric-coated microspheres
Ultrase MT12	Axcan Scandipharm	12,000	39,000	39,000	Capsules, enteric-coated microtablets
Ultrase MT18	Axcan Scandipharm	18,000	58,500	58,500	Capsules, enteric-coated microtablets
Ultrase MT20	Axcan Scandipharm	20,000	65,000	65,000	Capsules, enteric-coated microtablets
Viokase 8	Axcan Scandipharm	8,000	30,000	30,000	Tablet, no enteric coating
Viokase 16	Axcan Scandipharm	16,000	60,000	60,000	Tablet, no enteric coating
Viokase Powder	Axcan Scandipharm	16,800	70,000	70,000	Amount per ¼ tsp, no enteric coating

Numbers refer to content in USP units.

[a]Lipase, fat-digesting enzyme; most important for patients with cystic fibrosis; one capsule with 8,000 units of lipase is roughly equivalent to two 4,000-unit capsules of lipase (if all are enteric-coated or all non–enteric-coated).

[b]Protease, protein-digesting enzyme.
[c]Amylase, starch-digesting enzyme.
[d]Solvay (Marietta, GA)
[e]Ortho-McNeil (Spring House, PA)
[f]Digestive Care (Bethlehem, PA)
[g]Axcan Scandipharm (Birmingham, AL)

babies will gradually develop a need for enzymes over the first months or years.

How Much Enzyme Is Needed?

There is no rule for how much enzyme a patient will need, and the amount varies tremendously among patients, and even changes a bit for each patient depending on what is in the particular meal or snack. The amount of enzyme needed for a particular meal depends on several things, including

1. The person's age and size
2. Amount of pancreatic blockage
3. Amount of fat in the meal or snack

A tiny snack, or one with no fat, will require no enzymes, while enzymes will be needed for a meal or snack with fat in it, and more enzymes will be needed for an extra large meal or for one with a lot of fat. A plain potato is virtually all carbohydrate, and therefore doesn't require enzymes for digestion. However, if you eat your baked potato loaded with butter and sour cream, then you would need to take enzymes with it. Many patients know that for pizza or their dad's chili they will need more enzymes than for most meals.

How Do You Know How Much Enzyme to Take?

At first, it seems that it will be very difficult to learn how to adjust the enzyme dosages, but most families become experts very quickly. Here's how: Some people say that the digestive system is a long tube that leads from the kitchen to the bathroom (food in the top, bowel movements out the bottom). There is a certain truth here, and it's the key to knowing how much enzyme you need. Undigested fat ends up in the stool, making for frequent, bulky, smelly bowel movements that will sometimes have oil or grease droplets visible in them or leave an oily film on the toilet water. If you see bowel movements like that, you know that more enzymes are needed. Be careful not to make changes in the usual enzyme dosage on the basis of one messy stool; instead, make sure that there is a pattern. Everyone—CF or no—has a sloppy stool on occasion, whether it's because of a little virus, some bad food, a medication, or other cause. These common sloppy stools are nothing to worry about, and will get better on their own. Frequently, patients with CF get so used to increasing their enzymes for "sloppy" stools that they see a messy bowel movement, increase the enzymes, and find that the stools become normal quickly (which they might have anyway if it wasn't an enzyme problem that caused the one abnormal bowel movement in the first place). Then, since the stools have become normal, they keep the enzymes at the new higher dose. The next time there's another single abnormal stool, they increase the dosage again, and so on. In this way, many patients with CF end up taking much larger dosages of enzymes than they really need. So what? In most cases, the only problem with taking too much enzyme is the minor bother of swallowing extra pills, and cost: You're paying for more medicines than you need. For some people taking very high enzyme dosages, however, there is a small chance of a dangerous complication, with scarring of the colon (the large intestine), with the scary name *fibrosing colonopathy*. This condition almost always requires surgery (and is discussed in Chapter 4, *The Gastrointestinal Tract*). Fibrosing colonopathy almost never occurs in anyone taking less than 2,500 units of lipase each meal for each pound they weigh (and, in fact, the condition has been seen only rarely since the mid 1990s). A 25-lb child who takes five MT20s with each meal is probably taking too much:

$$5 \times MT20 = 100,000 \text{ units of lipase}$$

100,000 units for 25 lb of body weight: $100,000 \div 25 = 4,000$ units of lipase per pound

Most people can get by with much, much less. A reasonable starting dose of enzymes is more like 250 to 500 units of lipase per pound of body weight. For the same 25-lb child, this would be between:

$$25 \times 250 = 6,250 \text{ units of lipase, and}$$
$$25 \times 500 = 12,500 \text{ units of lipase}$$

This is between one and a half (1.5) and three MT4s.

[For those of you who prefer the metric system—the language most physicians and dietitians speak—the guidelines we just gave have been translated from the original: A good starting dose of enzymes is 500 to 1,000 units of lipase per kilogram (kg) of body weight, and there have never been cases of colon scarring in people taking less than 5,000 units of lipase per kilogram of body weight. The child in the example above weighs 11.3 kg, and was taking 8,850 units of lipase per kilogram of body weight.]

Even people whose enzyme dosage has crept up over the years to what might be a dangerous dosage can do well with a greatly decreased dosage.

Poor Response to Enzymes

There are several reasons that someone may not get the appropriate benefit from a usual dosage of enzymes. If stools continue to be loose, you should contact the CF center staff. Some causes of loose stools have to do with enzymes not working well, whereas others don't have anything to do with the enzymes. Some causes of loose stools are as follows:

• Excessive juice intake (very common with toddlers, no relation to enzymes)
• Introduction of solid foods to an infant (may need more enzymes)
• "Grazing" eating makes enzyme dosing difficult
• Not taking extra enzymes with "fast foods" or other high-fat meals
• Not taking extra enzymes with milk or other beverages with fat
• Not taking enzymes with snacks that contain fat (candy bars and peanuts are high in fat, for example)

- Lactose intolerance (inability to digest the sugar in milk) can cause malabsorption
- Chewing enzymes
- Excessive stomach acid
- Not taking enzymes
- Not taking enzymes in the beginning of the meal

HIGH-CALORIE NUTRITIONAL SUPPLEMENTS

Milkshakes and commercial high-calorie nutritional supplements can be prescribed if routine nutritional measures are not sufficient. Sometimes people who cannot eat enough calories in their regular diet can drink the supplements for enough extra calories to start gaining weight. Busy teenagers and active adults find the ready-to-drink nutritional supplements very convenient when away from home or in place of a meal. Examples of high-calorie supplements are presented in Table 6.5. Special high-calorie recipes are presented in Appendix D, *Some High Calorie Recipes*.

TABLE 6.5. *High-Calorie Oral Supplements*

Product Name	Serving Size	Calories per Serving
Boost	8 oz	240
Boost Breeze (juice)	8 oz	160
Boost Plus	8 oz	360
Boost Pudding	5-oz can	240
Carnation Breakfast	1 package and 8 oz milk	300
Deliver 2.0	8 oz	470
Enlive (juice)	8.1 oz	300
Ensure	8 oz	250
Ensure Plus	8 oz	355
Ensure Pudding	5 oz	240
Jevity	8 oz	254
Kindercal	8 oz	250
NuBasics	8.3 oz	250
NuBasics Plus	8.3 oz	375
Nutren Jr.	8.3 oz	250
Nutren 2.0	8.3 oz	470
Pediasure	8 oz	240
Peptamen 1.5	8.3 oz	360
Polycose Powder	As desired[a]	23 per tbsp
Pulmocare	8-oz can	360
Resource Fruit Beverage	8 oz	180
Resource Just For Kids	8-oz carton	237
Resource Plus	8 oz carton/can	355
Respalor	8-oz can	365
Scandical	As desired[a]	35 per tbsp
Scandishake	1 package and 8 oz milk	500
Two-Cal HN	8 oz	470
VHC 2.25	8.3-oz can	560

[a]The products whose serving size is listed as "as desired" are added to as much liquid (milk, for example) as you like.

HORMONES AND APPETITE STIMULANTS

If patients do not eat enough regular food and high-calorie supplements, they are sometimes given medications to increase their appetite. The most common of these are *growth hormone, testosterone, megestrol (Megace)*, and *cyproheptadine hydrochloride (Periactin)*. None of these have been studied in large groups of patients with CF, so their overall safety and effectiveness are still unknown. Growth hormone (somatropin) occurs naturally in the body, and is responsible for normal growth. Growth hormone injections have become popular as a way to cheat among strength and body building athletes. Patients with CF may have low levels of this hormone, and supplements with manufactured growth hormone have been shown in a couple of studies with a very few patients to be safe and effective in increasing body size. The drug is very expensive (as much as $500 per week), and needs to be given by injection, usually once a day. Testosterone is the most important male sex hormone in the body, and it too has been found to be low in some patients with CF. If testosterone levels are low, supplemental testosterone may be able to help restore normal growth. Like growth hormone, it is given by injection, and is very expensive. Some physicians worry that testosterone can hasten the aging of bones, which increases (height) growth initially, but prematurely closes the *growth plates* of the bones, shutting off the possibility of further growth. Megestrol is a female hormone, and it has been used successfully in recent years in a very few patients with CF as an appetite and growth stimulant. It may cause or worsen diabetes, and may suppress the normal activity of the adrenal gland, upsetting the body's own hormone regulation. Cyproheptadine hydrochloride (Periactin) is an antihistamine that can be useful in combatting allergic reactions, and has the *side effect* of increased appetite. Some physicians have prescribed it for patients with CF to take advantage of that side effect. It can also make you sleepy and cause a dry mouth. There is concern that it might dry lung secretions excessively as well, so it should be used very cautiously, if at all.

TUBE FEEDINGS

A few patients cannot take in enough calories by mouth to gain weight or to maintain weight. For these special patients, calories (in the form of liquid formulas) can be given by tube feeding while they sleep. The tube used reaches directly into the stomach or intestine. This has been done for patients with CF in a number of different ways. Some patients have used a nasogastric tube (or NG tube) that passes in through the nose, down the throat, and into the stomach. Some young children who found this idea repellent at first have quickly become used to the tube, and older children have learned to insert the tube themselves each night before bed. The improvement in growth and appearance and feeling of well-being has made this extra effort worth it to them.

A second—and much more common—method of tube feeding is through a gastrostomy (or G-tube). In this method a tube is placed through the skin of the upper abdomen and into the stomach during a minor operation. In some centers, it can even be done in the radiology department with the patient sedated, but not under general anesthesia. After the tube is placed, the patient is usually not allowed to eat large amounts for the first few weeks, while the small surgical wound heals. Once it has healed, the patient can eat as much regular food as he or she wants, and additional calories are fed through the tube while the patients sleeps. As with the NG tube, results from this type of feeding have been dramatic. See Figure 6.2 for an example of the kind of growth that can result from a G-tube. This tube has the advantage of not having to be replaced each night, and it does not involve the discomfort of a tube that goes through the nose. It also does not interfere with breathing or coughing. The G-tube is invisible under the clothes when it is not being used, and can be hooked up to the supplemental feeding at night. When it is no longer needed it can simply be removed without an operation. Jejunostomy (or J-tube) feeding is similar to gastrostomy feeding, except the tube goes into the second part of the intestine instead of the stomach. It is less commonly used, but has the advantage of protecting against gastroesophageal reflux of the tube feeding (see Chapter 4). Predigested formulas are often used for the gastrostomy and jejunostomy feedings. These formulas may not need enzymes for digestion or absorption (depending on exactly what makes up the fat source in the formula—if the fat is fully predigested, no enzymes are needed, but if the fat is *long-chain* or even *medium chain* fats, enzymes will still be needed).

No one likes the idea of tube feeding when they first hear about it. However, many people with CF have been converted when they see the dramatic growth that is often achieved with these tube feeds. Many patients have also felt a big burden has been taken off them: They have usually been trying to eat enough to gain weight, and their parents have certainly been "on their case" continuously to eat more; now with the food coming in by tube feeds, they don't have to force themselves to eat. It is important not to wait too long if tube feeds are to be tried: Someone whose nutrition and overall health are too bad may not benefit.

Problems with Tube Feeds

Tube feeds require either the discomfort of placing the tube each night and removing it each morning, or the discomfort and risks of a minor surgical procedure. Many people feel "full"—uncomfortably so for a few—in the morning after a night of tube feeds, and they may not want to eat breakfast. Some may even vomit from being overfull. These problems can usually be taken care of by slowing down the feedings toward morning. Some may not vomit, but may have increased *reflux* (see Chapter 4, *The Gastrointestinal Tract*). In these cases, a G-tube can be converted to a "G-J" tube by threading a smaller tube

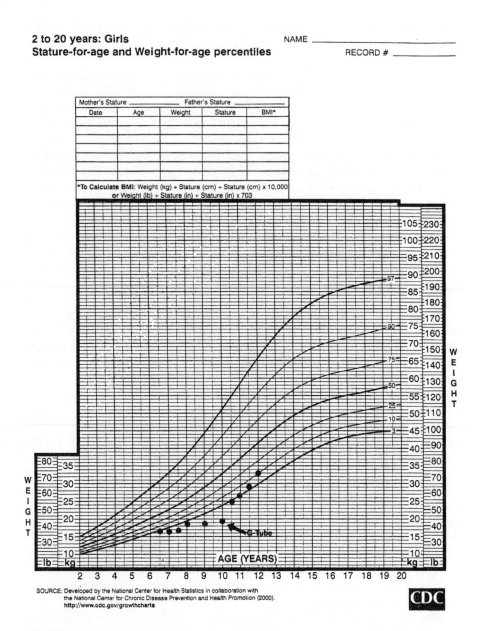

2 to 20 years: Girls
Stature-for-age and Weight-for-age percentiles

NAME _____

RECORD # _____

SOURCE: Developed by the National Center for Health Statistics in collaboration with the National Center for Chronic Disease Prevention and Health Promotion (2000). http://www.cdc.gov/growthcharts

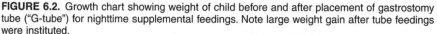

FIGURE 6.2. Growth chart showing weight of child before and after placement of gastrostomy tube ("G-tube") for nighttime supplemental feedings. Note large weight gain after tube feedings were instituted.

through the G-tube into the stomach and then into the duodenum and finally leaving its tip in the jejunum (Figure 4.1 on page 78). Occasionally the tubes will leak, causing some wetness and mess. This leaking can usually be taken care of by changing the tube. Finally, for many people, the weight gain is very good only while they get the tube feeding, and the benefits are lost if the feeds are stopped.

INTRAVENOUS NUTRITION

IV nutrition is rarely required, because nutritional supplements or tube feeding is usually sufficient to improve nutrition. IV nutrition (also called parenteral nutrition) can be given through a long-term IV into a large vein, usually in the upper chest. As with the supplemental nutrition by mouth and by tube, IV nutrition can be given at home, so that a person's life can be continued normally. This is a very expensive form of nutrition and should only be used if the patient is unable to tolerate tube feedings into the stomach or intestine. There is a slight risk of serious infection of the IV line. If the line does become infected, it needs to be removed, and another placed.

SUMMARY

In summary, there are three components of CF nutrition (high-calorie diet, oral pancreatic enzymes, and vitamin supplements). With aggressive application of all three components, most people with CF should be able to grow well and maintain nutrition that is adequate to support their overall health.

7

Hospitalization and Other Special Treatments

THE BASICS

1. Some patients need to be in the hospital, especially to treat worsened lung infection.
2. These hospitalizations often last 2 weeks, but can be shorter or longer.
3. During the hospitalization, patients get antibiotics through an intravenous (IV) line and have some blood tests.
4. There are ways to make the hospitalization less frightening than it might otherwise be.
5. Your CF center staff can help.
6. Some patients get IVs at home, usually after the IVs have been started in the hospital.

HOSPITALIZATION

In a given year, about 35% of patients with cystic fibrosis (CF) will have to be hospitalized. The most common reason for a hospital admission for someone with CF is for treatment of worsened lung infection (commonly referred to as a *pulmonary exacerbation* (see Chapter 3, *The Respiratory System*), especially with intravenous (IV) antibiotics and increased airway clearance. The time needed for IV antibiotics is the time it takes to get back to your usual state of health, most commonly about 2 weeks. This chapter reviews what happens during such a hospitalization, and includes general information about hospital routines and procedures, an explanation of the various treatments and tests, and an introduction to the different health professionals you'll see in the hospital.

131

Preparing for Hospitalization

Admission to the hospital upsets the daily routine of a family, and, can be confusing and frightening. With the help of staff from the CF center (especially CF nurses and social workers), children and families can cope with the stress, straighten out the confusion, and be much less frightened. In fact, both child and family can learn from the experience and come away from it as stronger, more mature individuals. In order to accomplish this, the family must be well informed about what to expect.

Parents should ask questions they may wonder about in order to know what to expect in the hospital. Here are some examples:

- What are the visiting hours?
- May I stay overnight with my child?
- May brothers and sisters visit?
- Is a "pass" allowed, so I can take my child out of the hospital for a break?
- Can I assist with my child's care (baths, feeding, treatments) if I would like to do so?
- Which doctor is in charge of my child's care? What other doctors will be working with him or her?
- Who are the other members of the health care team?

The best way to prepare your child for a hospitalization is to talk to him or her in simple, honest words about what will happen when he or she is in the hospital. What you say and *how you say it* are very important and will affect your child's understanding and comfort during his or her stay in the hospital. When possible, this should be done before admission. Some of the most common questions children may ask are

- How long will I be in the hospital?
- When will I go into the hospital?
- When will I come home?
- Will I get any needle "sticks"?
- What will the other kids be like?
- Can mom and dad stay with me?

As you answer these questions, you will acknowledge that there will be some painful procedures (IVs, blood tests). These things need to be mentioned, but do not need to be dwelt on. Similarly, you can and should point out the "neat" things about the hospital (playrooms, etc.), without implying that all will be wonderful fun. Some children may not ask their parents questions about the hospital. They may choose to discuss their worries with another trusted adult in an effort to spare their parents additional concern. Developing relationships outside the family circle is a normal part of growing up and this should be fostered as it occurs.

It is helpful for children to have descriptions of what the hospital rooms look like, and how daily life will differ from what they are used to. A prehospitalization tour is especially helpful so the children can see for themselves, and see that things may not be quite a scary as they feared and that some things can even be fun. These tours can usually be arranged through the CF staff (especially nurses and social workers).

Encourage your child to pack personal items from home (toys, blanket, clothes, pajamas, school books, cassette tapes and tape player) and perhaps pictures of family members. Parents should also plan to bring some things, including insurance information, a list of current medications, a list of allergies, important telephone numbers, money for parking and food (for parents), identification, legal papers (especially for adult guardians who are not the child's biologic parents).

Admission: Checking In

The following events occur just preceding most admissions to the hospital: The hospital admissions office will be notified by your physician of the date and reason for your hospitalization. The people in the admissions office will need to ask some general questions and get your insurance information. Your pediatrician or family doctor (or insurance company) will have to provide insurance authorization for the admission. This is done over the telephone before you come in or in the admissions office on the day of your arrival. After you "check in," in the admission office, you will be sent to one of the inpatient floors. A member of the staff will orient you to the floor (show you how to call for a nurse; how the bed, phone, and television work; and inform you of the usual floor rules and schedules, etc.).

Soon after you arrive on the floor, a nurse or patient care assistant will check your "vital signs" (pulse—how fast your heart is beating, respiratory rate—how fast you're breathing, blood pressure, and temperature), and will weigh and measure you. This person will usually ask you about what medicines you take at home, and whether you are allergic to any medications or foods. He or she will ask things like nicknames, food preferences, and where parents can be reached. These things will enable him or her to help plan for your care during your hospital stay.

The next step is usually to meet a doctor who will ask more extensive questions about your medical history and then perform a physical examination. In a small community hospital, the doctor may be your own physician; in a large university hospital, the doctor is likely to be an intern or resident (see below for an explanation of the "cast of characters"). After the questions and examination, the physician will write orders for treatment and the necessary treatment will begin. Whoever the doctor is who does your admission paperwork, examination, and orders, remember that you should always have the right to talk to your CF physician anytime during your stay in the hospital.

Daily Life in the Hospital

Most often when patients with CF are admitted to the hospital for treatment of a pulmonary exacerbation, they are not terribly sick or disabled. The reason for these hospitalizations is to *keep someone relatively well*, not to cure someone who is dreadfully ill. Some people, including young doctors or nurses, may not understand that and may even say, "You don't look sick enough to be in the hospital." They miss the point that your health is suffering and that the reason for the hospitalization is to get you back to your normal state of good health. While you probably won't be so sick that you need to be in bed all day, it is important to remember that you are in the hospital to improve your present and future health.

Most children's hospitals, and many general hospitals, encourage parents to participate in their child's care but to take care to remain *parents*, not *nurses* or *doctors* in the eyes of their child. Bathing, feeding, play, bedtime stories, and maintaining normal discipline standards are activities that promote normalcy in the hospital. While parents may want to be present as a source of support and consultation during painful or frightening procedures, some experts believe that they should avoid being enlisted to assist directly with such procedures (such as stabilizing an arm for blood test or injection). When this does happen, it may seem that the parent has given up his or her job as *protector*.

Different Ages, Different Needs

Hospitalized children need different things from their parents at different ages.

The infant and toddler are too young to understand what is occurring and cannot fully comprehend the parents' explanation. For an infant, the parents' trusted, nurturing presence can be comforting. Cuddling, rocking and singing, and playing are all familiar activities that bring security to a new, frightening environment.

As children advance to **the toddler and preschool years** they begin to understand more of what is occurring. Their primary fears in the hospital are abandonment and lack of mobility. They benefit from regular contact with parents and the presence of a stable group of caretakers when their parents cannot be there. They also enjoy active play, despite their IV lines!

Children in this age group have many fantasies and develop their own reasons for why things happen. They may interpret hospitalization as a punishment. New signs, smells, and sounds may be particularly frightening. They benefit from simple, concrete explanations immediately before the procedure about what they will sense (see, hear, feel, smell) during a new experience. They may also attempt to stall a nurse or doctor who is about to perform a painful procedure. As a rule, it is best to provide a simple explanation and then allow the staff member to proceed quickly and with confidence.

Preschool and school-aged children have an even greater understanding of events and benefit from explanations. They also benefit from participating in planning their daily care and being provided with choices about their schedules, meals, and therapy where applicable. They should be encouraged to maintain contacts with friends while in the hospital and to develop new friendships with other patients.

Teenagers with CF are faced with the complications of a chronic illness at a time when they are most concerned with a changing body, achieving independence from the family, and establishing relationships with the opposite sex. CF may thwart many of these goals by slowing growth and delaying puberty and by imposing a home-care regimen that perpetuates dependence on the parents. In addition, no teenager wants to be different from others, and the young man or woman with CF may appear different or have different needs, making it more difficult to establish new relationships. In the hospital, teenagers benefit from many of the same practices as their younger counterparts: explanations of what to expect, opportunity to participate in planning their care, making choices about some flexible areas of care, and contact with school friends. This assistance should be provided in the context of the special needs of the changing, developing adolescent who is seeking to establish some measure of independence.

What to Wear

Children will probably be up and around most of the day, so they should wear regular clothes. You might want to be sure they have roomy, loose sleeves to fit over IVs.

Activity

You should try not to let being in the hospital decrease your activity. Most hospitals, especially children's hospitals, will have playrooms and teen lounges, and you should take advantage of these facilities, while being careful about infection control at the same time (see section after next). You may be able to use a physical therapy gym or even to leave the hospital (on a pass) to get even more activity. This may be a chance to visit museums or other favorite places. You may be a bit tired, particularly at first, and you shouldn't push yourself too much, but you should try to be up and around most of the day. If you lie in bed all day, you will definitely get out of shape, and that will make it even *harder* to do stuff.

Schoolwork

Two or three weeks is a lot of time to miss from the school year, so it is very important to try to keep up with your schoolwork. Your doctor can help you arrange for work to be sent or brought to you in the hospital. Some hospitals have a schoolteacher on their staff to help students keep up with work. Some school systems have arrangements for home (or hospital) tutors for anyone who will be out of school a certain amount of time. It is very important that you do whatever is necessary to keep up with schoolwork while you're in the hospital.

Infection Control

Lung infection is of course one of the main things that cause deterioration of the health of people with CF. Worsened infection—particularly with bacteria like *Pseudomonas aeruginosa*, *Burkholderia cepacia*, and *Staphylococcus aureus*—is the main reason for hospital admission. We are not sure yet how people with CF become infected with these different bacteria (this topic is discussed at greater length in Chapter 3, *The Respiratory System*), but increasing evidence shows that *one* way is "person-to-person" transmission, meaning you can get some bacteria from other people. These other people include other patients with CF who might already have a particular kind of bacteria and could include health care workers. Because of the possible risks of getting new—and perhaps more dangerous and difficult-to-treat—bacteria from other patients, many hospitals and clinics now have rules that separate patients with CF from each other. These rules may include the following:

- No rooming together
- No visiting in one another's rooms during chest physical therapy (CPT) sessions or other times with heavy coughing
- The necessity to cover mouth and nose during coughing spells
- Careful disposal of tissues that have mucus in them
- No touching other patients with CF
- Perhaps requiring wearing masks
- And so forth

Some hospitals have set aside separate floors of the hospital for patients with and without certain specific bacteria (especially *B. cepacia*). These restrictions can be annoying, and perhaps even frightening, but they seem to keep to a minimum the number of cases in which patients come down with new bacteria, and therefore should be followed. In fact, you can help, by suggesting good hygiene to other people coming into your room: Ask other patients to cover their mouths when they are coughing and to wash their hands after coughing spells. Demonstrate that you're not "picking on" anyone else by doing the same things yourself. And, don't be shy about suggesting to your nurses, respiratory therapists, or doctors to wash their hands before they touch you.

The Hospital Cast of Characters

You will meet many different people in the hospital in addition to other patients, and it can be confusing as you try to figure out who everybody is. Remember, with any problems or major questions, your doctor is in charge.

Nurses and Patient Care Assistants/Partners

Hospitals could not run without *nurses* and *patient care assistants or patient care partners*. Nurses are licensed professionals who collaborate with the patient's attending physician and other health care team members to evaluate, plan, implement, and coordinate the child's care.

A patient care assistant (in some hospitals called patient care partners) is a trained caregiver who provides basic, direct patient care and will be "partnered" with your child's nurse. They are often assigned by the nurse appropriate aspects of your child's care such as taking vital signs, assisting with feeding and bathing, and other supportive tasks. The nurses and partners will help you to communicate your needs and concerns to the appropriate staff, and in general help to make your stay successful and pleasant. They may be able to answer many of the questions that arise regarding treatments, schedules, and so forth.

Physicians

You are likely to see a number of different physicians in addition to your own doctor. Especially if you are in a children's hospital and/or a teaching hospital (one that has students, interns, and residents), you will also be meeting a number of people at the various levels of medical training. It is helpful to know the different stages of medical training.

Medical students have gone to college for 4 years and are now enrolled in a 4-year medical school. The first 2 years consist of classroom and laboratory learning. In the third and fourth years, students spend time in the hospital, learning the various specialties such as pediatrics, general internal medicine, and surgery. After completing 4 years of medical school, students graduate and get their doctoral degree (M.D. or D.O.). They are now doctors.

The first step after becoming a doctor is internship. An *intern* is a doctor who is beginning to train in one specialty—pediatrics, internal medicine, family medicine, surgery, psychiatry, or obstetrics/gynecology. After the internship year, the specialty training continues with 2 to 4 years of "residency." (Most programs no longer call first-year trainees "interns," but rather, "first-year *residents*.") After a resident has finished the 3-year residency, he or she is qualified to set up practice as a specialist (family doctor, pediatrician, etc.).

Some physicians choose to get even more specialized training, and take 2- or 3-year subspecialty *fellow*ships. Subspecialties include pulmonology (respiratory problems, including CF), cardiology (heart), and neurosurgery (brain and nervous system surgery). Some of the "trainees" you meet might be young students, whereas others may have had 4 years of college, 4 years of medical school, 3 years of pediatric or medicine residencies, and several years of fellowship.

As we've already mentioned, interacting with many different people at various levels of training and understanding can be difficult for patients and families, especially when several people ask you the same questions. It may also be frustrating to realize that you know more about CF than some of the nurses and physicians who will be taking care of you or your child. Remember, though, that your own physician is knowledgeable about CF and is in charge of your (or your child's) treatment.

In addition, you can view this as an opportunity to help in the education of the people who will be the nurses and physicians in the community. Many families with a child with CF have had the very frustrating experience of going from doctor to doctor trying to find out what was wrong until they found one who knew about CF. One of the best things that anyone can do to help future children with CF is to make a contribution to the education of physicians who will be seeing those children, so that eventually all family doctors, pediatricians, and even adult medical specialists will be knowledgeable about CF, will be able to recognize it, and will have an idea of how to begin treatment.

Consultants

Occasionally, your physician may ask a colleague to give an opinion about a problem or a possible treatment. The other physician will probably look through your (or your child's) chart, ask some questions, and do a physical examination. This colleague is likely to be a specialist or subspecialist, possibly a *gastroenterologist* (stomach, liver, and digestive system specialist), *surgeon*, or *cardiologist*. These colleagues who are called in to give an opinion about one part of the treatment plan are called consultants. It is the job of the consultant to give an opinion and perhaps make suggestions. It is not the consultant's job to carry out treatments or order tests without your physician's approval.

Other Health Professionals

In addition to nurses and physicians, you are likely to have contact with other professionals, including *respiratory therapists* and *physical therapists*, who may be involved with aerosols and postural drainage treatments. Some hospitals will have *child-life workers* to help make the hospitalization a more positive experience. These people are trained in child development principles, and are frequently clever at finding just the right kind of entertainment for a child in the strange environment of the hospital. More important, they are sensitive to the signals children give through their play and talk about things that are upsetting or threatening to them. Child-life workers and *child development specialists* often can give parents, nurses, and physicians important insights into what is going on in the minds of hospitalized children.

Nutritionists or *dietitians* may help with menu selection, recommendations about high-calorie supplements, special diets that might be needed (for example, for someone with diabetes), adjustments to enzymes. *Social workers* will be available to help with a variety of problems, from very tough family adjustment problems (these are discussed in Chapter 12, *The Family*) to the day-to-day worries of insurance and transportation expenses. Other people you may come in contact with include people from a television service, hospital maintenance people, and janitors.

Parents play an important part in their child's health care and contribute their intimate knowledge of their child. Health care providers have experience with many different children over a span of years. Together, in a cooperative, positive attitude, parents and health care providers can educate one another about the needs of this child and effectively plan and carry out hospital care.

TREATMENTS AND TESTS

Intravenous Antibiotics

One of the main reasons for being admitted to the hospital is to get powerful antibiotics (especially those that kill *Pseudomonas* organisms) that are effective only when given directly into the bloodstream. A short, soft, plastic tube or catheter is inserted in the vein with a needle; the needle is then removed, leaving the soft catheter in place. (Some children seem to like to know that the dreaded "N-word"—needle—will be thrown away, leaving just a tiny strawlike tube in.) The end of the catheter is taped to the skin, and its end is closed off with a rubber cap or attached to more tubing through which fluid can be administered. When the needle is first inserted, it will hurt a little as it pierces the skin, but once it is removed, leaving the plastic catheter in place, it is rarely painful. Babies, children, and older patients alike can usually carry on their daily activities with an IV in place. There is a medicated cream (EMLA cream) that can be used to numb the skin where the IV will go. The only problem with this cream is that it needs to be in place for 45 minutes for it to work, so putting it on will delay things a bit while you wait for it to take effect.

The veins that are most often used are those on the back of the hands and on the forearms, but if these veins are difficult to find in an infant (as is often the case with a chubby baby), foot veins or veins in the scalp may be used. Foot veins should not be used in anyone who can walk, unless there is no other choice. Scalp vein IVs look as though they'd be very uncomfortable, and most parents are bothered by the idea of them at first, but they are no more painful than an arm vein IV and have the advantage of not requiring the immobilization of an arm. If a hand or arm vein is used, an arm board (which looks like a splint) helps to keep the hand or forearm stable, which in turn helps keep the IV within the vein. A plastic or cardboard cup may be taped over the needle to protect it and prevent it from being bumped.

When the IV is about to be started, it's a good idea to tell the person starting it if you have preferences about which hand or arm to use: If someone is right-handed, it's better to leave the right hand alone, so it can be used for writing, playing Ping-Pong, and so forth. Similarly, it's better to pick a spot that will leave the elbow free to bend. If a baby has favorite fingers or thumb to suck, he or she will be much happier if those fingers or that thumb is not taped out of mouth's reach.

IVs last only for a limited period, for they eventually go bad ("infiltrate") and need to be replaced: Antibiotics are powerful chemicals, and may irritate the vein, eventually weakening its wall so that it starts to leak, making the arm swell and become tender. When this happens, it is time for a new IV. Although IVs may occasionally last a couple of weeks, a few days is closer to the average. Fortunately, there is another kind of IV that can last safely and comfortably for a long time.

Intravenous Lines for Prolonged Use: The Central Line

In patients who require very long courses of IV treatment and, in fact, in patients who are getting the standard 2 or 3 weeks of IVs, it is not convenient or comfortable to keep using regular hand or arm vein IVs, which only last a few days before they have to be changed. In these cases, a "long line," or a "central line," can be lifesaving, or at least much more convenient. These lines are a special kind of IV that has its end in a very large vein or in the heart (the "central" from "central line" refers to the fact that the end of the tube, and therefore where the medicines go, is in the central part of the body—near or in the heart—compared to the regular old IVs—also called "peripheral" IVs, because they are in the *periphery*, or outside surface, of the body). When this IV is used, the medication runs into an area of very large blood flow, so that even powerful chemicals will be diluted quickly and will not irritate the veins the way they do with a hand vein. Long lines are either tunneled under the skin (and in some cases, placed entirely under the skin) or held in place with a stitch or two so that they will not become dislodged by accident.

The main types of central lines are (a) Broviac and Hickman catheters (permanent—or very long-lasting—central lines, with exit tubing tunneled under the skin, exiting through the skin on the chest); (b) Mediports, Infusaports, and Portacaths (also permanent—or very long-lasting—central lines that are *totally* under the skin); (c) Hohn catheters (placed in the same way as a Broviac or Hickman, but much easier to remove); (d) and "PICC" lines [percutaneously inserted central catheters, which are designed for temporary use for up to several weeks—"percutaneously inserted" means they're put in by sticking a needle through the skin; this is to distinguish them from the other lines, which usually require a bigger operation, with an incision (cut) made in the skin].

The Hickman and Broviac catheters are similar to each other and are lines that are inserted through a small incision, usually in the skin of the neck or by the collarbone, with one end being placed in one of the large veins in the neck, and threaded down into the *superior vena cava* (the largest vein bringing blood back to the heart from the upper part of the body) or into the heart itself, while the other end may be tunneled under the skin of the chest. In this way, the only part of the catheter that is in contact with the external environment (air, clothes, bath water, etc.) is the tip, which comes out from under the skin on the front or side of the chest. Once the original incisions have healed completely, it's safe to bathe, play sports, and pursue normal activities with the line in place. You should avoid getting hit directly in the chest, and some surgeons prefer that you not swim with one of these long lines in place, but everyone agrees that most normal activities are perfectly safe.

Mediports, Portacaths, and Infusaports are used much more commonly nowadays than the Hickmans and Broviacs, mostly because of their greater safety and convenience: They are inserted similarly to the Hickmans and Broviacs, with the tip ending in the *superior vena cava* or the heart, but the end through which medicines are infused is *under the skin*, with no tubing sticking out. This means any activity (other than those in which the area would be hit hard) is safe with these devices, and the risks of infection are much less, since the end is not exposed. These totally implanted devices have a small reservoir just under the skin. It's the rubber top of this reservoir that is punctured with the needle for hooking up to antibiotic infusions. For most of the time, these devices—which can be placed under the skin of the chest, upper leg/groin, or arm—are just left in place and are out of the way. When antibiotics are needed, a small needle can be put into the rubber cap at the beginning of the 2- or 3-week antibiotic course, and the infusion tubing hooked to it. The skin does not need to be punctured for each dose of antibiotics. The skin will need to be punctured about once a month for flushing the tubing with saline and heparin, to make sure the line does not become blocked with blood clots. PICC lines are very similar to regular IVs except that the tubing is much longer, and can be pushed into the vein far enough that it follows the vein back to the large veins in the chest (such as the superior vena cava) or even back to the heart. These lines can stay in for weeks at a time.

Placement of Long Intravenous Lines

Most of the long lines are placed by surgeons; but some particularly skillful pediatricians, internists, or radiologists might also do the line placement. Broviac, Hickman, Mediports, Portacaths, and Infusaports are intended for very prolonged usage—months or even years—and are usually placed in the operating room, with the patient under general anesthesia. Recovery from the procedure is very rapid.

For PICC lines, general anesthesia is virtually never needed, since their placement is not very much different from a regular IV; they just are longer, get gently pushed farther into the vein, and last much longer than a regular IV.

Removing Long Lines

Central catheters may be removed when they are no longer needed; they may *need to be* removed if they become infected or damaged. Mediports, Portacaths, and Infusaports, Hickmans, and Broviacs require a formal operative procedure for removal. The Hohn catheters and PICC lines do not stick as tightly to the tissue under the skin, so they can be removed easily, just by pulling (after removing any stitch that might have been used!). For this reason, they can be used in situations where they will be needed for just a couple of weeks.

Equipment

Some special equipment is needed for the proper care and use of the central lines, especially when they are used out of the hospital. Supplies for keeping them sterile are essential. Special pumps are helpful to push medications in at the proper rate, because problems could develop with medications running in too fast or too slowly. Special needles and tubing are needed to attach the central lines to the bottle or plastic bag holding the medication. For Hickman, Broviac, and Hohn catheters, the needles pierce the rubber cap at the end of the line, but for the Infusaports, Portacaths, and Mediports, special needles are required to pierce the skin and stay firmly in the reservoir under the skin for the days or weeks of the course of antibiotics. Solutions must be on hand to flush the lines after use (these typically contain saline and heparin to keep blood clots from forming in the line while it's not being used).

Care of Central Lines

Exquisite care must be taken so that these lines do not become infected. Infection in these lines nearly always means that they must be removed. If they need to be replaced, another procedure is required and perhaps another session under general anesthesia, entailing additional risks. More important, these lines are in the heart or close to it, and infection in the lines means serious bloodstream infection in the patient. People can get extremely ill from bloodstream infection. Fortunately, with proper care, these lines seldom become infected, even out of the hospital, perhaps because the people who take care of the lines at home are usually the patients themselves or a close family member. Whenever the small dressing (often little more than a Band-Aid) is changed, and medications begun, the technique used must be sterile (allowing no germs to enter). Sterile gloves are worn, the area is cleaned according to strict guidelines, using strong antiseptic solutions, and all tubing ends that would touch the end of the central line are kept scrupulously clean.

Care must also be taken to see that the lines are not pulled out or bumped hard. This protection is easy to provide: The tubes are quite thin and only a short portion sticks out of the skin, so the tubing can be coiled and covered with a small amount of gauze and taped in place. Care of the central lines that are totally under the skin (Mediports, Infusaports, Portacaths) is much easier between courses of medication than care of the lines with ends sticking out from under the skin. In fact, other than avoiding direct hits to the site of the implanted device, very few precautions need be taken; It's fine to swim, surf, and so forth. Unfortunately, every course of antibiotics does require that a needle pierce the skin to enter the central line whose reservoir lies just beneath the skin, and such a needle stick is also needed about once a month *between* courses of antibiotics, to keep the tubing open. Usually, people with these central lines do not mind the inconvenience of these few needle sticks, particularly compared to the many sticks they would have had with traditional IVs.

In deciding whether to have one of these lines, you have to decide where you'd like to have it. As with so many things, each location has advantages and disadvantages: On the chest, the reservoir is probably the most stable, and easiest to enter with the needle, but may interfere with CPT treatments. In young women, the surgeon must take care to avoid breast tissue when he or she places a reservoir under the skin on the chest. The upper leg has been a convenient place for many patients, and a few young women have given the surgeons strict instructions that it be hidden by a bikini-bottom for their time on the beach. Some patients are a little shy with the placement meaning that any manipulations of the reservoir (like the every-month "flushing" of the line), done by a stranger, are in what is usually a private part of their body. Many others have liked the fact that lines placed in the upper leg are hidden from public view virtually all of the time. One patient couldn't have this kind of line because it would have hit on the lower "uneven bar" when she did her vigorous gymnastics practice and competitions. Some patients have liked the convenience—despite a small lump—of having these ports (reservoirs) in their arm.

Complications

Infection is the most common serious complication that can occur with a central line. A central line infection can be a medical emergency, and at best usually means removing the infected line and replacing it with another one. There is a limit to the number of times this can be done, because once a long line has been in a particular vein, it can be difficult to put another line back through the same vein.

A very rare complication, air embolism, can be fatal. This happens when the central line has been opened to the air (rather than clamping it before connecting it to the medication tubing) and the patient takes a big breath, allowing air to rush into the line, and then into the heart. A small amount of air in the line will do no harm, but a large amount can be extremely dangerous. This can be guarded against by not leaving the line open to air; older children and adults can be careful to hold their breath for the short period of time that the line might be open. The danger of air accidentally entering a central line does not exist with the Mediport, Portacath, or Infusaport systems, since they are not uncapped when hooked to the bottle or bag of medication. In rare cases, a piece of the catheter has been known to break off and travel through the veins and lodge in a dangerous position, where it can block blood flow to an important part of the body.

Bleeding from accidentally uncapping the central line can be serious, since the tip of the line is in an area of very high blood flow.

Fortunately, most of these complications are quite uncommon when central lines are taken good care of.

Once the IV is in place, the medicines can be given through it. The medications are mixed with saline (salt water) or dextrose (sugar) water and then either allowed to drip through tubing into the IV under the force of gravity or are pushed through the tubing by electric pumps that regulate precisely how much goes in and how fast. It usually takes 30 to 60 minutes for antibiotics to run into the vein. When the medications have finished going into the vein, the IV may then be connected to tubing through which simple saline or dextrose mixtures are passed until it is time for the next antibiotic. A much more convenient procedure is to flush the IV with a small amount of saline and heparin (a drug that prevents blood clots from blocking the needle) and then to leave a cap on the end of the IV. Once the IV line is flushed with heparin and capped, it can safely be left alone for many hours and will be ready for use when it's time to give the next dose of antibiotics. This means that the person does not have to be tied continually to the IV pumps, tubing, and bottles, and will be free to move about.

Two different antibiotics are commonly used. Each of the antibiotics must be given on its own schedule. Schedules range from every 4 hours to every 24 hours, with the most common intervals being every 6 or 8 hours. If blood levels are checked, they may indicate that the dosage or schedule needs to be changed, for example, from every 8 hours to every 6 hours.

OTHER TREATMENTS

Other aspects of the treatment will vary at different CF centers, but will often include *CPT* (postural drainage or other form of airway clearance; see Chapter 3,) two to four times a day (or even more), and *aerosol treatments* (with bronchodilators, antibiotics, or both—also discussed in Chapter 3. It is not unusual for a patient (especially a teenaged patient) to get a bit cranky when he or she is awakened in the morning for an aerosol or chest PT. It's important to remember that these treatments are a big part of the reason for the hospitalization, and the people who are giving you the treatments are trying to help you get better. *Antiinflammatory medications* (e.g., prednisone) may be included in the treatment. *Exercise* may or may not be prescribed, and on admission, patients may be feeling a bit "under the weather" and need more rest than usual. In most cases, after the first few days, patients should be up and out of bed most of the day. In some hospitals, you may be able to attend school (your own school or an in-hospital school room) or work, on an altered schedule built around the medication schedules.

Nutrition is also an important part of in-hospital treatment, including *vitamins*, *pancreatic enzymes*, and plenty of *calories*. Food can sometimes be an issue, because the hospital food is seldom as good as home cooking. Most hospitals give a choice of foods, and many even allow inpatients to order from a hospital cafeteria menu if they don't see something they want on the regular patient menu.

TESTS

The effectiveness of the antibiotics probably relates to the peak level of the drug (the highest level that is reached), and their toxicity (harmful effects) most likely relates to the "trough" (lowest level). Since the peak usually occurs within 30 to 60 minutes after the medication enters the vein, and the trough is hours later (just before the next dose), careful monitoring of drug levels will necessitate a double test, one just after the drug has gone in, and one just before the next dose. If the levels are too low or too high, the physicians will know that they must adjust the dosage. In this way, it is possible to get the maximum benefit from the medications and the minimum toxicity. This is good, but at the same time, it's a bother, since blood levels may need to be checked again with the new dosage. (An idea that occurs to many patients is, "Why not draw my blood from my IV, so you don't have to stick me?" This can be done for some tests, but not for antibiotic levels. The reason it can't be done for the antibiotic levels is that, since the antibiotics were given through the tubing, there is often some extra left within the IV tubing itself, so the level within the tiny length of tubing will be higher than the real level in the rest of the bloodstream.) Once the right dosage is found, it is not necessary to recheck the levels frequently.

Other Blood Tests

When someone is admitted to the hospital, several kinds of blood tests are usually done. Almost always, these admission tests can be done with one needle stick, even if several tubes of blood are needed (the total amount of blood needed will seldom be more than 1 tbsp). Different tests may be done, including blood counts and measurement of blood electrolytes (chemicals such as sodium, chloride, and potassium). It is also common to check the blood levels of chemicals that reflect kidney function, because many antibiotics can affect kidney function.

Some of the tests are done only at admission, but others are repeated periodically through the hospitalization. For example, kidney function tests might be repeated once or twice a week to make sure that the drugs have not caused a problem. As we've already discussed, blood may be taken several times to measure antibiotic levels.

Other Tests

Chest radiographs ("chest x-ray") and *pulmonary function tests* (PFTs) may also be done shortly after admission and at intervals during the hospitalization to monitor the progress you are making (see Chapter 3, *The Respiratory System*, for a discussion of these tests). *Electrocardiograms* (ECGs) and *echocardiograms* are often performed to determine the heart's condition and see if it's showing evidence of having to do extra work. Other tests might also be done, depending on the circumstances. A *hearing test* might be performed if drugs are being used that might affect hearing. As always, if you do not understand what a test is, or why it's being done, ask.

Length of Intravenous Antibiotic Treatment

The ideal length of time to get IV antibiotics to fight bronchial infection is the time it takes to get you back to your baseline pulmonary function, that is, the amount of time needed to get you back to your usual state of health. Most often, this is about 2 weeks, but it can easily take 3 weeks. It is rarely more than 3 weeks or less than 2. Most CF experts feel that it is a mistake to let the calendar determine the length of treatment without regard to the patient's progress; rather, it is the patient's response to treatment that should dictate the length of hospitalization. PFTs and a physical examination can often help in determining the length of stay, but often it is the patients themselves and their families who contribute most to this decision. They are the people who know best, for example, just how much the patient is coughing. The observations of the patient and family are very important in this regard. While several weeks on IVs can seem like a very long time, and it may be tempting to try to arrange stopping as early as possible, it is wise to remember that the time invested in achieving good health is time well spent. It is quite possible that a few extra days at the end of a hospitalization or course of IV antibiotics may mean several more weeks or months of good health.

BRINGING THE HOSPITAL HOME

There are many ways that complex kinds of treatment can be carried out at home, thus avoiding prolonged hospitalization. These include home IVs, various kinds of tube feedings, and different ways of giving oxygen.

Home Intravenous Lines

In years gone by, IV treatments were usually done in the hospital. In recent years, partly because of pressure from insurance companies, IV antibiotics are frequently used at home, either after progress has begun in the hospital, or in some cases even starting at home. Whether you can do these treatments at home will be determined by your physician, in consultation with you. Insurance companies and HMOs (health maintenance organizations) are putting increasing pressure on families and physicians to use IVs at home instead of the hospital, since it may be cheaper for these companies, whether or not it is as effective as the hospital. Families may push for home treatment as well, for obvious reasons: Travel back and forth between home and hospital to visit a hospitalized child is difficult and time-consuming. If there are other children at home, it's that much more difficult. Patients like the idea of being at home with family, friends, and pets, too. Families need to be absolutely clear about the disadvantages as well as the obvious advantages of home treatment. Several things must be taken care of before someone can be sent home with an IV: There must be someone at home to take care of the IV—to connect the tubing to the needle for infusing the antibiotics, to flush the tubing after the antibiotics have run in, and to keep the IV from clogging. The medications must be mixed and stored properly, and they must be run in at the right speed. Someone must be available who knows what to do if the IV comes out or goes bad. Arrangements also have to be made for regular checkups, including blood tests (antibiotic levels, etc., as would be necessary in the hospital) and physician examinations. This can be extremely tiring and—depending on how well the IV is working, and what schedule is needed for the particular antibiotics—time-consuming. For example, a common combination of two antibiotics includes one that needs to be given every 6 hours and another that is given every 8 hours. This is a schedule that leaves little time or energy for the parent (or adult patient) to do anything else, including good CPT for airway clearance.

Who Takes Care of the Intravenous Line?

In many metropolitan areas, home medical care companies or IV infusion companies have taken on many of the tasks of visiting homes, helping to restart IVs when necessary, working with families to run the IV medications, supplying electric pumps to regulate the speed at which the medication is run in, drawing blood for tests, working with pharmacies to supply the medications, and so on. If such a service is not available, public health organizations, such as visiting nurses, may help with these details. In other cases, families and physicians have been able to piece together a team of people to do the various things. Some emergency department nurses have volunteered to restart IVs when necessary, and helpful pharmacists may take care of preparing the antibiotics. Your CF center staff can help you make these arrangements. It is very important to check whether home IVs will be covered by your insurance.

Checking Up

Once someone is freed from the constraints of the hospital, by being sent home on IVs, it is easy to forget that if he or she were in the hospital, there would be physicians to monitor the progress of the treatment and to check for evidence of drug toxicity at least once a day. It is important to maintain close contact with your physician after hospitalization, particularly if you're still taking the powerful drugs that traditionally have been given only under supervision in a hospital. Checkups once a week, or more or less frequently, may be necessary.

Ending Hospitalization or Home Intravenous Treatment

When leaving the hospital or finishing a course of home IVs, it is important to get written instructions about home care and whom to call with questions and when to return for a checkup.

Parents may notice some temporary changes in their child's behavior after hospitalization. Children may have nightmares, fear of strangers, fear of the parent's absence, or tantrums or may become aggressive or rebellious, or may try to avoid returning to school. Some children have "regressive behavior"—that is, they act babyish even though they had been quite "grown up" for their age before the hospitalization. These reactions are not unexpected, but should be brought to the attention of the pediatrician or cystic fibrosis center team for recommendations.

SUMMARY

A several-week course of IV antibiotics, whether in the hospital or at home, can cause anxiety and disrupt a patient and family's life. Yet, with cooperation among patient, family, and health professionals, these treatments can be carried out with a minimum of discomfort and can help improve and sustain health for a long time.

8

Transplantation

THE BASICS

1. Transplantation is taking a healthy organ from one person and putting it in another person, usually to replace a damaged organ. This has been done with the lungs for hundreds of people with cystic fibrosis (CF). (It has also been done rarely with the liver.)
2. Transplantation is very difficult and expensive, and requires as much or more care afterward than CF itself. Getting a transplant is much like trading one disease for another.
3. Some patients with CF have done very well after lung transplantation, some have had months or years of problems, and some have died.
4. Medicines to prevent the body from attacking the transplanted organ are important after transplantation; getting too little of this type of medicine can cause rejection, while too much can allow infection to set in.
5. About 75% of patients with CF who get a lung transplant will be alive 1 year later, about 50% to 60% after 2 to 3 years. Longer survival is certainly possible. More than 80% of children with CF who receive liver transplants will be alive 3 to 5 years later.

The term "transplantation" is commonly used in the daily newspapers as well as in the medical literature. Transplantation is surgically removing an organ from one person and placing it in another person. The person receiving the transplanted organ is known as the *recipient*. The person from whom the organ is obtained is known as the *donor*. In virtually all cases, transplantation is designed to replace severely damaged organs with organs that are healthier. In almost every case, the damaged organs are removed from the recipient at the time the new organs are put in.

The donor organ is removed from someone who doesn't need it. In the case of a kidney or a bone marrow transplant, this is often a living relative of the recipient. We have two kidneys, but can live healthy lives with only one kidney. Part of the bone marrow can be removed and the remaining marrow will grow back with no harm to the donor. In each case, the living donor can spare the transplanted organ for a sick relative. In most cases, though, the organ needed for transplantation is one we can't live without—such as the heart, lung, or liver. In this case, the person from whom the donor organ comes is most often someone who is dead, particularly someone who has had severe brain damage from trauma (car crash, etc.), but whose lung (or liver or heart) has not been damaged. Later on, we'll discuss this further.

Several different types of organ transplants have been performed, dating back as far as 1906 when the first attempt was made to transplant a pig's kidney into a person. The first human-to-human kidney transplant was done in 1936, and the first successful kidney transplant was done in France in the early 1950s. (Some of the organs for these early transplants in France came from prisoners right after they had been executed by guillotine.) Since then, attempts have been made—with varying degrees of success—to transplant the liver, heart, pancreas, intestines, bone marrow, and lung.

The first human liver transplantation was performed by a team directed by Dr. Thomas Starzl on March 1, 1963. At that time, there were only a few drugs available to prevent rejection of a transplanted organ. Dr. Starzl persisted in his pursuit of liver transplantation, despite the fact that it was not until 1969, some 6 years after the first attempt (!), that a patient lived for more than 1 year after a liver transplantation. In June 1963, only 3 months after the first liver transplantation, the first human lung transplantation was carried out. That first patient survived less than 1 month after the transplant. Rejection of the transplanted organ and infection were both major problems in the early days of transplantation. They still are formidable challenges to successful transplantation and will be discussed later in this chapter.

A major advance in transplantation was the discovery of the powerful antirejection drug cyclosporine in 1978, which improved the ability of physicians to prevent rejection of transplanted organs. Recognizing this new drug as one that would be useful for organ transplants, Dr. Bruce Reitz of Stanford University successfully carried out the first combined heart–lung transplantation in 1981. Only a couple of years later, in 1983, the first heart–lung transplantation in a patient with CF was performed at the University of Pittsburgh by a team headed by Dr. Bartley Griffith.

The number of successful liver, lung, and heart–lung transplantations increases every year, but there are many more people awaiting transplants than there are available organs.

Some patients with CF may be faced with the possibility of a transplant because of their disease. In most of these cases, it will be a lung transplant; in a very few cases, it will be a liver transplant. The total number of patients with CF (adults and children) who received lung transplants between 1992 and 2002 in the United States is 1,748. The total number of patients with CF (adults and children) who received liver transplants in that same decade is 241. At the end of 2002, there were 591 patients with CF in the United States who were waiting for a lung transplant, compared with 156 who received lung transplants during the preceding year. At the end of 2002, there were 43 patients with CF in the United States who were waiting for a liver transplant; 17 received liver transplants in the previous year. When compared with the total number of patients with cystic fibrosis (20,000 to 30,000 in the United States), these are relatively small numbers of patients. Of this small group of patients who are thought to need a transplant, many more are waiting for transplants than organs are available for transplantation.

In this chapter, we'll describe transplantation, explain the reasons some people with CF might benefit from a transplant, and identify some of the more important problems with transplantation. In addition, we'll try to explain why transplants may sometimes have to be considered even if the patients don't feel sick enough to think they need a transplant. First, we'll discuss transplants in general, then, matters that are specific to lung transplants, and, finally, matters that pertain especially to liver transplants.

WHO NEEDS A TRANSPLANT?

With a treatment as new and hazardous as transplanting an organ, it is difficult to say that anybody *needs* it. With a broken arm, it's easy to say, "you need to have that bone set, and the arm put in a cast," because we know that you will have much less pain, suffering, and long-term disability if the break is treated that way. With organ transplantation, particularly lung (or liver) transplantation for someone with CF, it's much harder to be certain of the outcome with or without the treatment. This uncertainty is related to the difficulty in predicting what will happen to patients with CF who do and don't get transplants. We will discuss this later in this chapter. Despite the uncertainties, most CF doctors agree on some broad guidelines for which patients should be considered for transplantation. These guidelines assume that in order to be a "good candidate" for a transplant, you need to be sick enough, but not too sick. If you're not very sick, it doesn't make sense to get a transplant because your chances of doing well for a long time are better without a transplant, and you would be using organs that could otherwise be used for someone who might die without them. On the other hand, if you are too sick, or have certain medical conditions that we'll discuss later, the chances of success with the transplant are small, and you and your family will have been put through a very hard (and expensive) ordeal, again using organs that would have had a better chance of helping someone else.

LUNG TRANSPLANTATION

Who Should Be Considered for Lung Transplantation?

For lung transplantation to be worth the risks, most experts believe that the patient's quality of life must be intolerable, with difficulty breathing and an inability to carry out the daily tasks of living (school, work, recreation activities). The experts also believe that lung transplantation should not be done if the person is likely to survive for more than 2 years without a transplant. One difficulty here is that there are no good tests to tell us when someone's life is intolerable or when someone with CF will die. People are amazingly different from each other in their ability to function under what seem to be the same circumstances. This is certainly true for people with CF and their lung function. Two patients with CF with equally good (or bad) lungs, as measured by their pulmonary function tests (PFTs) (see Chapter 3, *The Respiratory System*) may have very different lifestyles: One may be nearly bedridden, while the other carries a full load of college courses and works part-time in a pizza shop. So, the PFTs cannot tell us if someone's quality of life is good or bad. One yardstick that is sometimes used is that if someone needs to use oxygen all the time in order not to feel short of breath, he or she should consider lung transplantation.

What about knowing when someone with CF will die from his or her lung disease? Just as the PFTs don't tell us exactly how well someone feels or what he or she can do, they also can't tell us how long he or she will live. As is discussed in Chapter 15, *Death and Cystic Fibrosis*, there are some rough statistics that say someone with CF with a PFT [specifically, the forced expiratory volume at 1 second (FEV_1)] below 30% of what it should be has a 50 : 50 chance of being alive in 2 years. Many physicians have taken this information to mean that if someone has PFTs that low, he or she should consider lung transplantation. Recent studies have suggested that using other factors such as weight, the presence or absence of diabetes, and the type of bacteria in sputum may all be useful at predicting survival. However, a lot of work must still be done before physicians can use this information to decide who should receive a transplant. Later in this chapter, we'll talk about how to make the final decision about whether or not to go for lung transplantation.

Who Should Not Be Considered for Lung Transplantation?

Just because certain organs, such as the liver or the lungs, can be transplanted, it does not mean that every patient will benefit from a transplant. For some people, the modern medical approach of "if it's possible, we should do it!" does not fit with their view of the world. For these people, the very high-tech (and high-cost) modern medical procedures are not appealing, especially if it means that they might lose control of their own destinies. Some patients have felt that, although a transplant might be the only way to prevent dying within the next few years, dying may not be the worst thing possible. There is no question that the possibility of transplants has changed the way people with CF die. In the past (or now, if someone is not considering transplantation) when patients' lungs had reached a certain point, and it was likely that a patient would die in the near future, the physicians', patient's, and family's efforts generally were directed at trying to keep the patient comfortable while providing care that might help make the patient better if that were possible. If there were ever a conflict between patient comfort and a treatment, the treatment would be skipped and patient comfort emphasized. Now, if someone is waiting for an organ to become available, there is often a level of desperation: We need to wait for the organ, so stay alive at all costs! Thus, a patient and family may not be able to deal with their own thoughts of losing each other and may not be able to say or do things that need to be done. Instead, all efforts are put into survival at all cost until the call comes saying that lungs are available. Losing the little peace and calm that previously was possible in contemplating death seems too high a price for some patients, and they choose not to consider transplantation. Patients, families, and physicians also now realize that getting new lungs does not guarantee that everything will be perfect afterward. Instead, many patients have as much trouble, and spend as much time in the hospital after transplantation as they did before the transplantation. So, some patients and families choose not to be considered for new lungs.

In some other situations, the likelihood of success of transplantation is very small and the known risk of the procedure is quite large. Such situations are known as *contraindications* to (reasons not to do) transplantation. Physicians must take into account all such factors before deciding whether a transplant procedure is indicated. Certain factors are associated with such a poor outcome that they are considered *absolute* contraindications to transplantation. Other factors may be associated with an increased risk, but this risk may be acceptable in a sick patient; these factors are considered *relative* contraindications to transplantation. A single relative contraindication usually does not prohibit transplantation, but the presence of several relative contraindications may be adequate to disqualify a patient from receiving a transplant. Not all transplant centers agree on relative or absolute contraindications, although all transplant physicians must confront such issues in each patient they see. The decision to "list" someone for transplantation (see below for more on the transplant list) is often made by a group of physicians, and their view of the relative or absolute contraindications in each patient becomes the basis for their final decision to proceed or not proceed with transplantation.

There are several absolute contraindications to lung transplantation. A severe infection that has spread into the bloodstream and caused alterations in the function of other organs, such as the kidney, heart, and brain, is one of the most important contraindications to transplant. A cancer that is not confined to the organ for transplantation is a second absolute contraindication. In many centers, severe kidney or liver disease is a contraindication to lung transplantation.

Because patients with CF commonly have bacteria such as *Pseudomonas* or *Staphylococcus* organisms in their airways, the mere presence of these bacteria is not a contraindication to transplantation. However, as will be discussed in the next section, bacterial infection of the transplanted lung is a common complication in patients with CF. Over the years, several transplant centers have reported that airway bacteria that are resistant to antibiotics are a problem following lung transplantation. In several of these reports, a specific type of bacteria known as *Burkholderia cepacia*, particularly if it was resistant to all antibiotics ("panresistant"), was associated with a very high mortality. Studies that are more recent have shown that the bacteria present in CF sputum before lung transplantation are the same organisms that cause lung infections following transplantation. This means that if a patient with CF has panresistant organisms (*B. cepacia* or others) before transplantation, then the infections after transplantation will be very difficult to treat. Because of the risk of severe and untreatable infections following transplantation, many centers now consider the presence of panresistant strains of bacteria in the airway an absolute contraindication to lung transplantation.

There are numerous relative contraindications to lung transplantation. These include previous chest surgery or pleurodesis (discussed in Chapter 3, *The Respiratory System*), poorly controlled diabetes, or a history of a psychiatric disorder. Malnutrition is a relative contraindication to transplantation, and many transplant centers are unwilling to consider performing transplantation in a patient who is too thin. As you will see, the surgery involved in transplantation is very extensive and there is a long recovery period. Patients who are weak because of malnutrition may not have the physical strength to recover from the operation. Most transplant centers suggest feeding tubes such as nasogastric (NG), gastrostomy, or jejunostomy tubes to provide enough nutrition to allow the patient to be strong enough to survive the surgery.

Another relative contraindication is a history of what is referred to as "noncompliance." This means not taking prescribed therapy such as antibiotics or pancreatic enzymes, not doing regular chest physiotherapy, or failing to be seen regularly by a CF physician. The importance of a patient and family being able to take medications, do treatments, and show up regularly for their appointments cannot be overstated. Transplantation is a complex process, and the treatments and medications following transplantation must be done exactly as prescribed. Because there are many more people who need new lungs than there are lungs available, it is important that the organs be transplanted into patients who will take care of them. Patients and families must be able to cooperate with the transplant team in order to maintain good function of the transplanted lungs; transplant physicians are less likely to believe that a patient will do what he or she is told after transplantation if the patient is unable (or unwilling) to follow instructions before the transplantation.

The Transplant List

There is no shortage of people whose doctors believe they need a transplant. There is, however, a big shortage of donor organs to use for these patients. There are several reasons for the shortage, beginning with the fact that most donor organs have to come from people who have died—and died in a way that has not damaged the organ in question (for patients with CF, this means lungs or liver). In some circumstances, the donors have decided while they were alive that in the event of their death they wished to be organ donors. They may have signed a "donor card" and informed their families and clergy. Unfortunately, relatively few people have expressed such a desire. More often, the families of potential donors must be approached at the tragic and upsetting time when their loved one is dying. It is difficult for many families to agree to organ donation at such a time; therefore, many organs that would have been suitable for transplant are not made available.

Organs must be taken for transplantation before they are too damaged to help the transplant recipient. Once the heart stops beating and blood is no longer flowing into organs such as the lungs or liver, those organs rapidly become damaged. For this reason, organs are removed from the donor before the donor's heart has stopped beating. Many of us were taught from childhood that the heartbeat is the true sign of life, and life continues until the heart actually stops beating. Medicine, however, has advanced to the point of having ventilators that breathe for us and medications that stimulate the heart to beat strongly. The availability of transplantation as a science has raised the question of what constitutes life and what constitutes death. Most physicians, scientists, and clergy now believe that the true measure of life lies not in the heart beating or in breathing, as these can be artificially stimulated, but in the presence of brain function. Now, people with severe brain injuries, who are being kept alive with machines such as ventilators, can be tested to see if they have any brain function. If they don't have brain function and are not receiving medications that affect brain function, they can be considered "brain dead." This term means that their brain will not recover any function and, although the machines may keep them "alive," they are not experiencing life, are not thinking, and have no brain function. (It may be more appropriate to think of the machines that keep air moving in and out of their lungs, and blood circulating, etc. to be "organ support," and not what they're usually called, "life support.") Such patients could serve as donors of organs for transplantation if those organs (heart, lung, liver, etc.) still function normally. This is the reason for the timing of when organs are taken from donors. It also helps to explain why many families find it difficult to agree to organ donation: Their loved one appears asleep, rather than dead.

Once the organs are removed from the body of a donor, they are cleared of all blood by washing a salt solution through the blood vessels that go to the organ. This preparatory phase before transplantation is known as preservation and allows the organs to be transported to the recipient's hospital. A liver can be preserved for up to 24 hours after it is removed from the body, while lungs become hopelessly damaged within 4 to 8 hours. So, even if there is no difficulty with a family's agreeing to donate the organs from their family member, the organs do not keep very long at all. If they are to be transplanted, it needs to be within a matter of hours. You can't call the central supply department in the hospital to order up a lung or liver.

Soon after transplantation became a widespread medical technique, it was apparent that there were many more people who were waiting for transplants than there were organs available. Because physicians and politicians were worried that organs might actually be sold or not given to the most needy recipient, The Transplant Act of 1984 was passed by Congress to make sure that organ donation is fair and equitable. A private, nonprofit national organization known as the United Network for Organ Sharing (UNOS) was set up to keep track of transplant recipients and donors. As a part of their job, UNOS maintains a computerized list of patients awaiting transplantation and matches donor organs with appropriate recipients. In the UNOS system, the country is divided into regions served by local Organ Procurement Organizations (OPOs), which in turn are responsible for helping local physicians identify potential organ donors and helping transplant centers obtain the organs for transplantation.

Getting on the Transplant List

The first step in being considered for transplantation and getting on the transplant list is being referred to a transplant center by your regular physician. In the case of patients with CF, this physician would most likely be your CF physician. The referring physician sends information about you to the transplant center, and the transplant physicians then decide whether you should be seen and evaluated. The information your physician will send to the center will include your recent PFTs, chest radiographs (x-ray films), results of your sputum cultures, and laboratory reports about your kidney and liver function. In addition, your physician will usually speak with one of the transplant physicians about your illness, how many hospitalizations you've had, and how well you follow the physician's advice. The transplant physicians will look at the information, including the sputum culture results, and decide whether you should be evaluated more fully to see if you should be listed for transplantation. If the decision is made to evaluate you, then you travel to the transplant center and undergo more tests (radiologic tests, blood tests, exercise tests, etc.). You are seen by a number of physicians, usually including a transplant surgeon, a pulmonary specialist, an infectious disease specialist, and (in the case of liver transplantation) a gastroenterologist. You and your family are interviewed by social workers and, in many centers, a psychiatrist. This latter point is important and emphasizes the fact that transplantation is not only a difficult surgical and medical procedure, but is also a highly stressful circumstance for patient and family. If all the members of the transplant team agree that you are sick enough to require a transplant and that you do not have one of the absolute contraindications to the procedure (such as the presence of panresistant *B. cepacia* in your sputum), then you are "listed" on UNOS's computer as an "active" candidate for transplantation.

Your Spot on the List

The main reasons for UNOS to keep a transplant list are that there are more people waiting for transplants than there are organs to go around, and it is necessary to decide as fairly as possible who should get an organ when it becomes available. There are separate lists for different organs, and, although it may seem a bit odd, the "rules" governing the different lists are different.

The List for Lung Transplants

Where you are on the list waiting for lungs depends on very few things: your size (since lungs that are either too big or too little are more difficult to transplant successfully), your blood type, and, most important, the length of time you've been on the list. If two people on the list are the same size and blood type, and one has been on the list for 2 years and the other has been on for 1½ years, the one with the 2-year wait will be offered the next set of lungs, even if she or he is not as sick as the other one. In some ways, this system seems unfair, but UNOS decided that anyone who was sick enough to be accepted onto the list was sick enough to deserve organs, and the fairest way to allot available organs is on the basis of the total waiting time a potential recipient has accumulated.

The assignment of lungs solely on the basis of waiting time has had an unexpected effect. The wait for lungs now is often 2 years or longer in most U.S. transplant centers, and this has led to the earlier "listing" of patients. In other words, the long wait for lungs means that in order to get a set of lungs when you need them, it's probably necessary to get on the list before you're actually sick enough to need them. So, if you're not sick enough now to need new lungs, but might be that sick in 2 years, now is the time to start the evaluation process to get on the list. Another problem that has arisen because of the long wait for lungs is that patients who delay being considered for lung transplantation may find themselves very sick and not able to receive lungs. One of the painful lessons learned at many lung transplant centers is that between one fourth and one third of the patients waiting for lungs will die before lungs become available.

Waiting on the List

Once the patient is "listed" for transplantation, the patient must wait until he or she has moved to the top of the list and until an organ becomes available. As we've just discussed, this can be as long as 2 or more years for patients waiting for lung transplants. In most cases, routine follow-up care is done by the refer-ring physician (your usual CF physician and family physician), but the transplant physicians will often want to see you at their center at regular intervals (usually every 6 to 12 months). The visits to the transplant center will allow the transplant physicians to examine you, to look at your sputum cultures, PFTs, and radi-ographs, and to get an idea of how sick you are.

Some transplant centers require candidates for transplantation to become involved in specific exercise and nutrition programs, which are designed to strengthen the patient and improve his or her ability to withstand the stresses of surgery and recovery during the postoperative period. Several centers require that patients and their families move to the city where the transplant will take place. Some of these demands on patients may improve their chances of surviv-ing until the transplant can be done, and some of the demands placed on both patients and their families will show the transplant team that these prospective recipients are able to follow directions, take medications, and comply with all therapeutic measures. While this may seem unfair, we should remember that organs for transplantation are rare and valuable commodities. There are many more patients seeking transplantation than there are available organs. A patient who does not take care of himself or herself after transplantation not only hurts himself or herself, but has also "taken" a donated organ away from someone else—someone who might take better care of themselves (and the new organ). Many centers doing transplantation are less willing to transplant organs into patients who have shown that they are not able to take care of themselves prop-erly before transplantation.

"Active" and "Inactive" Patients on the List

The list of candidates awaiting transplantation is divided into *active* and *inac-tive* status. The status of any candidate can be changed from active to inactive (or vice versa) depending on a variety of factors that we'll discuss below. People who are "active" move up toward the top of the list as people ahead of them go off the list (because of getting a transplant, dying, deciding against transplanta-tion, or becoming inactive). Once the patient reaches the top of the list, the active candidate will be offered the next organ that becomes available.

People who are inactive will not be offered an organ (even if they are at the top of the list), nor will they be given credit for the time they are waiting, as long as their status is inactive. They can move up the list as people ahead of them come off the list, but other active candidates can pass them on the list as the active candidates receive credit for the time they are waiting for organs. How-ever, candidates who change their status from active to inactive do not lose credit for the time they've already waited as active candidates. So, if someone has been an active candidate on the list for 22 months and then becomes inactive, he or she still has 22 months of waiting time to his or her credit if the patient goes back on the active list later.

There are several reasons that a patient might change from active to inactive on the list. First, a candidate may be at the top of the list and receive a call to be transplanted at a time that he or she doesn't feel sick enough to have the transplant, or the candidate might be too frightened. The candidate may then turn down the offered organ. The lung will then be offered to the next person on the list, and the first candidate will not be penalized. If this happens several times, however, the transplant team can suggest that the candidate be changed to inactive for a while. If some time later the patient is ready to be considered for a transplant, he or she will become "active" again and the place on the list will be determined by the amount of time he or she had accumulated waiting while on the active list.

A second major reason for changing a candidate from active to inactive may be a change in the candidate that is an absolute contraindication to transplantation. An example of this might be the finding of a major new infection outside of the lungs, such as an infection in a Mediport central line (see Chapter 7, *Hospitalization and Other Special Treatments*). This would have to be treated before the patient could get a transplant. Most of the time, the patient is not put on the inactive list while such an infection is being treated, but if organs became available during the treatment of the infection, those organs would have to go to the next person on the list. If the infection proved difficult to treat, the candidate might have to change his or her status to inactive at that time.

Sometimes the problem may not be in the patient's overall health, but in his sputum cultures. As we've already discussed, some centers will not allow transplantation in patients who have panresistant bacteria in their sputum. An example of this would be a patient who starts to grow *B. cepacia* in his or her sputum after being listed as active. If someone's culture begins to show those bacteria, the patient may be inactivated until the culture clears up. In many centers, such patients are not inactivated, but they will not undergo transplantation. This allows them to continue to move to the top of the list while efforts are made to get rid of the resistant bacteria in their sputum.

In some instances, candidates have been made inactive when they have not been able to follow through with their medical therapy. For example, patients who refuse to do prescribed chest physiotherapy treatments or who fail to be seen regularly by their CF physician are more likely to be inactivated by a transplant center.

The Technique of Lung Transplantation

General Considerations

Transplantation surgery is complicated and difficult. It is done in specialized medical centers by highly skilled surgeons and anesthesiologists. The surgery involved in lung transplantation requires large incisions (cuts) through the skin and other tissues that make up the wall of the chest, which permit the surgeons to inspect, remove, and replace the damaged organs. The removal of the organ from the recipient must be done carefully, leaving the arteries, veins, and (in the case of the lung) airway (trachea and main bronchi; see Chapter 3, *The Respiratory System*) in place, for these must be attached to the donor organs in such a way as will allow the new organ to function normally. Each of these new attachments, in which a donor artery, vein, or airway is joined to the native (recipient's) artery, vein, or airway, is known as an *anastomosis* (pronounced a-nass-to-mo-sis) and is a crucial part of the surgery. The site of the anastomosis may be weaker than the rest of the donated organ and can come apart more easily. This breakdown of an anastomosis, known as *dehiscence* (pronounced *de-hiss-sense*), can result in severe bleeding or (in the case of the airway) sudden respiratory difficulty. Anastomoses are also subject to narrowing, known as stricture or stenosis. In blood vessels, this can lead to blood clots at the site of stricture. Stenosis of the anastomosis in an airway can result in difficulty breathing.

Although the transplant surgery is done while the patient is deeply anesthetized, there is a lot of pain and discomfort during recovery from these operations. While many patients do very well right after lung transplantation, full recovery from these procedures may take weeks or even months.

Specifics of Lung Transplantation Procedures

Until the late 1980s, most lung or heart–lung transplantations were done through what is called a median sternotomy, in which the breast bone is cut from top to bottom and the chest is opened by pulling the cut sides apart. Now, most lung transplant operations are done using what is known as an *anteroinferior transthoracic incision*, also known as the "clamshell" approach. This means the surgeon cuts across the lower part of the chest wall from one side to the other, allowing the entire upper part of the chest wall to be lifted up, much as you would raise the hood of a car (or open a clamshell). This gives the surgeon a better look at both lungs and makes the surgery somewhat easier. A good view inside the chest is especially important if the recipient has CF, because patients with CF often have scarring of the thin membrane (the *pleura*) that covers the surface of the lung. This scarring may also involve the lining of the chest wall, which is also a thin membrane and is also called the pleura. Normally, the space between these two membranes (called the *pleural space*) is lined only with a tiny amount of fluid, and the lungs can be pulled out of the chest cavity relatively easily, but in CF, there can be a lot of scar tissue between the pleural surfaces, making it difficult to remove the lungs. Furthermore, scar tissue bleeds easily when it's pulled apart.

The earliest operations for lung (and heart–lung) transplantation involved removing the donor lungs together, still attached to the lower part of the donor trachea. (In the case of heart–lung transplantation, the lungs still had their attachments to the heart, and the heart and lungs together, known as the "heart–lung block," were removed from the donor.) For those early lung transplants, the recipient lungs were also removed together, leaving behind most of the recipient's trachea, along with the pulmonary arteries coming from the right side of the heart and the pulmonary veins leading back to the left side of the heart. The top of the donor trachea was attached to the lower part of the recipient trachea and the donor and recipient arteries and veins were joined. This is known as double-lung transplantation, because the two lungs are placed into the donor as a single unit.

As you can imagine, this is very exacting, tedious, time-consuming work. The surgeons must use many tiny stitches in these delicate tissues, making sure there is not even a small hole left behind that would allow blood to leak out of the veins or arteries being sewn together or air to leak out of the ends of the trachea which were sewn together. The surgery takes hours, during which time the patient has no functioning lungs (and in the case of heart–lung transplantation, no beating heart). In order for this surgery to be possible, the patient's blood must be rerouted outside the body through plastic tubing to a "heart–lung machine," also called "cardiopulmonary bypass." This machine takes blood and oxygenates it, then pumps it back into the body. Blood going through cardiopulmonary bypass machines has the danger of clotting within the plastic tubing, or in the patient when it returns, so it needs to be treated with "anticoagulants," drugs that interfere with clotting. Like so many other things done in medicine, this can be a double-edged sword: Along with preventing the bad clotting that might take place within the bypass machine or the patient's blood vessels, these medicines can also prevent good clotting that is needed to stop the bleeding of surgical wounds. Some of the early patients with CF who had this kind of surgery for lung transplantation had a lot of bleeding into the pleural space around their new lungs and many of them died because the bleeding would not stop. This is one of the reasons that previous *pleurodesis* (see Chapter 3, *The Respiratory System*) is considered a relative contraindication to lung transplantation at many centers. Another problem with this form of double-lung transplantation is that the anastomosis of the trachea may not receive good blood supply and the tissue may die, leading to dehiscence of the anastomosis, which can lead to sudden respiratory difficulty and death. In addition, the tracheal anastomosis is more likely to become narrowed (stenosed) if the tissue is damaged at the junction.

There is a newer technique for lung transplantation that has become more widely used. It is called "sequential single-lung transplantation." In this technique, each donor lung is removed as a separate entity, with its attached artery, vein, and airway. Each recipient lung is also removed one at a time, leaving behind small lengths of the artery, vein, and airway that can be joined to the corresponding donor artery, vein, and airway. One donor lung is transplanted into the recipient while the patient is breathing with the remaining lung. Once the first lung is transplanted, the recipient breathes with that new lung while the second lung is removed and the second donor lung is transplanted into position. The technique of sequential single-lung transplantation is considered safer and has a better survival record than double-lung transplantation. In many cases, cardiopulmonary bypass is not needed during sequential single-lung transplantation, so the risk of bleeding during and after the transplant surgery is much less. (A few patients with especially poor lung function may still have to go on bypass during the surgery because they don't have enough functioning lung tissue left in one lung to support them with that lung alone while the other lung is being removed and replaced.) By reattaching each airway near the lung instead of reattaching both lungs as a unit to the trachea, this technique leads to a lowered risk of dehiscence of the airway anastomosis. However, the risk of stenosis of the airway with sequential single-lung transplantation is increased, because the airway near the lung is smaller than the trachea.

At the time of surgery, several plastic drainage tubes are placed through the skin into each side of the chest. These tubes will drain any air or fluid around the transplanted lungs and will help keep them inflated. They are usually removed within the first 2 weeks after surgery.

"Living Donor Lobar" Transplantation

A relatively new and exciting development is the technique of "living donor lobar" transplantation for lung recipients. This procedure uses two live donors, each of whom donates a part of one lung. The donors are usually (but not always) related to the recipient. The part donated is one of the sections of the lung known as a "lobe" and serves as an entire lung for the recipient. Living lobar transplantation offers several potential advantages over transplantation using organs from people who are unrelated or who have died. First, since the donor organs are being given specifically to the recipient, there is no competition for those particular organs, and therefore no need to be on a waiting list. This means that someone who is too sick to survive the long waiting list time might be able to get a transplant anyway. Second, the operation can be scheduled, and can be done during the day with everything relatively calm and prepared. All too often, organs for the usual lung transplant recipient arrive on very short notice, in the middle of the night, perhaps when the chief surgeon is out of town or when the patient and family are not fully prepared to take the huge leap necessary for transplantation. Yet decisions must be made within minutes or hours to "go" or not. Finally, if the donors are closely related to the recipient, there may be a lowered risk for severe rejection. While the risk for rejection is always present (unless an organ is transplanted from an identical twin), transplantation under this circumstance may mean that the recipient will require lower doses of immunosuppressive medications.

There are, however, several potential disadvantages to living related donation. First, it involves three people who have major chest surgery: the recipient and two donors. All surgical procedures have some risk involved, and although the risk is greatest for the recipient, there is some risk to the donors. Second, there is the possibility that a donor might feel undue pressure to donate part of his or her lung even though he or she is not sure about doing it. In families with more than one patient with CF, the decision to consider living lobar transplantation can be agonizing: If you donate a lobe to one patient, you will not be able to do so for anyone else.

PROBLEMS (COMPLICATIONS) ASSOCIATED WITH TRANSPLANTATION

General Considerations

Transplantation is a science that is still in its infancy. There are many problems associated with organ transplantation, and complications of transplant procedures are common. Several of these complications can occur with any type of transplant, and we shall discuss these, and the care necessary to prevent and treat them, in this section. Specific problems with lung or liver transplantation will be discussed separately.

One problem that many people with CF wonder about is whether their transplanted lungs or liver will develop CF. They will not. CF is a part of the cells that make up the actual tissue of each organ, and if you get a new organ, that organ will not develop CF. There are many other problems that can develop, some of which are related to the fact that the patient still has CF, even though the transplanted organ does not. Patients with CF who receive a new lung or liver will still have to be seen regularly by their CF doctor in addition to their transplant doctor. Many other problems are complications of the transplant itself, and we will discuss these problems now.

Immunosuppression: Too Much or Too Little (Infection or Rejection)

The saying, "each one of us is unique," has special importance in relation to transplantation. Each of us has built-in systems designed to protect our body from attack from bacteria, viruses, and fungi. These complex defense systems, known as our immune system, work together to kill invading germs and keep them from harming us.

But our immune system can do more than protect us from germs that may try to invade our bodies: It can recognize and destroy cells or organs from another person. When a new organ is transplanted into someone, the immune cells of the recipient will know that the new organ is from someone else, and they will set about to destroy it. This destruction of the transplanted organ is known as *rejection*.

Rejection is one of the major problems following transplantation, and medical researchers have struggled for years to understand it and try to prevent it from destroying transplanted organs. There are a couple of ways to do this. The first way is to transplant an organ or tissue that is not foreign. That can be done if the organ comes from oneself (as can be done with bone marrow transplants in some cases of cancer treatment: A person donates some of his or her own bone marrow for storage, and then that same bone marrow is transplanted back into the person after the cancer treatment). It can also be done if the organ comes from the recipient's identical twin, since these two people are immunologically identical. Such transplants have been done very successfully; but of course this option is open to very few people, because most of us don't have an identical twin, and the bone marrow, a kidney, or a single lobe of a lung is about the only tissue or organs that a living donor can safely contribute.

For people who don't have an identical twin to donate an organ or who need an organ (like lungs or liver) that a living twin can't do without, we must interfere with the immune system's ability to recognize and attack foreign tissue. In other words, we must suppress the immune system. The most common way of doing this is by giving the recipient medicines that weaken the immune system, making it incapable of rejecting the transplant. Such drugs are known as *immunosuppressive agents* (or immunosuppressive drugs or *immunosuppressants*) (Table 8.1).

Few immunosuppressive drugs were available at the time of the first transplants. Steroids, such as prednisone, were used to decrease the function of certain white blood cells known as lymphocytes. An anticancer drug known as azathioprine (Imuran), which interferes with the ability of any cell to divide, was also used. Unfortunately, it decreases the production of good cells as well as potentially harmful cells. Steroids and anticancer drugs like Imuran were somewhat effective, but they could not prevent rejection completely without causing severe side effects.

With an improvement in our understanding of the mechanisms involved in rejection came the development of new immunosuppressants that were more powerful in their actions on the immune system, yet didn't have as many side effects. Table 8.1 describes the major types of immunosuppressive medications now in use at most transplant centers, how they work, and what major side effects they have. We will discuss them in the next several paragraphs.

A revolution in transplantation occurred in the early 1980s with the development of a drug called cyclosporine, which was the first of these more specific and powerful agents. The improved success of liver and lung transplantation is a direct result of the development of new antirejection drugs like cyclosporine. Cyclosporine and other modern immunosuppressive drugs (including FK506, which is now known as tacrolimus, or Prograf) are more effective than earlier drugs, and have fewer side effects. Unfortunately, fewer side effects does not mean *no* side effects, for all drugs (even aspirin) have side effects. We'll discuss several of the more important side effects of each class of immunosuppressive drugs in the next section (see also Appendix B, *Medications*).

Probably the most important "side effect" of the immunosuppressive drugs is that they might work too well. Remember, the immune system's primary job is to protect us from infections, and weakening it too much with immunosuppressants will result in an increased risk of developing infections. As we might expect, transplant recipients who take immunosuppressive agents are at increased risk for developing infections, in either the transplanted organ or elsewhere. Some of these infections may be life-threatening. Infections can be caused by bacteria, such as *Pseudomonas* species, or by viruses or fungi. Viral infections can be particularly difficult to treat and may have further complications, which will be discussed later.

Two particular viral infections deserve special mention here. These are *cyto*megalo*virus, known as *CMV*, and *E*pstein–*B*arr virus, called *EBV*. CMV is a common virus, which many of us have been exposed to (often without realizing it) by the time we are adults. If we've been exposed to CMV, we have built up immunity to it and don't usually get sick if we are reexposed to it, even if we take immunosuppressive drugs. CMV is a very clever virus, however, and seems to be able to hide in lungs, liver, or blood of people who have had the virus. It can stay there, not causing any trouble as long as the person's immune function is normal. If the lungs of a donor who had CMV in the past are transplanted into someone who has never had CMV (and therefore doesn't have any immunity to CMV), and the recipient has to get immunosuppressive drugs, the CMV can cause serious disease in the transplanted lung as well as in other sites such as the eye, the intestines, or the liver. Another situation can lead to CMV disease in a transplant recipient: If neither the recipient nor the donor has ever had CMV, the recipient can still be exposed to CMV after the transplantation. This can happen simply by coming into contact with someone who has CMV (remember, a lot of healthy people have CMV and don't know it) or—as was common up until recently—through blood transfusions from someone who has had CMV. Transplant recipients now get blood only from people who have no evidence of ever having had CMV. Children may not have had CMV disease (and therefore have no CMV immunity), and if they undergo transplantation and are exposed to CMV while they receive immunosuppressive medicines, they may become quite ill. Fortunately, there are new medicines to treat CMV, but it is still a major problem, particularly in lung transplant recipients, and we shall discuss this a little more, below.

EBV is the virus associated with mononucleosis ("mono"). Like CMV, it seems to have the ability to "hide" in the tissues (and possibly blood) and cause severe problems in people who receive immunosuppressive drugs. Also like CMV, many adults have had EBV, even though they may not have had an illness like mononucleosis. Children, however, are less likely to have had EBV. They may become infected with EBV after transplantation and become ill with a disease that is similar to mononucleosis. Of more concern, however, is the association of EBV infection in transplant recipients with a special complication, which is a tumor of lymphatic tissue (lymphoma). This lymphoma is called *post*transplantation *l*ymphoproliferative *d*isease, or PTLD. If PTLD occurs after transplantation, it usually is treated by decreasing the immunosuppressive medications. On rare occasions, PTLD may require other special forms of therapy. Although PTLD often responds to treatment, it doesn't always and can be fatal.

Another problem with immunosuppressive drugs is that they may not work well enough. When this happens the immune system recognizes the transplanted

TABLE 8.1. *Immunosuppressive Medications*

Type of Drug	Brand Name	Generic Name	How Given	How it Works
Corticosteroids *Decrease inflammation and can treat or prevent acute rejection.* The exact mechanism of action of corticosteroids is not understood. They are able to decrease lymphocytes (the cells that are involved in rejection) directly. Corticosteroids attach to proteins called receptors; the steroid–receptor combination then goes into the nucleus (control center) of cells, where it affects the activities of the cell. Corticosteroids also interfere with the activation of lymphocytes by other cells.	Deltasone (and others)	Prednisone	Oral	See Column 1
	Medrol, Solumedrol	Methyl-prednisolone	Oral; IV	See Column 1
	Prelone	Prednisolone	Oral	See Column 1
Lymphocyte-specific Drugs *Decrease the ability of lymphocytes known as T-helper cells to function properly.* These T-helper lymphocytes are central to the immune system's ability to reject foreign tissue such as a transplanted lung or liver.	Sandimmune	Cyclosporine	Oral/IV	Attaches to a protein called cyclosphilin inside lymphocytes. This inhibits the ability of the lymphocyte to make proteins called interleukins, which stimulate other cells to attack the graft.
	Neoral	Cyclosporine/micro emulsion	Oral	Works like cyclosporine, but may be absorbed better from the gastrointestinal tract.
	Prograf	Tacrolimus	Oral/IV	Similar to cyclosporine, except that it has a different binding protein and is more potent in its action.
	Rapamune	Sirolimus	Oral	Similar to cyclosporine and tacrolimus, but with a different binding protein and acts on a different part of the lymphocyte cell cycle

Antimetabolites
Interfere with the ability of cells to manufacture normal DNA, which is essential for cell division. This decreases the number of cells available to reject foreign tissue.

Imuran	Azothioprine	Oral/IV	Metabolized in the body to a compound called 6-mercaptopurine, which interferes with DNA production
CellCept Oral	Mycophenolate mofetil	Oral	Metabolized in the body to a mycophenolic acid, which interferes with DNA production

Antilymphocyte Antibodies
Preparations of antibodies that can bind to and attack proteins on the surface of lymphocytes. This will inactivate or destroy those lymphocytes.

Atgam	Anti-thymocyte globulin	IV	See Column 1. This antibody preparation is derived from horse serum. The horses are "immunized" with human cells.
Orthoclone OKT3	Muromonab-CD3	IV	See Column 1. This antibody preparation is "bioengineered." It is produced by mouse cells in cultures.
Zenapax	Daclizumab	IV	"Bioengineered" antibodies directed against a specific protein on the surface of lymphocytes
Simulect	Basiliximab	IV	"Bioengineered" antibodies directed against a specific protein on the surface of lymphocytes

IV, intravenous.

organ as being foreign and tries to destroy it, leading to rejection. There are two major "types" of rejection: acute and chronic. Rejection, along with infection, remains a major problem for transplant recipients, and is discussed later in this chapter.

In summary, the transplant doctors try to use immunosuppressive drugs in just the right amount. Too little immunosuppression leads to the threat of rejection; too much immunosuppression leads to the risk of infection or PTLD. Transplant physicians and scientists are constantly trying to widen the distance between the extremes of rejection and infection that can cause severe illness in the recipient. As more research is done, it is likely that safer yet more powerful immunosuppressive drugs will be discovered, allowing for better control of both rejection and infection.

Side Effects of Immunosuppressive Drugs

As we've already said, the major "side effect" of immunosuppressive drugs is either having too much immunosuppression, which leads to infection or PTLD, or too little, which leads to organ rejection. Immunosuppressives are medicines that can have other true side effects, that is, effects that are unrelated to the main reason you take them in the first place.

The main side effects of cyclosporine, tacrolimus, and similar drugs are kidney damage, high blood pressure, diabetes, seizures, increased growth of the gums in the mouth, and excessive body hair. Despite this long list of possible side effects, many of the most serious ones can be minimized by measuring the blood levels of the immunosuppressive drugs and adjusting the dosage as required. In some cases, however, where the immunosuppressives are harming the kidneys, it may not be possible to lower the drug without causing or worsening lung rejection. In those few cases, it comes down to a choice between saving the lungs and saving the kidneys. The lungs always win, because you can live (with treatments several times a week from a kidney dialysis machine) without kidneys, but you cannot live without lungs. Some patients have even received kidney transplants after a heart or lung transplantation because of the kidney damage caused by the immunosuppressive drugs. Some of the recipients who develop diabetes from the immunosuppressive medications may need to receive insulin shots.

The other immunosuppressants that have been used for the prevention of rejection also have side effects. Azathioprine (Imuran), as we've already discussed, interferes with the development of blood cells. Because of this, anemia and a low white blood cell count, which can increase the risk of infection, are the main side effects of Imuran. In addition, nausea and diarrhea are fairly common with the use of this drug. Steroids such as prednisone may lead to high blood pressure, diabetes, obesity, cataracts, ulcers of the stomach and bowel, excessive bruising, and some decrease in the ability to fight off infections. Our body normally makes its own steroids similar to prednisone, and these naturally occurring steroids are important in helping us withstand stresses like infection, surgery, or exposure to cold temperature. Taking prednisone for a long time can decrease the body's ability to make these natural steroids and lead to an increased risk if we encounter any of these stresses.

Surgical Complications

Transplantation—as we've seen—involves very complex surgery. During any such procedure, it is possible that something (a blood vessel, nerves, the organ itself, etc.) could get cut that shouldn't get cut. This can cause problems after surgery.

Complications of Lung Transplantation

Aside from the general complications of transplantation that we've mentioned already as "side effects" of the immunosuppressive drugs, most important, infection and rejection, there are several complications specific to lung transplantation. These complications include organ failure, bleeding in the chest, damage to nerves in the chest, blood clots in the veins going from the lung to the heart, and narrowing of the airway where the donor lung is attached to the recipient. Some of these complications happen soon after transplantation (early complications), while others happen later (late complications).

Early Complications of Lung Transplantation
(Hours-to-days After Transplant)

Organ Failure

Any organ that does not have a healthy blood supply can be damaged. This can happen to a donor lung when it is removed from the donor or when it is still in the donor, if the donor's illness or injury has interfered with the blood supply to the lung (or harmed it in any other way). Once the organ has been removed from the donor, it is washed free of blood with a special solution designed to keep it healthy for the trip to the operating room, where it will be put into the recipient. If the trip takes too long, or if the preservative solution doesn't work perfectly, there can be damage to the organ. Any one or combination of these factors can damage the transplanted organ badly enough that it may not be able to function. This kind of problem shows up in the early hours or days after transplant, and is referred to as "preservation injury." This injury is believed to be the result of either inadequate blood supply to the lung for too long a time, poor preservation of the lung, or both. A severe form of this injury results in damage to the air sacs throughout the lung and can lead to respiratory failure soon after transplantation. While this injury may resolve, it may leave scarring in the lung that will limit the amount of recovery.

Bleeding in the Chest

The surgery for lung transplantation involves opening the chest by making an incision across the front of the chest wall (the "clamshell incision"). As we've already mentioned, one of the important reasons this incision was developed was because of the problem of bleeding from the lining of the chest wall (pleura) following surgery, bleeding that is common in patients with CF because of frequent scarring of the pleural space that has resulted from chronic lung infections. This can be a problem when a surgeon tries to remove the lungs from a patient with CF in order to put new lungs in. The clamshell incision, by allowing better access to the lungs, helps the surgeon find and stop the bleeding, but bleeding after surgery (after the chest is closed again) is still a problem in patients with CF following transplantation, particularly in those patients who had to go on heart–lung bypass during their surgery.

Blood Clots

Blood clots can form in the veins leading from the transplanted lungs to the left side of the heart, and can greatly interfere with heart and lung function right after a transplant procedure. In order to find such clots, the physicians usually use a technique known as *transesophageal echocardiography*. In this technique, a plastic probe about as big around as a finger is passed through the mouth, down the back of the throat, and into the esophagus. The probe contains a miniature echocardiograph machine, similar to the machines used for ultrasound. Because the esophagus is behind the heart and because the veins from the lungs enter the backside of the heart, the physicians can see them better with this approach. Transesophageal echocardiography is usually done with the patient heavily sedated.

Nerve Damage

When lungs are transplanted, the nerves that usually accompany them are cut and not reattached. Although this might seem to be quite dangerous, it usually has a relatively small effect on recovery and this will be discussed later in this chapter. There are, however, several other important nerves that run through the chest rather than into the lungs, and these may be damaged accidentally during surgery. The most important of these nerves are the *phrenic nerves*. These nerves go to the diaphragm, which is the main muscle involved in breathing; damage to these nerves may decrease the ability of the diaphragm to contract, which limits the ability to breathe. Damage to one of these nerves may lead to the diaphragm on that side being too high in the chest. Although the nerve may regrow, this can take a very long time. Treatment of this injury involves surgically "pulling down" the affected diaphragm.

Narrowing (Stenosis) of the Airway

It sometimes happens that the one or both of the main bronchi become narrowed following transplantation. This is most often right where the donor and recipient airways are joined (the bronchial anastomosis). If the narrowing is severe, it can be hard to breathe and hard to move mucus past the narrowed area, setting the stage for hard-to-control infection. The narrowing can be caused by the surgeon's having sewn the bronchi too tightly, by the bronchi simply being too small, or (and this is by far the most common) by the formation of scar tissue at the anastomosis.

Rejection

Despite the use of immunosuppressive drugs, rejection remains a major problem following lung transplantation. Rejection, which is the result of the recipient's cells trying to destroy the "foreign" lung tissue from the donor, takes two major forms, called *acute* and *chronic* rejection.

Acute rejection is especially common in the first weeks to months following transplantation, but may occur years after transplant. Episodes of acute rejection tend to occur abruptly and cause breathing difficulties, cough, lowered blood oxygen levels, and changes in the chest radiograph. If acute rejection is diagnosed and treated promptly and aggressively, it usually responds well to treatment, and the patient improves. The usual treatment of acute rejection is with high doses of steroids given through an intravenous (IV) line. The other immunosuppressive drugs, such as cyclosporine or tacrolimus, are often given in higher doses to prevent acute rejection from coming back. If the steroids don't work (they usually do), some other treatments may be used and are often effective. These more specialized treatments are designed to attack the specific kind of blood cells (lymphocytes) that are causing the acute rejection. The two major treatments are known as OKT3 and ATG (which stands for *anti*thymocyte globulin). Both of these must be given, in the hospital, by IV over several days.

Chronic rejection is less well understood than acute rejection and is more difficult to treat. It tends to have a slower onset, and last longer, with more subtle symptoms of shortness of breath with exercise, cough, or a fall in PFTs. We will discuss chronic rejection in more detail under the section that deals with the late complications of lung transplantation.

The diagnosis of rejection is made with certainty only by examining a piece of lung tissue under the microscope. The piece of tissue, known as a *biopsy* specimen, is usually obtained with a procedure called *bronchoscopy*, which will be discussed later in this chapter. Acute rejection is easier to diagnose than is chronic rejection with this type of biopsy. At times, the biopsy specimen must be fairly big to diagnose chronic rejection, and this may lead the transplant physicians to recommend an "open" biopsy, in which the chest is opened surgically and a piece of lung removed by a surgeon.

Infection

As we've seen, immunosuppressive medicines increase the risk of infection in transplant recipients. This risk is greatly increased in the lungs of patients with CF. In fact, the major cause of death following lung transplantation in patients with CF is infection. The windpipe (trachea) and sinuses of the patient with CF still "have" CF, even though the new lungs don't. Bacteria such as *Pseudomonas* or *Staphylococcus* organisms will remain in the airways (sinuses, trachea, and bronchi) of these patients and can cause infection in the transplanted lung. The combination of immunosuppression and *Pseudomonas* organisms, particularly if the *Pseudomonas* organisms are resistant to antibiotics, can prove deadly for the recipient. Because of this risk, some centers decrease the immunosuppression as much as possible in CF lung transplant recipients. More important, virtually all transplant centers look closely at the bacteria in their patients with CF before transplantation. As we've already discussed, organisms that are resistant to all antibiotics are considered by many centers to be a contraindication to transplantation. Infections can be an early or late complication of lung transplantation. Infections can occur in the transplanted lungs, or elsewhere.

The new lungs are the most common targets for infections after transplantation, for several reasons. First, the lungs are the only major transplanted organs in direct contact with the outside world after transplantation. Every time we breathe, air enters our lungs; the very air we breathe is often contaminated with materials that can harm us. Bacteria, viruses, small particles of dust or dirt, or certain toxic gases may be in that air. Our lungs normally have a set of barriers or ways to deal with many of these dangerous materials. Scientists and physicians refer to these as the lung defenses. Transplanting lungs directly affects lung defenses, and this makes the lungs more susceptible to infection. Some of these have been discussed in Chapter 3, *The Respiratory System*, but we'll review the affected lung defenses in the next few paragraphs.

Since the nerves supplying the lungs are cut and not reattached during transplantation, the new lungs do not have any sensation. One important sensation that we all normally have in our lungs is what we call the *cough reflex*, which is the stimulation to cough that is brought about when any material like increased mucus builds up in the airways. This urge to cough is lost at least for the first months after transplant, meaning that mucus can build up in the new lung without the recipient's feeling the need to cough. Of course, some people—who have coughed all of their lives up to the time of the transplant—might think that the lack of cough is wonderful. But, we must remember that cough is one of the lung's most effective ways of getting rid of bacteria and excess mucus. Thus, this loss of the cough reflex adds to the risk of developing infections in the lung. Lung transplant recipients can still cough, but they must actually *decide* to cough because, without the cough reflex, coughing won't happen on its own.

Another of the lung's usual defenses that is altered by a transplant is *mucociliary clearance*. Normally, secretions such as mucus help to trap unwanted small particles such as bacteria and keep them from damaging the lung. Because the airway cells are continuously making mucus, a way to move the mucus out of the lung is needed. This movement is the responsibility of the cilia, which are very small, hairlike tufts that project out from airway cells and are in contact with the mucus. Normally, these cilia move in a regular way that slowly but surely moves the mucus up the airways to the trachea, from which it can be coughed out, or to the back of the throat, where it can be swallowed. For unknown reasons, even though the cilia are still present on the airway cells following transplantation, they just don't move as well, allowing mucus to build up in the lung.

Finally, for reasons that we don't yet understand, the white blood cells that fight infection in the lungs do not seem to be able to get into the lung as well as they should following lung transplantation. All of these defenses and their status following lung transplantation are the subject of intense scientific study. It's likely that we'll have better ideas on how to improve the lung defenses and decrease the risk of infection following lung transplantation as we learn more about the way the lungs defend themselves normally.

Late Complications of Lung Transplantation (Weeks-to-months After Transplant)

Infection

As we just mentioned, infection can be an early or late complication of lung transplantation. Infection can be caused by bacteria like *Staphylococcus* and *Pseudomonas* organisms that the patient with CF has had in the sinuses and trachea for months or years before transplantation. These bacteria can infect the new lungs at any time.

Although we discussed it earlier, the problem of CMV infection deserves special mention when discussing the late complications of lung transplantation. Once CMV has infected a person, that individual will make antibodies to CMV, which is one of the body's ways to try to fight off infection: Antibodies attack specific targets; antibody to CMV fights CMV. The virus is a clever one, however, and it may not be eliminated from the body, and instead may lie dormant in the lung, intestines, kidney, or liver, temporarily not causing trouble. We can determine whether antibodies to CMV are present in the blood of a lung donor and a lung recipient. If the donor is positive for the antibodies (meaning the donor at one time had a CMV infection), then CMV may be lying dormant in the donated lung. The immunosuppression given to the recipient will allow the CMV that has been lurking in the donor lung to become free to cause a new infection, particularly if the recipient is negative for the antibodies (meaning that the recipient has probably not ever been infected with CMV and has no antibodies to help fight CMV). CMV infection in this setting can be an especially bad infection, causing fever, sore throat, or other symptoms. In addition, it now seems that CMV disease in the lung recipient may increase the risk for the development of chronic rejection, which we mentioned briefly before and will discuss further below.

Several approaches have been used to try to prevent and/or treat CMV disease and chronic rejection in lung transplant recipients. In some transplant centers, recipients and donors are now "matched" whenever possible, so that lungs from CMV-positive donors are transplanted into CMV-positive recipients, while lungs from CMV-negative donors are reserved for CMV-negative recipients. Another approach is to treat CMV-positive recipients and CMV-negative recipients who have received CMV-positive lungs with an anti-CMV medication known as ganciclovir. A third approach is to give CMV-negative recipients a special antibody preparation that is high in antibodies directed against CMV. These approaches are not all always feasible (particularly the method of "matching" donors and recipients) or completely effective. Physicians and scientists are working on new approaches to try to minimize the effects of CMV in transplant recipients.

Chronic rejection (long-lasting), which was mentioned earlier, is a poorly understood form of lung rejection. While it is clear that chronic rejection is a way that the recipient's cells try to attack and destroy the new lung, the part of the lung that is attacked is usually the small airways. This leads to a very serious form of airway damage known as *bronchiolitis obliterans*, which is characterized by scarring of the small airways. We don't yet know the reason for this pattern or the exact cause of chronic rejection. Chronic lung rejection is sometimes associated with CMV infection in lung transplant recipients. Several other factors, including recurrent episodes of acute rejection, especially severe episodes of acute rejection, and stenosis of the airway anastomosis, have also been associated with chronic rejection. Approximately 25% to 35% of all lung recipients develop some form of chronic rejection, and it remains a major cause of death in transplant recipients. Of those lung recipients who develop chronic rejection, approximately 35% to 50% will die, and most of the remaining 50% to 65% of patients will have some degree of compromise of their airway function. As is the case for acute rejection, steroids as well as medications like OKT3 and ATG have been suggested for the treatment of chronic rejection. Several experimental treatments are being tested for the treatment of chronic rejection. We hope that as more is learned about chronic rejection, we will get better at preventing and treating it in lung transplant recipients.

Other Late Complications of Lung Transplantation

Although infection and rejection are the most common and usually most serious complications of transplantation, there are some others.

Narrowing (stenosis) of the airway was discussed under the section *Early Complications* above, but actually is more likely to be a problem weeks to months after the transplant. A little bit of narrowing of the airway usually causes no problems. More severe narrowing can cause difficulty in breathing, difficulty moving mucus, and therefore worse problems with infection beyond the narrowed area. Sometimes the physician can open the stenosis with bronchoscopy (we'll describe bronchoscopy later in this chapter). This can happen in several ways: Sometimes just pushing the bronchoscope through the narrowed area can stretch it open. Instead of a bronchoscope, surgeons or radiologists may be able to pass a special deflated balloon to the narrowed anastomosis, inflate the balloon with a lot of pressure, making the now-rigid balloon stretch open the stenosis. Sometimes the extra scar tissue that is blocking the airway can be cut away during bronchoscopy. A third way of dealing with stenosis is to use a special laser beam (again during bronchoscopy) to "burn off" some of the scar tissue. Finally, in very severe cases, a surgeon or radiologist may be able to place a plastic or metal *stent* in the airway. This device is stiffer than the airway and props it open. This is a difficult procedure, and is used only when there seems to be no other choice. If the length of narrowed bronchus is short and the stenosis is severe, in rare cases the surgeon may reopen the chest and cut out (resect) the narrowed portion, sewing the open ends of the normal-sized bronchus back to each other.

Psychological, Social, and Financial "Complications" of Transplantation

Transplantation is very expensive. Figures from one major transplant center for 1995 show that pretransplant care for a patient with CF averaged $80,000. These costs have not changed very much since. The transplantation itself (and the hospital stay afterward) cost $200,000 to $250,000, and the costs for the first year after transplantation were about $100,000. Most, but not all, insurance companies will pay for transplantation, but some still consider the procedure (and some of the medications used afterward) experimental and therefore not covered.

A lot of care is required after transplantation and, in addition to costing money, this adds to the inconvenience and discomfort of the process. Many patients will have one or more of the complications of transplantation and will require further testing and care. All this may increase the time spent in the hospital and away from work, school, family, and friends. Often these hospitalizations are at the transplant center, which may be hundreds (even thousands) of miles away from home.

Transplantation is stressful for patients, their parents, and their physicians and nurses. Even for someone who does very well, there can be emotional challenges: It is often not easy for someone who has had trouble breathing for months or years to adjust to not needing oxygen, and to trust in his or her newly gained energy.

As in any new field of medicine, difficult lessons about transplantation are learned all the time. Unfortunately, many of these lessons are taught by the patients who develop problems related to the transplantation or to the medications given to prevent rejection. The history of transplantation (particularly for lung transplants) is short, and the length of survival following a new lung or liver is impossible to predict. The uncertainty of the course someone will take after transplantation adds to the stress of the procedure. Transplantation is probably not a good treatment for someone who needs assurance that "everything will be fine." We'll discuss this further in the section entitled "Making the Decision."

CARE AFTER TRANSPLANTATION

General Considerations

During any transplantation, the patient is unconscious, under general anesthesia, with his or breathing being done by a machine (a ventilator) through a tube that goes in the nose or mouth into the trachea (endotracheal tube). The patient will have other tubes in as well: drainage tubes from the chest, a urine tube in the bladder, and several different catheters in blood vessels, including IVs, sometimes a tube in an artery (an "a-line") for easy measurement of the oxygen and carbon dioxide levels in the blood, and sometimes a long tube that goes into the heart to be able to measure blood pressure very accurately. Immediately after the transplant surgery, the patient is cared for in the intensive care unit (ICU) until strong and healthy enough to breathe on his or her own, and to withstand the removal of the various tubes. During this time in the ICU, tests will be done to make sure that the new organs are working satisfactorily and that there haven't been any immediate problems associated with the surgery, like bleeding or formation of large blood clots. Once it seems that there are no major postoperative problems, and the patient is ready to breathe on his or her own, the endotracheal tube can be removed (we say the patient is "extubated"). Getting to this point usually takes a few days, but can take longer. There are a couple of different approaches to extubation of a patient after surgery: One approach is to get the tube out absolutely as soon as possible, since the tubes are very uncomfortable, and the patient cannot talk while the tubes are in place. The other approach is more conservative, and delays extubation until it is absolutely clear that the patient is ready because an extubation that is done too early can fail (if the patient isn't strong enough yet, he or she could tire and must then be reintubated). Reintubation may be harder for patients than a slightly longer single intubation.

In the ICU, the patient will usually need a lot of pain medication and sedatives. While a patient is on the ventilator, medications are often given that paralyze the patient, to make it easier for the ventilator to "breathe" for him or her. Once the patient is breathing on his or her own, is relatively alert and not requiring large amounts of sedatives and pain medication, and all organ systems are working satisfactorily, he or she can be moved to a regular hospital room. This usually takes several days to a week or so, but in some cases can take weeks or even months.

After transplantation of any organ, that organ requires a lot of care and close monitoring to be sure that it continues to function well. Rejection of the organ and infection (of the transplanted organ and of other parts of the body) remain dangers forever after transplantation. The posttransplantation care is at least as time-consuming, bothersome, and important as regular CF care is. Because of the health risks, and because of the care required after transplantation, we often say that getting a transplant is like trading one disease for another (the new lungs or liver don't have CF anymore, but they will have other problems that need to be treated). And of course, someone with CF who has new lungs or a new liver still has CF, even if the new organs don't. So digestive enzymes, vitamins, and so on, continue to be important. Care of the lungs remains essential after transplantation of any organ in a patient with CF.

Testing a patient for rejection is necessary on a regular basis following transplantation of any organ. PFTs can give early hints that there might be a problem with the transplanted lung, but any kind of problem, not just rejection, can make these tests abnormal. The most accurate way to see if rejection is present in a transplanted organ is to examine a small piece of it under the microscope. The technique of taking a small piece of an organ is known as a *biopsy* procedure, and the small piece itself is referred to as a biopsy specimen, or sometimes just a "biopsy." For liver or lung transplant recipients, it is not uncommon for five to ten biopsies to be done in the first year after transplantation.

Tests After Lung Transplantation

After lung transplantation, several kinds of tests are done in the ICU, in the regular hospital room, and afterward when the patient has gone home.

The most common tests that help to monitor the health of transplanted lungs are PFTs and chest radiographs. PFTs are described more in Chapter 3, *The Respiratory System*, and are no different from the PFTs used for most people with CF who have not undergone transplantation. In addition to regular PFTs at the clinic, most patients are given small electronic PFT machines to take home with them, which they are asked to use two or three times per week. If the results of these home PFTs get worse, the patient notifies the doctor for further testing. The radiographs are no different from the usual chest x-rays that CF patients have had for years. The types of problems that might show up on PFTs or radiographs can be different from the pretransplantation CF lung problems, and might prompt the physicians to recommend specific treatment or further testing, which will almost always mean a special test known as *bronchoscopy*, *bronchoalveolar lavage* (called BAL for short), and *transbronchial biopsy*. We'll describe this test, which is commonly done for lung recipients, in the next several paragraphs.

Bronchoscopy is a way of looking into the trachea and bronchi of the lung, using a tube called a *bronchoscope*. There are different kinds and sizes of bronchoscopes. In most cases, the kind used for patients who have had lung transplants is flexible, so it can be passed through the nose, bend around curves down the back of the throat, through the vocal cords, and into the trachea and bronchi. It has a light and lens at the end, so the physician doing the procedure can see into the dark bronchial tubes. In most transplant centers, the bronchoscope is connected to a video camera, and the physician doing the bronchoscopy (the "bronchoscopist") moves the bronchoscope while watching the television image. (The patient can watch the procedure "live" on the television, too, if she or he likes, or afterward on a video playback.) There is also a hollow suction channel running the length of the bronchoscope through which liquids can be squirted in or sucked out, and through which thin, flexible wire instruments can be passed.

BAL means, quite simply, that a liquid, usually saline (salt water) like that used for an IV solution, is washed ("lavaged") into an area of the lung through the thin channel of the bronchoscope and then sucked back out into a sterile container. The total amount of fluid used is often several ounces, given a small amount at a time, with suctioning done after each individual amount of fluid. As the saline washes into the lung, it mixes with the cells and fluid in the lung. When it is sucked back, it carries with it some of those cells and fluid. In addition, if there are bacteria or viruses in the airway, some of them will be in the suctioned fluid as well and can be cultured in the laboratory. Cultures of the fluid for bacteria, viruses, or fungi take several days to weeks to give definite answers, however. The laboratory can determine the number of cells taken out of the airway and the type of cells removed. These tests will help tell the physicians if there is evidence of an infection in the lung or if there might be rejection. To diagnose rejection most accurately, the physician will also want to do a biopsy through the bronchoscope (see below).

Within the first day or so after lung transplantation, one of the physicians might perform a bronchoscopy for a quick look at the bronchial anastomoses (the places where the donor bronchi are sewed to the recipient bronchi). For this procedure, the bronchoscope can simply be passed through the endotracheal tube into the trachea and bronchi, and the procedure should not be much of a big deal for the patient.

Beyond the first days, bronchoscopies with BAL and biopsy are performed every few weeks at first, then every few months if things are going well. Bronchoscopies will also be performed if there is any hint that there is a problem. These "hints" might come from symptoms, like increased cough or sputum production or laboratory test results, like lower oxygen level, worsened PFTs, or some new findings on the chest x-ray.

A biopsy done through the bronchoscope is known as a *transbronchial biopsy*. There are other types of lung biopsies, and we'll describe those later in this section. For a transbronchial biopsy, the physician using the bronchoscope will pass small forceps through the bronchoscope. These forceps are at the end of a long thin wire and are a tool that has small jaws with tiny teeth. The jaws of the forceps can be opened and then closed to take biopsy specimens ("bites") of the small bronchi and surrounding lung tissue. These samples are also sent to the laboratory for examination under the microscope. It usually takes a day or so for the biopsies to be prepared and examined. The biopsies can give some information about possible infection, but their main use is to tell if there is rejection. The more pieces of tissue the physician obtains, the better the chances that they will give a true representation of the situation in the lungs. However, the more pieces taken, the greater the chances of a complication of the procedure, too (see below).

Complications of Bronchoscopy

There are several important possible complications of bronchoscopy, but fortunately, complications are relatively rare. The most important of these complications are oversedation, nosebleed, cough, bleeding within the bronchi, and pneumothorax (collapsed lung). These will be discussed in the next several paragraphs.

The usual bronchoscopy procedure is done by passing the bronchoscope through the patient's nose, down the back of the throat, through the vocal cords, and into the trachea and bronchi. The procedure sounds brutal, but is surprisingly easy to tolerate. The bronchoscope itself is soft and flexible, and the procedure, while a bit uncomfortable, is not painful. To minimize the discomfort, several things are done. Most patients are given sedatives through an IV. This will help the patient relax and make it easier for the physician to do the bronchoscopy. Notice, we didn't say the patient had general anesthesia: Most flexible bronchoscopies are done with the patient sedated and breathing on his own. This is important, because the patient has to breathe around the bronchoscope. The usual bronchoscope is about as big around as a pencil, and most patients breathe around it without any difficulty. Occasional patients don't want any IV medications, and actually watch the procedure being done on the same TV screen that the bronchoscopist watches. Others prefer to see the video afterward, while others want nothing to do with the bronchoscopy, preferring to be asleep for it. As much or as little sedation as the individual patient needs can be given.

Whenever sedative (or any other) medicines are used, there is a small chance that dosing errors can happen, and the patient can get too much. In this case, that could cause the patient to be oversedated and fall so deeply asleep that he or she doesn't breathe. In order to prevent this complication, sedative doses are checked carefully and are usually given in relatively small amounts, with extra being given as needed. Furthermore, the patient is monitored carefully for any signs of not breathing enough (a pulse oximeter, or "pulseox," is attached to the finger to give a continuous reading of blood oxygen levels). Finally, medicines are readily at hand to reverse the effects of the sedative medicines. The sedatives are usually very effective in keeping patients comfortable, without their needing general anesthesia as they would for painful surgical procedures. The sedatives used most often have the added benefit of causing what is known as retrograde amnesia, which means the patients forget what happened while they were sedated.

As soon as the patient is comfortable, the nose and back of the throat are numbed with Xylocaine drops (like the dentist uses, but not injected with a needle), Xylocaine jelly on the end of a cotton swab, or even Xylocaine aerosols. As the bronchoscope is passed through the nose and to the back of the throat, the vocal cords are also numbed with Xylocaine dripped through the suction channel of the bronchoscope. The nose is the narrowest part of the patient's body that the bronchoscope has to pass through, and it can sometimes bleed from the rubbing. These nosebleeds are not serious and not common (about one of every 20 or 30 patients).

The bronchoscope is then passed through the patient's vocal cords into the trachea. The trachea also gets some Xylocaine, not really to prevent pain (it doesn't hurt), but to prevent cough (the body's natural reaction to an "invader" like a pencil-sized tube at the vocal cords or in the trachea is to try to expel it with cough). In some patients with CF, it is difficult to numb the vocal cords and trachea completely, and they do cough a bit during the procedure. Once the bronchoscope reaches the bronchi of the new lungs, the need for anesthetizing the airways has lessened, since the new lungs do not have nerves connected to them. The new bronchi do not have any feeling or cough reflex.

Once the bronchoscope is in the small bronchi, it is pushed gently so that it is firmly sealed into the airway (this is known as "wedging" the bronchoscope). When the bronchoscope is wedged into place, blocking off the bronchus, the physician performs the BAL (that is, she or he washes in the saline, and sucks it back out again, saving it for culture and microscopic examination). Sometimes, just pushing the bronchoscope down bronchi, especially bronchi that are inflamed because of infection or rejection, can cause bleeding. Usually this bleeding is not serious, but occasionally it can be.

After doing the BAL, the physician repositions the tip of the bronchoscope so that it's well placed to obtain biopsies. Most often, the physician uses a radiograph screen (fluoroscopy or just "fluoro") to show the exact position of the bronchoscope and the forceps. The physician then passes the forceps through the suction channel and takes a few "bites" of tissue for the biopsies. One would think that the taking of biopsies would be painful, but it is not. Taking bites from the lung (or any living tissue) usually causes some bleeding, as you might expect. Usually the bleeding stops very quickly, but on occasion, particularly if the lungs are inflamed (infection or rejection), the bleeding can be difficult to control and can be dangerous. In extremely rare cases, it has even been fatal.

Taking a bite of tissue can also cause a hole in the outside of the lung, allowing air to leak outside the lungs. The air that escapes through a hole in the lung is still trapped within the chest, and can accumulate around the lung, press in on the lung, and cause it to collapse. This condition is called a *pneumothorax*, and is discussed a bit more in Chapter 3, *The Respiratory System*. A pneumothorax is much more likely to occur in a patient who is breathing with the help of a ventilator, since the ventilator works by blowing air into the lungs under pressure. This added air pressure can open up a small hole and prop it open, preventing it from sealing itself shut, and allowing air to escape with each breath in. If someone develops a pneumothorax, he or she will usually need to have a tube placed through the skin, between the ribs, and into the chest in order to let the air escape and allow the lung to reexpand. These tubes are called chest tubes, for obvious reasons. A pneumothorax is usually painful, and chest tubes are always painful, so pain medications are given if this problem develops.

There are some situations where a biopsy with the flexible bronchoscope (a transbronchial biopsy) might not be possible, but a biopsy of the lung is needed. For example, the patient may be too small to breathe around the flexible bronchoscope, the patient may be too sick to have flexible bronchoscopy, or the physicians believe that the bites taken with biopsy forceps are likely to be too small to give an accurate diagnosis. In these cases, an *open* lung *biopsy* might be necessary. An open biopsy is done in the operating room, under general anesthesia. The surgeon makes an incision through the chest to expose part of the lung under his direct vision, and cuts out a small piece of the lung, sews the hole, and closes the chest. This procedure is more involved, requires general anesthesia, and takes more time to recover from, but, in a very sick patient, is probably safer than the transbronchial biopsy, and guarantees a bigger piece of tissue, which is more likely to allow for a correct diagnosis.

Ongoing Care

After transplantation, as you've heard many times already, continuing care is absolutely essential and never-ending. Treatment with immunosuppressant (anti-rejection) medications is essential. Other CF treatments, like enzymes and nutritional supplements, are also important. Many patients will still need to do chest PT, or use their Flutter valve, vest (or other airway clearance techniques) for clearing mucus from their new lungs. Some patients may have to have special treatment for their sinuses, if their physicians feel that infected sinuses have been causing problems in their new lungs. In most cases, care can take place at your regular CF center, but with periodic visits back to the transplant center. Your physician and the transplant team will work together to make sure your overall care is as good as it can be.

RESULTS OF LUNG TRANSPLANTATION (PROGNOSIS AFTER TRANSPLANTATION)

Lung transplantation for patients with CF is still a relatively young science and art. The first procedure, you'll recall, was in 1963, and for the first several years of lung transplantation, patients did not live more than a few weeks. Although we have improved a great deal since then, we are certainly not at the point where it's simply a matter of ordering a set of new lungs, getting them hooked up, and going on about our business. Now, and for the foreseeable future, lung transplantation, perhaps especially for patients with CF, will be a very difficult procedure, with many deaths and with much suffering for many of those who survive. In fact, starting in 1994, "transplant complications" moved into second place in the list of reasons for death of patients with CF (whereas CF pulmonary disease used to account for 95% of the deaths of patients with CF each year, in 2001, the lungs are listed as the cause of death in 79.7%, and transplant complications in 9.1%).

Nonetheless, many patients have done spectacularly well, with full resumption of work, school, recreation, and family life, some of them 9 or 10 years after transplantation. As transplant centers gain more experience, and as scientists develop better ways to preserve lungs outside the body and better and safer immunosuppressive drugs, we can expect the results to improve. It is worth keeping in mind that the first kidney transplant recipients did not survive long, and liver transplantation had no long-term survivors for the first several years that the procedure was performed. Now, both of those procedures are accepted as standard care for many conditions, and the outcome is excellent. As experience with lung transplantation increases, the results will almost certainly improve.

At the writing of this book, most centers report about 50% to 60% 2-year survival after lung transplantation for patients with CF. That means that if 100 patients get a transplant, 50 to 60 will be alive 2 years later; 40 to 50 will be dead. Let's look at some other numbers that don't have anything to do with transplants: Patients with CF with the worst PFTs have about a 50% 2-year survival (without transplant). So, of 100 of those patients, 50 will be alive and 50 dead in 2 years. Transplantation may allow up to ten more out of a hundred of these sickest patients to survive for 2 years than would have survived without transplantation. Other factors need to be considered too: Of those who survive, about half will develop bronchiolitis obliterans, a severe condition seen in transplanted lungs. Bronchiolitis obliterans causes progressive difficulty breathing and is ultimately fatal in about one third to one half of the patients who develop it.

In one recent report from England, 76 patients with CF were referred for lung transplantation. Of those 76 patients, 36 died waiting on the transplant list, and 15 were alive (still waiting for transplant) at the time of the report; 25 patients received their transplants, and of those, ten died and 15 were still alive. So, of the original 76 patients put on the transplant list, 46 died (ten after transplant, 36 waiting for organs) and 30 were alive, 15 of them still waiting for transplant and 15 of them after getting their new lungs. Of the 15 alive after the new lungs, we can assume that seven or eight will likely develop bronchiolitis obliterans, and become sick. The seven or eight others are likely to be doing well. Although such numbers make lung transplantation appear too risky for many people, we should stress that scientists and physicians continue to improve the outlook for lung transplant recipients, and we have reason to expect that more and more patients will do well after the procedure in the future.

MAKING THE DECISION

The decision to proceed with transplantation is always a difficult one. Most patients express disbelief when told that they should consider a transplant; often they just don't feel sick enough to require a transplant. This is especially true for lung transplant candidates. Because there is a long wait for lungs, patients must get on the list early if they are going to get credit for waiting time. In addition, the idea of transplantation can be frightening. It is, after all, an unknown procedure to the patient, and this can be especially difficult for patients (and families) who are used to a routine of treatment for CF. Deciding to undergo a transplantation often means the patient and family will have to get used to a whole new set of physicians and nurses (the transplant team); adding this new care team may interfere with the patient's ways of dealing with his or her original CF team. Finally, a patient who is very sick with CF may be able to accept his or her illness and decide to be comfortable and in control of his or her destiny. Such a patient may not want the uncertainty of transplantation, and may feel it is better to die peacefully rather than be expected to fight to stay alive long enough to receive lungs that may never come. This last point is one of the most difficult aspects of a family's decision in "going for" transplant.

When your CF doctor suggests that a transplant may be the best thing to do, you must first find out why he or she feels that way. Is it because your PFTs are very bad? Have you gotten worse quickly over the preceding year? Ask your own CF physicians; they will tell you.

Your family can often help you with your decision. For a major procedure like transplantation, particularly one that will surely require lots of care after the procedure, you will need help and support. Any form of transplantation is something that should be viewed with both eyes open. The more you and your family understand the procedure and the risks involved, the better you and your physicians will be able to deal with the consequences of transplantation.

Finally, remember that no one can really make your decision about transplantation for you. In addition, *there is no right or wrong decision when and if you are asked to consider having a transplant.* Many patients are eager to have a transplant, many others don't want to consider one under any circumstances. Both groups of patients (and all of those patients whose feelings are in between the two) are right. You must be comfortable with your decision, for you will have to live with the results of your decision.

Deciding to be considered for transplantation, however, does not mean you have to actually undergo transplantation. This is an extremely important point. It is possible, in other words, to be evaluated for a lung transplant, to get on the list for the transplant, to move up to the top of the list, and *then* decide that you really don't want a transplant. Obviously, if you do this, you will have to have the tests needed for evaluation, and you may have to go on the "inactive" transplant list if you decide not to have a transplant. On the other hand, if you decide *not* to have an evaluation for a lung transplant and change your mind a year later, you will have lost a year of time on the list and you will have to wait that much longer for a set of lungs. Unless you are opposed to a transplant, you should at least discuss it with your physician when it is suggested to you. After you have all the information available, it will be possible for you to make an informed and responsible decision about proceeding or not proceeding with the process of transplantation.

LIVER TRANSPLANTATION

Who Should Be Considered for a New Liver?

Liver transplantation is usually considered in two situations (see Chapter 4, *The Gastrointestinal Tract*, for more details): (a) when there is liver failure, with buildup of toxic chemicals that the liver normally clears from the body, and low levels of chemicals (including protein and factors that help blood clot properly) that the liver normally makes; and (b) when there is uncontrollable bleeding from esophageal varices (the details of this problem are spelled out in Chapter 4).

Who Should Not Be Considered for a New Liver?

Just as there are some people who feel that they don't want any part of the high-tech world of lung transplantation, with its many unknowns and its possible complications, some people make the same decision about liver transplantation. There also are some situations in which there are medical contraindications to (reasons not to do) liver transplantation. A widespread bloodstream infection carries such a high risk of death after transplantation that it is considered an absolute contraindication for any transplant, including liver, by most transplant centers. *Very severe* lung disease is also believed by many to be a contraindication to liver transplantation alone. There have been many patients with CF with mildly or even moderately affected lungs whose PFTs have stayed the same or even improved after liver transplantation (see below). There have even been a couple of patients with CF who have received lung and liver transplants during the same surgery.

The Transplant List for Liver Transplants

The system for determining your spot on the liver transplant list takes into account the time on the list and how sick you are. Each patient is assigned a "patient status" that affects where you are on the list. The status ranges from status 1 (patients in ICUs, on life support) to status 4 (stable, not hospitalized). Those patients who are status 1 are automatically moved to the top of the list by UNOS and receive the first available organ. In some ways, this system may seem to be fairer than the lung waiting system, which is based solely on the length of time waiting, but there have been instances where patients have been hospitalized or put in an ICU, not because they were sicker, but in order to move them higher on the list. The wait for a liver is not as long as for lungs, partly because livers can be preserved longer than lungs and therefore can be brought from farther away, and partly because the liver is less delicate than the lung and more likely to have acceptable function despite the injury or illness that has killed the donor or the treatment the donor has received in attempting to save her life.

The Technique of Liver Transplantation

The liver is located in the upper portion of the right side of the abdomen, just below the diaphragm. Its blood supply comes from an artery (the hepatic artery), and a vein (the portal vein). Blood leaves the liver in a vein known as the hepatic vein. The liver is also connected to the gallbladder, which releases bile into the small intestine through the bile duct. To transplant a liver, the surgeons must make a very large incision across the upper part of the abdomen of the recipient, carefully remove the liver, and then attach the blood vessels to the blood vessels going to and coming from the transplanted liver. The bile duct from the new liver may not be reattached at the time of surgery, and instead is often allowed to drain directly into the small intestine. Because of the difficulty in taking out the damaged liver and replacing it with the transplanted liver, it is not unusual for a liver transplant operation to take more than 9 hours. Because of the many blood vessels that must be attached and because the liver contains a large amount of blood, many transfusions are often needed during the surgery. In addition, some patients have their blood diverted away from the abdomen using an artificial pump to take blood from the lower part of the body and return it directly to the heart while the liver is being replaced.

Because bleeding in the abdomen is fairly common after the surgery, several drainage tubes are placed in the abdomen at the time of surgery. These tubes go out through the skin into small plastic reservoirs, which can hold blood or other secretions that come out of the abdomen. This will allow the surgeons to see if there is a large amount of bleeding in the abdomen following surgery. The drainage tubes will also help with the healing process by removing excess blood from the abdomen. They are usually removed within the first 2 weeks after surgery.

Complications of Liver Transplantation

The most worrisome complications specific to liver transplantation are organ failure, bleeding, and blood clots in the artery or vein to the liver. As with any organ transplantation, rejection of the transplanted organ and infection (of the new organ or elsewhere in the body) are also major concerns, and necessitate very careful dosing of the immunosuppressive medications.

As is the case with any transplanted organ, the liver must be obtained from a donor and then must be kept alive long enough for the surgeon to place it into the abdomen of the recipient. Over the years, the technique of organ preservation has improved, but it is still not perfect. The liver, once removed from the donor, has its blood washed out in order to prevent the donor's blood from clotting within the vessels and to prevent the donor's white blood cells from damaging it. The blood is washed out of the liver through the blood vessels, by rinsing a large amount of a special solution that contains minerals and special sugars that will allow the liver to remain alive even though the blood is gone. Sometimes, despite the best efforts to preserve the function of the liver, it is injured, because of liver damage while still in the donor or because the preservation process is inadequate. If this occurs, then the liver will not work after transplantation, and the patient will suffer from liver failure. In some instances, the liver damage may be so severe that the patient dies as a result. In other cases, the liver may recover enough function to allow the patient to survive and ultimately do well.

As mentioned before, bleeding is a fairly common problem during the liver transplantation procedure itself. Bleeding can also be a dangerous problem in the hours and days following transplantation. The drainage tubes placed into the abdomen at the time of surgery can alert the surgeons to bleeding after surgery. Although blood and clotting factors given to the recipient after surgery may stop the bleeding, there are instances in which the only way to stop the bleeding is for the surgeon to reopen the abdomen and find the blood vessels that are bleeding and stop the bleeding directly.

Blood clots can form and block the blood vessels to the transplanted liver. In some cases, these clots can decrease blood flow to the liver, leading to liver damage. At times, such clots must be removed surgically, by opening the abdomen, locating the clot in the blood vessel, opening the blood vessel, removing the clot, and then surgically closing the blood vessel. Clotting within major blood vessels to the liver, unfortunately, does not always resolve or may lead to irreversible liver damage before the clots can be removed.

Care After Liver Transplantation

Tests After Liver Transplantation

As with lung transplant recipients, liver recipients must undergo regular tests to make sure the new liver is functioning well. Blood tests of liver function (usually abbreviated as LFTs) are followed on a frequent basis, but if rejection is thought to be likely, biopsies are necessary.

A liver biopsy is done by cleaning and numbing the skin over the liver and then inserting a special needle directly into the liver. This needle is designed to cut into the liver and hold a small piece of the liver inside the needle as the needle is removed. The biopsy can then be sent to the laboratory and examined. As with the lung biopsies, liver biopsies are usually performed after the patient has been given some IV sedative medication.

Complications of Liver Biopsy

Most liver biopsies are performed with no ill effects. But, as with any procedure, there is a small chance of problems. Beyond the risk of oversedation, the biggest risk of liver biopsy is bleeding. The liver has a rich supply of blood vessels, and it is possible to tear one of these and cause bleeding. In most cases, the bleeding isn't serious, but, particularly if the liver isn't working well and not making blood clotting factors normally, it can be difficult to control.

Ongoing Care

After liver transplantation, as with lung transplantation, continuing care is absolutely essential and never-ending. Treatment with immunosuppressant (anti-rejection) medications is essential. Other CF treatments, like enzymes and nutritional supplements, are also important. Patients will still need to do chest PT, or use their Flutter valve or vest for clearing mucus from their lungs. In most cases, care can take place at your regular CF center, but with periodic visits back to the transplant center. As in the case of lung transplantation, it is important that your CF physician and the transplant team work together to deliver the best care possible to maintain good liver function as well as to preserve lung function.

Results of Liver Transplantation

The results for liver transplantation for people with CF are a little harder to know for certain than those for lung transplantation, because there have been far fewer liver transplantation procedures done in patients with CF. Nonetheless, it appears that the outcome is somewhat better at this point than for lung transplantation, probably because there is more experience with liver transplantation in general (in non-CF patients) than with lung transplantation and because the liver can survive longer out of the body. In one large CF and transplant center, approximately 92% of the patients with CF who received liver transplants survived 1 year after the procedure, and 75% survived 5 years.

One surprising result has been that patients with CF who have received liver transplants do not have an immediate worsening of their lung infection, as many people worried they would. The reason for the worry, of course, was that these patients have to take immunosuppressive medications to prevent liver rejection. Immunosuppressive medicines decrease the body's ability to fight infection, and there already is infection in the lungs of people with CF. So most physicians assumed that lung infection would worsen as soon as someone with CF was started on immunosuppressive medicines. Instead, what happens is that in most cases the lung function of patients with CF either doesn't change or actually gets a bit better in the weeks to months after liver transplantation. The reasons for this are not completely clear, but one possible explanation is that the immunosuppressive medicines cut down on the inflammation within the airways. As you've seen in Chapter 3, antiinflammatory medicines, like steroids, can sometimes be helpful in patients with CF. It may be that this antiinflammatory action of the immunosuppressives helps more than the increased risk of infection hurts.

THE FUTURE OF TRANSPLANTATION

Transplantation is a young science, and many physicians and research scientists are working to unravel its secrets and solve its many problems. With the development of newer antirejection medications and an improved understanding of the ways to prevent and treat the complications of transplantation, the future of transplantation is bright. It remains, however, a major medical and surgical commitment for any patient who wishes to pursue this avenue of treatment. Confidence in the transplant physicians, a willingness to undergo special tests, and an ability to cooperate with the transplant team will increase the chances for any one patient to undergo transplantation successfully. It is clear that there is much to learn about transplantation, but many patients with CF who are alive following liver or lung transplantation are a testimony of the promise inherent in this form of therapy.

9

Daily Life

THE BASICS

1. Most patients with cystic fibrosis (CF) should be expected to live a very normal daily life (except for treatments): They go to school, do homework, have friends, play sports, grow up, many marry, and so on.
2. Children with CF should have the same expectations and responsibilities as other children.

There are many aspects of daily life that are altered very little by having cystic fibrosis (CF): Babies cry and laugh, and children still sleep through the night, wake up, go to the bathroom, have breakfast, go to school, play with friends, play sports, do homework and chores, watch television, and go to parties. They may go on trips with or without their families. They grow up and finish school; they take jobs; many marry, and may decide to raise a family. It is very important for a child's emotional well-being, and that of the family, that daily life be approached with these expectations. The emotional aspect of living with CF is discussed in Chapter 12, *The Family*, and the issues that relate specifically to teens and adults are addressed in Chapters 13 and 14, respectively. This chapter addresses the few areas in which CF does have an effect on the patient's (or family's) daily life.

In most stages of life, having CF requires some form of airway clearance therapy, anywhere from one to four times a day. Approximately 90% of people with CF must remember, or be reminded, to take digestive enzymes with each meal and usually with snacks. Most patients will also have to take vitamins each day, and many will need to take antibiotics by mouth fairly frequently.

Clinic visits for checkups will be required anywhere from one to eight times a year, depending on your physician's approach and your health. These visits are very important for health maintenance (see Chapter 3, *The Respiratory System*).

During periods of pulmonary exacerbation (see Chapter 3), it may be necessary to come into the hospital for 1 to 3 weeks, or to receive intravenous antibiotics at home (see Chapter 7, *Hospitalization and Other Special Treatments*). This treatment may be necessary one to three times each year for as many as one in every three or four patients.

Patients who have more severe lung disease may need to adjust the intensity of their physical exertion, and a very few may even need to wear oxygen tubing while they are up and around and perhaps during sleep, but this is a very small proportion of patients.

Mealtimes should not be too different for people with CF than it would be if they did not have CF, except for remembering to take the enzymes. If someone has had trouble putting (or keeping) weight on, there may be meals with added fats and calories, or even nighttime tube feedings to help with growth (see Chapter 6, *Nutrition*).

MEDICATIONS AND TREATMENTS: WHO IS IN CHARGE?

During a child's early years, the parents are responsible for the medication and must know which medicines should be taken when, why they are needed, and what additional treatments are required. By the time a young adult leaves home, he or she must be in charge of these areas. Most experts believe that a good time for the transition in this responsibility from the parents to the young patient is early in the teenage years. Before the teen years, many youngsters are simply not emotionally mature enough to take on these responsibilities, no matter how smart they are, no matter how well they do in school, and no matter how much their parents want them to be "grown up." Conversely, if a parent refuses to begin the peaceful transfer of control well into the child's teenage years, it can be harmful for a teen's ability to function independently later on, and it may well fuel parent–adolescent battles.

Adolescence is both a good and a bad time for accomplishing the transition in responsibility for medical care. It is a good time because the teenager wants very much to become independent of the parent and is looking for ways to assert that independence. Teenagers welcome the trust that accompanies responsibility as well as the absence of nagging that results when they have learned all their medications and take them faithfully.

Adolescence can be a difficult time, however, for the transition in responsibility, because in normal teenage rebellion against authority there is a strong urge to ignore what the parents want. When the teenager has CF, what the parents want is for the teenager to take the prescribed medications and treatments in order to stay well. This may be an area where the teenager is able to exert some control, and the relatively common feeling of invulnerability ("nothing will happen to me") may just add to the appeal of not taking medications. As with so many other aspects of the teenager's life, the best solution is to encourage him or her to take full responsibility for medications and treatments, but to be aware of what is and is not being done, and to encourage the best cooperation possible. To encourage this self-care and independence, the physician may choose to meet with the patient alone and to have the parents sit in the waiting room during clinic visits.

DAYCARE

Daycare has become very common for many families with babies, especially if both parents work. Babies in daycare get more colds than babies kept at home. Babies with CF will get neither more nor fewer colds than the other babies, but some of these colds may develop into bronchial infections (*pulmonary exacerbations*). This fact has made some families try to avoid daycare. For the first months of an infant's life, when the bronchi are very tiny and when infants with CF may have more trouble keeping the bronchi clear, it may be advisable to delay daycare. However, if this is financially difficult, it should not be considered a major setback. Remember that the goal of avoiding all colds is impossible to achieve, especially if there are other children in the family, and that careful attention to an infant's health, with quick treatment for any pulmonary infections, is likely to result in very good maintenance of health.

Occasionally, a misguided daycare supervisor, parent, or even physician may be concerned that the presence of an infant with CF will pose a danger to the other children in daycare. *CF is not contagious.* Even if a baby with CF is coughing a lot, the bacteria in the lungs of someone with CF are not dangerous to children without CF. Of course, a baby with CF can get a regular cold, just like any other baby, and pass that cold on to anyone else, but babies with CF should not be excluded from daycare just because of having CF or cough.

SCHOOL

School is very important for all children, and virtually all children with CF should be able to go to school and carry a full load, including homework and extracurricular activities. When a child has a lung infection, he or she may not feel as well as usual, but in most cases this should not interfere with education. Children should be encouraged to go to school, even if they are coughing more than their usual, as long as they are receiving the appropriate treatment (antibiotics and increased airway clearance treatments).

Teachers may need to be educated about CF to make a very few special considerations for the child with CF. They need to be aware that the child with CF is likely to have more cough than other children, and should never be discouraged from coughing. The child with CF may also need to have more frequent bathroom privileges. Most CF centers have a very good booklet designed for teachers (see Appendix F, *Bibliography*).

Homework should be required from the child with CF, just as from his or her peers. There should be almost no exceptions to this rule. Even if a child has to be hospitalized, he or she should keep up with schoolwork. If a child is hospitalized, the school district should provide tutoring to enable the child to keep up with the class.

Physical education class is as important (or even more important) for children with CF as for other children. Physical education class should not be graded on the basis of athletic performance for any child, especially those who might have a physical reason for lower than average performance, as a child with CF and lung disease might have.

COLLEGE

See Chapter 13, *The Teenaged Years*, for a discussion of going to college—going away or staying home.

SPORTS AND EXERCISE

In general, there is no reason for children, adolescents, or adults with CF to avoid exercise. Exercise is good for most people, including people with CF. Everyone, with CF or without it, needs to adjust the amount and intensity of exercise to his or her own abilities and needs, but this can be done fairly easily. (Exercise and sports are discussed more in Chapter 10, *Exercise*.)

VISITS WITH FRIENDS

Visiting with friends, either at their houses or your own, is an important part of growing up, learning to get along with others, and learning to become independent away from home. Children and adolescents with CF should have these same opportunities as anyone else. In most cases, special arrangements will have to be made to be certain that medications are being taken and that treatments are being done. In some cases, for a single overnighter for a grade-school child, it might not be a problem to skip a single day's treatment, but this should not become a habit. Adolescents who give themselves their own treatments should be able to do this anywhere. If either part of the visiting pair is sick, changes may have to be made, but this is no different from what would be done if neither child had CF. All experts now advise against close contacts (like overnights) between patients with CF, to avoid the possibility of their sharing potentially harmful lung bacteria. Although the bacteria that patients with CF may cough out or have on their hands present absolutely no danger to people without CF, there is a small but real risk of harm to someone with CF (see Chapter 3, *The Respiratory System*, for more discussion of the issue of *person-to-person transmission* of CF bacteria).

SMOKING

People with any form of lung disease should not smoke, nor should they inhale other people's smoke. This is certainly true for people with CF. Smoke is harmful to children's lungs, even if the lungs are normal. Someone who has abnormal lungs, especially if asthma is part of the condition, has a greatly increased risk of complications if he or she must breathe cigarette smoke. Smoke from cigarettes can be harmful to a child's lungs even if the person smoking the cigarette loves the child very much. Parents whose child has CF should stop smoking immediately, and smoking should not be allowed in their homes. Most people, including smokers, know that smoking is very harmful to the smoker; not everyone realizes that it is also harmful to the lungs of children who are forced to breathe in the second-hand smoke. **It has been shown unequivocally that being exposed to parents' cigarette smoke causes worsened lung function in children with CF**.

Many parents who have been unsuccessful at stopping smoking are able to stop when they realize that it is not just for their own health but for the children's as well. If you cannot stop right away, it is essential that you stop smoking in the house. If you are smoking in the same house, the baby will get the fumes. You must especially never smoke in the car, since that is an enclosed space where smoke can get very thick and irritating. If you need help stopping, your physician may be able to help. For someone who is truly addicted to cigarettes, the addiction is every bit as serious as—and *harder to break* than—a heroin addiction. (Some people feel it's even worse than heroin, since with heroin it's mostly the person directly taking the drug whose health is impaired, while with cigarettes, it's also the "innocent bystanders.") Nicotine chewing gum and patches have been helpful for people who are dedicated to stopping smoking but cannot do it on their own.

TRAVEL

Patients with CF can travel, just as people without CF can travel. There are a few practical considerations for the traveling CF patient.

Remember to Take Your Medicines

Some medications used for patients with CF (especially enzymes) may not be carried in every pharmacy, so it may be difficult to replace medications while you are away from your regular pharmacy. If you travel out of state, you may find that a pharmacy will not accept your doctor's prescription if he or she is not licensed in the state you are visiting. In most cases, pharmacists are very helpful, and will do what they can to provide you with the service you need, but it is better to be prepared for a problem.

Remember to Take Any Equipment You Might Need for Aerosols or Postural Drainage Treatments

If you are going on a short trip, it may be possible to bring less bulky equipment than you use at home. For example, if you use the vest for airway clearance, your doctor might approve the Flutter for your trip; you might be able to user inhalers instead of nebulizer treatments for a short time (see Chapter 3, *The Respiratory System* for more details). If you are traveling to a different country, you may need to bring special electrical outlet adapters for whatever electrical equipment you use, because different countries use different power sources. Adapters are available to enable you to convert the power source to fit your own equipment.

High Altitude

If you live at or near sea level and travel to higher altitudes, you may experience difficulty because of the lower oxygen pressures at altitude. The air in Denver, for example, has only 80% as much oxygen as that in San Diego or Boston. Someone whose lungs are in excellent condition should have no trouble in these places, but someone who has serious lung involvement may be comfortable and safe at sea level, but develop problems in the mountains. It is a good idea to discuss travel plans with your doctor before going.

Airplane Travel

Commercial airlines pressurize their cabins to 5,000 to 8,000 feet. That means that the oxygen level inside the cabin is comparable to Denver's or a place even higher. The large majority of patients with CF and mild or even moderate lung disease can fly in commercial airliners with no problems. If you need oxygen at sea level, you will need more in an airplane, and if you are close to needing it at home, you may need it while you fly. The major airlines are used to dealing with requests for oxygen during flights, and usually are very helpful, but *most insist that you contact them well in advance* to let them know about your plans and needs (usually there is a special medical department to contact at the airline).

SUMMER CAMP

Summer camps can provide valuable experience for children and adolescents, and most children and adolescents with CF should be able to attend camp if they want to. Most children whose lungs are in good shape and whose digestion is fairly well controlled with enzymes should be able to attend any kind of camp, as long as arrangements for medications and treatments can be made with the camp physicians and nurses. Many areas used to have CF camps, especially for kids with CF. These have now all disappeared, because of the risk of infection (see Chapter 3, *The Respiratory System*).

WHERE TO LIVE

People often wonder if there are areas of the country that are better than others for children (and adults) with CF. From what is known now, the answer is no.

In individual patients, it is possible that they might do better in one geographic location than another, but so many factors influence how someone will do, and patients are so different from each other, that no one place has the perfect combination of factors that make for good health for all people with CF.

Cities and states differ in the amount of pollution, cold, wetness, and allergens, and in the availability of good medical care. While one might think that the cold, wet, polluted, industrial, northeastern cities (Cleveland, Pittsburgh, Boston, Toronto, etc.) would be the worst places for CF patients to live, national survival statistics, which measure how long people live, have previously shown that it is exactly these cities that have had the best CF survival. The explanation almost certainly lies in the fact that these cities have had excellent CF centers for the longest time. Excellent CF centers now exist in most regions of the United States, Canada, Europe, and Australia, and the survival statistics now reflect this change. Most CF physicians believe that ready access to a good CF center is important, but other than this criterion, there is very little basis for recommending one geographic area over another for someone with CF.

10

Exercise

THE BASICS

1. Exercise is good for virtually all people with cystic fibrosis (CF).
2. People with CF lose more salt and drink less fluid than normal when they exercise in the heat.
3. Physically fit patients with CF live longer than those who are not fit.
4. Children with CF should be encouraged to be active from a very young age, and that active lifestyle should continue all their lives.

Everyone is interested in exercise these days. People with cystic fibrosis (CF) are no exception. Exercise done properly, in the right amount, the right intensity, and with the proper safety precautions, can be fun and beneficial for nearly everyone. Again, people with CF are no exception. There is even evidence that the more physically fit people with CF are, the more likely they are to stay alive for the next 8 years and beyond!

EFFECTS OF EXERCISE ON PEOPLE WITHOUT CYSTIC FIBROSIS

Single Sessions of Exercise

When someone begins muscular exercise, the body has to make some fast adaptations, most of which relate to supplying the exercising muscles with considerably more oxygen than is needed at rest. These adaptations help the muscles remove excess carbon dioxide, which is produced when they are active. Muscles are able to contract and move the body without oxygen, but this is much more difficult than muscular work performed with adequate oxygen. Work that is performed without adequate oxygen being supplied to the muscles is called *anaer-obic* work; work that is performed with enough oxygen is called *aerobic* work. Anaerobic exercise can only be carried out for a period of seconds or minutes, whereas aerobic exercise can be sustained for many minutes or even hours. Anaerobic exercise is not only more difficult and less efficient than aerobic exercise but also results in the production of lactic acid in the muscles, and in the production of considerably more carbon dioxide, which then has to be removed.

Since oxygen is supplied to the exercising muscles (and carbon dioxide is removed) by circulating blood, one of the first changes at the beginning of exercise is an increase in blood flow to the active muscle. Since the heart has to pump more blood, it has to pump faster, and the heart rate (pulse) increases. The heart rate reaches a maximum which can be predicted accurately from the person's age: maximum heart rate = 220 – age (in years). Thus, a 20-year-old person would have a predicted maximum heart rate of 220 – 20 = 200 beats per minute. It is also necessary to increase the amount of oxygen available to the blood, and, especially with anaerobic exercise, to increase the disposal of carbon dioxide. The increase in oxygen supply and carbon dioxide removal are both accomplished by increasing the amount of air that is breathed each minute. The accuracy of these adjustments is astounding, as you've already seen in Chapter 3. During heavy exercise, the heart may increase its output five- or sixfold, and the lungs may bring in (and exhale) five to ten times as much air as they do during naps, and yet, the levels of oxygen and carbon dioxide in the bloodstream remain nearly constant.

It takes anywhere from a few seconds to 1½ minutes to adjust the amount of blood the heart pumps to the exercising muscles. Therefore, during the first seconds of exercise, the muscles are undersupplied with oxygen. In other words, the first seconds of any form of exercise are anaerobic exercise. Exercise that is strictly "stop-and-go," in which you exercise, rest, and then exercise again (for example, racquet sports) is anaerobic exercise. Exercise is also anaerobic if it is very heavy work and the muscles demand more oxygen than can be supplied (for example, heavy weightlifting, running, or riding a bike up a steep hill). In contrast, aerobic exercise is a low intensity, rhythmic type of activity, such as walking, swimming, easy jogging, and bike riding.

Exercise in the Heat

The more someone exercises, especially in hot weather, the more heat the body produces. If the body temperature becomes too high it can be dangerous, so there has to be a way for body temperature to remain relatively constant. This is accomplished through several mechanisms. The first is that a greater amount of blood than usual is sent to the skin, especially the scalp and hands. This is a way of bringing the warmth of the body close to the surface, where it can be given off to the surrounding air (unless the air is hotter than body temperature). If all of the blood stayed in the heart and other internal organs, it would be insulated by the skin, muscles, and fat, and the heat would build up. The other way of giving off excess heat is through sweating. As sweat evaporates, it cools the surface of the body. This is why you sweat when you exercise, especially in the heat.

Exercise Tolerance

When someone is given a test on an exercise cycle, it becomes progressively more difficult to pedal and, eventually, *everyone* will get to the point where he or she can no longer pedal. In most healthy people, the point at which this occurs is determined by two factors. The first is that the heart reaches a point at which it can no longer increase the amount of blood it pumps to the muscles, so the muscles become relatively undersupplied with blood and oxygen and become fatigued. This usually happens when the heart rate has reached the maximum limit. If a 20-year-old person is exercising so hard that the heart rate is 200 beats per minute, it will not be able to go much faster, so the amount of blood being pumped out will not be able to increase any further.

The second limiting factor may be the muscles themselves: There is a limit to how much oxygen the muscles can process, so they may become fatigued even though enough oxygen has been delivered. In someone with normal lungs, the lungs are never the limiting factor in exercise. Even at total exhaustion, the lungs have considerable reserve. Recall from Chapter 3 that the maximum voluntary ventilation (MVV) is the measurement of the largest amount of air someone can move in and out of the lungs in a minute. During exercise, even at the point of total exhaustion, most people don't use any more than 70% of their MVV; that is, their lungs could still deliver another 30% effort. But this wouldn't help, since other factors would have impeded the exercise before the extra breathing reserves were needed.

Repeated Sessions of Exercise (Exercise Programs)

If you exercise each day, or at least 3 days a week, for a certain minimum time (10 to 30 minutes a day) and at a certain minimum intensity (hard enough to raise your heart rate to approximately 75% of its maximum, which is around 150 beats per minute for adolescents and young adults), after a few weeks (6 to 12 weeks), you will become more fit, that is, you will be able to do more of the same kind of exercise with less stress on your body. If the type of exercise you were doing each day was aerobic, then you will increase your *aerobic fitness*. If it was anaerobic exercise, then your *anaerobic fitness* will increase. Jogging 30 minutes each day will make it much easier for you to jog, but it will not make you able to lift 200 lb, whereas lifting weights every day may make your muscles stronger (and bigger) for weightlifting tasks, but will not improve your endurance or your ability to carry out prolonged walks or bike rides.

With repeated aerobic exercise sessions involving walking or jogging, one of the ways in which you become more fit is that your heart is able to pump more blood with each beat, and therefore you need fewer heart beats to deliver the same amount of blood to the muscles. You can see this change by checking your heart rate for a certain workload before you start an exercise program, then rechecking it after a few months of exercise. The easiest "work load" to check is no work at all, that is, measure your resting heart rate. The more fit someone is, the lower his or her resting heart rate. You may know runners who brag about having a resting heart rate of 45 or 50 beats per minute.

Another change that occurs with a training program and increased fitness is in the muscles themselves: They become able to process much more oxygen and to put that oxygen to use in performing work.

One change that does not occur with an exercise-training program is in lung function. Most scientific studies have shown no important changes in lung function in healthy people after they train and become very fit. Because lung function doesn't have much to do with one's exercise ability if the lungs are normal, this doesn't make much difference to most people.

There is increasing evidence that people who engage in lifelong exercise live longer than sedentary people and have lower risks for various diseases, especially heart disease and some kinds of cancer.

Exercise-training programs have long been felt to be valuable to people's emotional health as well as their physical health, with decreased depression and stress levels and increased work productivity. Many large corporations have installed impressive gym facilities for their employees because they have felt that fit employees were happier, healthier, and more productive.

Heat Training

Another change that comes with an exercise program, especially if it's been carried out in the heat, is that you become heat-acclimatized, that is, you can withstand exercise and heat stress better than you could before you got in shape. Several changes account for this improved heat tolerance. The first is just that exercise itself is easier because of being more fit (lower heart rate, etc.), without regard to the heat. But additional changes occur that are related specifically to increased heat tolerance. People who train in the heat begin to sweat earlier during an exercise session, thus cooling themselves earlier through evaporation. In addition, and quite remarkably, when someone without CF trains in the heat for several weeks, the sweat that is produced contains less salt. This may be the body's way of preserving salt, since much salt can be lost when someone sweats excessively. (People running a marathon can easily lose 5 to 10 lb of sweat in 3 or 4 hours.)

EFFECTS OF EXERCISE IN PEOPLE WITH CYSTIC FIBROSIS

Single Sessions of Exercise

The responses to exercise in people with CF are generally similar to those of people who don't have CF. To meet the increased oxygen needs of exercising muscles and to remove carbon dioxide, both the heart's output and the amount of breathing are considerably increased. If the person's lung function is normal or nearly normal, he or she will have exactly the same responses to exercise as anyone else. However, there are some differences in the response to exercise in someone with CF whose pulmonary function is not normal. One difference is that people with CF frequently stop exercising before their heart rate has reached the maximum predicted based upon age. In these cases, the minute ventilation (the amount of air being breathed each minute) may be very large in comparison with the person's capacity or reserve. Remember that people with normal lungs seldom breathe more than 70% of their MVV, even during strenuous exercise. People with CF often use more than 80% of their MVV (in some cases, more than 100% of their "maximum" capacity is used!). Even as you can't expect a person with a normal heart to make the heart beat faster than its maximum, you can't expect *anyone*—with or without healthy lungs—to be able to use more than 100% of the lungs' capacity.

Most patients with CF maintain their blood levels of oxygen and carbon dioxide during exercise. In some patients, the blood oxygen level actually increases with exercise. However, in people with severe lung disease, the blood oxygen level may fall during exercise, and in some of these patients, the carbon dioxide level may increase. [This decrease in oxygen level does not occur in anyone whose forced expiratory volume in 1 second (FEV_1) is greater than 50% of their forced vital capacity (FVC) (see Chapter 3, *The Respiratory System*), and it doesn't occur even in most people whose FEV_1 is that low.] This means that for the amount of oxygen being used and the amount of carbon dioxide being produced by the exercising muscles, the person is not breathing enough. It is not known if this is harmful, but most CF physicians recommend that patients avoid this situation. That does not mean to avoid exercise altogether. Specific exercise guidelines are discussed later in this chapter.

Some people with CF also have asthma, particularly in response to exercise (*exercise-induced asthma*, or EIA). This is a common condition, and one that need not curtail your exercise program—about 10% of the United States Olympic team had EIA! I mention this not to guarantee you a spot on the Olympic team, but just to let you know that people with EIA may still be able to exercise and compete at a very high level. People with EIA will experience cough, wheeze, chest tightness, chest pain, or a combination of these symptoms when they exercise—typically, it's a few minutes *after* they exercise. The exercise that is most likely to bring on these symptoms is vigorous exercise—especially running—lasting 6 to 8 minutes, and especially in the cold air. The problem can be prevented in most people with a couple of puffs from a bronchodilator (like albuterol) metered-dose inhaler about 15 minutes before exercise.

Many people with CF (whether or not they have asthma as well) cough during or after exercise. This may be distressing to someone who is watching, if he or she doesn't know about CF, and may be somewhat uncomfortable to the person coughing, but it is not dangerous. In fact, it is probably helpful in bringing mucus up out of the lungs.

Exercise in the Heat

Having CF should not prevent someone from exercising in the heat. People with CF have the same ability as people without CF to keep their body temperature down while exercising in hot weather. However, since they have the same mechanisms for doing this, including sweating, and since CF sweat is so much saltier than any other sweat, athletes with CF lose much more salt than their non-CF friends. They may lose so much that the blood levels of sodium and chloride drop. In most cases this does not cause a problem. Young people with CF also have a very accurate salt "thermostat" that enables them to know how much salt they need to take after exercise to replace what they've lost during exercise. Replacing salt is something that can be done over a period of hours and does not have to be done immediately after it's lost.

Replacing lost fluid is quite another matter, though, for anyone, with or without CF. It is very important for all people who exercise in the heat to drink plenty of fluid, but it is particularly important for children and adults with CF to drink while they exercise in hot weather, because while their salt "thermostat" works very well, their fluid "thermostat" is a little sluggish. *All* children tend to drink less fluid than they lose during exercise in the heat, but children with CF are especially bad at drinking as much as they need.

Exercise Tolerance

Many children and adults with CF who have good lung function are limited in their exercise capacity by the same factors that limit their classmates; namely, the heart reaches a limit to how much blood it can pump, and/or the muscles reach a limit to how much oxygen they can process. These factors will be especially limiting if someone has not exercised much and is out of shape. But those whose lungs are affected more extensively by their CF are likely to be limited by the lungs before the heart and muscles are pushed to their limits. This does not necessarily mean that their blood oxygen levels will fall, but rather that the work of breathing may just become too great and they will need to stop because of that discomfort. Even in most people whose oxygen level does fall, it is probably the discomfort of hard breathing and not the lowered oxygen level that forces them to stop running or pedaling. There are certainly a few people who benefit from using oxygen during exercise and who are able to do considerably more exercise if they use extra oxygen when they are active.

Although coughing may be severe, it seldom limits exercise.

Exercise Programs for People with Cystic Fibrosis

Exercise programs have the same benefit for people with CF that they have for people without CF, namely, increasing their fitness and sense of well-being, and probably improving their overall outlook on life. "Increased fitness" is defined as being able to do more physical work and having a lower heart rate for the same workload. Some studies have shown better lung function after a CF exercise-training program, and other studies have shown no change in lung function. A very important study showed that fitness levels of patients with CF corresponded more closely with their survival (how likely they were to be alive 8 years later) than any other factor did. So, although it hasn't yet been proved that becoming more fit means you'll live longer, it's tempting to think so, and act as if that's so by working to get and stay in shape!

For people with normal lungs, strenuous aerobic exercise programs should raise the heart rate to 75% of its maximum, or about 150 beats per minute. Many people with CF will not be able to exercise this hard, because their breathing will stop them before their heart rate has risen that high. This does not mean that someone with CF cannot become more fit. In fact, it seems that patients with CF can become more fit by exercising hard enough to raise their heart rates to 75% of their *own* maximum, and not the maximum that you'd predict on the basis of their age. Thus, if someone with CF has a maximum heart rate of 150 beats per minute (that is, the pulse goes up to 150 during the most strenuous exercise he or she can tolerate), that person will be able to benefit from regular exercise sessions with the heart beating around 115 beats a minute (roughly 75% of 150).

Fortunately, it's not necessary to measure the heart rate precisely during all exercise sessions to know if you're working hard enough to bring about improvements; instead, you can strive for a *pleasantly tired* feeling. If you're not at all tired, you are not working hard enough. On the other hand, if you're so tired that you don't feel at all good, you're pushing yourself harder than you need. That becomes important in planning a long-term exercise program because human nature is such that no one wants to do unpleasant things, and exercise is no exception: If your exercise sessions leave you exhausted and feeling bad, you will be much more likely to find excuses to skip them than if they are enjoyable. In the section after the next, there will be an introduction to the nitty-gritty of carrying out an exercise program.

Heat Training in Cystic Fibrosis

Like everyone else, people with CF can become adapted to exercise in the heat. If you exercise in the heat every day for a week or more, at the end of that period, your heart rate and body temperature will be lower when you exercise than they were at the beginning.

When you have CF, you are likely to lose large amounts of sodium and chloride during each exercise session in the heat. If you allow yourself to eat and drink without restriction, you will find that you automatically select items that will completely replace the lost salt. This is very important because a major difference between the normal response to heat training and the CF response is that CF sweat glands cannot decrease the salt content of sweat. This means that even though you have greater tolerance for exercise and heat stress, you still lose much more salt than is normal. In addition, after you've trained for a while, you will begin to sweat earlier in the exercise session (this change occurs in everyone during heat training) and you will be able to exercise for a longer period, thus losing even more salt after you've become adapted to the heat.

GUIDELINES FOR AN EXERCISE PROGRAM

General

Most CF physicians now believe that exercise is beneficial for all patients with CF and that an active lifestyle should begin early in childhood, well before a formal "program" is prescribed. In most cases, more activity is better than less, and parents should encourage activity from very early on. As with any child, parental encouragement is good; parental aggressive pushing is probably not. Parents can often help establish the exercise habit in their children by example: If they exercise, their children are likely to. And the family that exercises together is most likely to maintain the exercise longer than those who don't. As children get older, they may want to participate in sports, and this is fine. There are virtually no limits to what sports or activities they can engage in. Patients' bodies will usually tell them when they need to stop, so they need not be limited by parents or coaches. However, for patients with some degree of lung disease, their coaches must be aware of their condition and must allow the patients to limit themselves: The patients should not be pushed beyond their comfort/tolerance. Teenagers and adults may want to have some guidelines for setting up their own exercise program. Read on.

Medical Advice

Check with your doctor before you start. If your lungs are severely affected by CF, your doctor may recommend an exercise test first to check your oxygen level. If your FEV_1 is less than 50% of your FVC (or 50% of the predicted normal level—that's about the same as 50% of FVC), it's a particularly good idea to see if your oxygen level falls during exercise, and if so, at what intensity: If your oxygen level is good until your heart rate reaches 150 beats per minute, it's relatively easy to keep your exercise program light enough that your heart rate stays below 145. Your doctor might even want to prescribe some oxygen for you to use while you exercise. For most people with CF, this will not be necessary.

Time Allotment

Set aside a time to exercise. This should amount to about 30 minutes a day, three to five times a week for the exercise itself, plus whatever time you need to shower and dress. You should guard this exercise time jealously and keep it for yourself. It doesn't matter what time of day you exercise. Some people prefer to exercise in the morning, whereas others prefer to wait until they've been awake and active for several hours. Of course, if your exercise is in gym class or with a team, you won't have much choice as to timing.

Type of Activity

Pick an activity that is a good aerobic conditioner. These activities are ones that are continuous, not stop-and-go; they are light enough that they can be carried out for many minutes at a time, without causing total exhaustion. Typical aerobic activities that are discussed in this chapter in greater detail include running, swimming, and biking. Others include rowing, skating, stair-stepping, "elliptical trainers," aerobic dance, cross-country skiing, indoor "skiing" on a NordicTrack or similar equipment, and vigorous walking. Brisk walking (including race-walking) is excellent, and has recently become one of the most widely practiced forms of regular exercise.

Activities that are *an*aerobic include weight training, most racquet sports, and volleyball. These activities are also beneficial, and many are fun; some may make you stronger and build your muscles, including the chest muscles that you use for breathing. Anaerobic activities will probably not help your endurance. For most patients with CF, it's probably ideal to include a hefty dose of aerobic exercise, whether or not you also do anaerobic exercise.

Boxing is too dangerous even to be mentioned as an activity, except to condemn it.

Regular daily activities should not be overlooked in planning a more active lifestyle. If you usually walk the dog around a short block, try going around a long block instead; walk or ride a bike to the corner store when you run out of milk instead of getting a ride; take the stairs instead of the elevator whenever possible; and so on. Try cutting down on television time in favor of exercising time. It does you a lot more good to walk or run around the block than to watch someone else doing it on television.

PACING YOURSELF

Getting Going

Whatever activity you pick, remember not to overdo it, especially when you first begin to train. Listen carefully to what your body is telling you about how hard, fast, or far you're going. It's much better to take a few days, weeks, or even months to work your way up to the desired amount of exercise than to get injured or discouraged by trying too much too soon. If you haven't been particularly active, limit your first exercise session to no more than 10 minutes. Continue to exercise for 10 minutes each day for the first week. With each successive week, try adding 2 minutes to each session. By the time several months have passed, you'll find that you're exercising for as long as 30 minutes.

Listen to Your Body

If you're getting winded, go slower until you've caught your breath, and then continue at an easier pace. If you feel as though you've hardly exerted yourself after 10 minutes, you can push a little harder for a little longer.

Injuries

Minor injuries can occur with most forms of exercise. Don't ignore them. While you can continue to exercise with some discomfort, real pain is a signal to stop. Let a few days pass without exercising, and if your pain persists, inform your doctor.

Medications, Food, and Drink

If you have asthma or if you take any inhaled bronchodilators, it's advisable to take an inhalation before you exercise. It is not wise to exercise after a heavy meal; in fact, waiting several hours after a meal before you run or swim will make your exercise more pleasant.

Exercise in the Heat

If you're exercising in warm weather, you should drink *while you exercise—even more than you think you need.* You do not need to take salt pills, but sports drinks like Gatorade are especially helpful for people with CF, as they help replace the sodium and chloride that you lose.

RUNNING

Equipment

The only special equipment you need for running is a good pair of running shoes. Gym shoes or tennis shoes are not appropriate for regular running. A long-term running program involves a lot of pounding of your feet on the pavement. If you don't have the proper shoes, this pounding travels from your feet to your shins, knees, and hips and can cause an injury. It is advisable to buy your shoes in a store that specializes in runners' supplies. When shopping for running shoes, pick a shoe that feels good on your foot. Do not expect an uncomfortable shoe to "break in" after a while the way a leather shoe might (most running shoes are made of synthetic materials that do not change their shape with time and wear).

Clothes

You can run in clothes that you probably already have. For summer running, dress as lightly as possible. Nylon shorts and shirts are light and dry out quickly, but cotton is more absorbent. Some newer synthetic materials like "polypro" help wick sweat away from the skin for better evaporation and cooling. For running in colder weather, you are more likely to overdress than underdress. When the temperature is below freezing, cotton socks and sweat pants or stretch tights are the best. Cover your chest with several light layers rather than one heavy layer. On the coldest days, a T-shirt, cotton turtleneck, and hooded cotton sweatshirt should be enough. If it is very windy, a thin nylon shell suit over your running clothes will insulate you and keep the wind out. Gore-Tex and similar high-tech fibers are expensive, but are impressive in their ability to keep you dry: They don't let rain or snow in, but they do let sweat out. Be sure to cover your head with a wool cap or the hood from your sweatshirt or jacket, because much of the body's heat is lost from the head. A scarf or mask over your nose and mouth may make breathing easier, particularly if you have exercise-induced asthma. Your feet are working hard, so they won't get very cold, but your hands will. To keep your hands warm, mittens or socks are better than gloves, since they let your fingers keep each other warm. Some petroleum jelly on your lips and cheeks will reduce the sting of the cold.

Starting to Run

Remember not to push yourself too hard, especially at first. You should be exercising to make yourself feel good; if you push so hard that you feel bad, you've missed the point. Start with a 10-minute run/walk session. Run slowly, and when you get tired, start walking. When you are ready, run again. Continue this for three or four sessions during your first week, trying to run for most of the 10 minutes. As the weeks go by, you should gradually add time to your run/walk sessions. Add 2 or 3 minutes each week, so that, after 7 to 10 weeks, you are running for most of each 30-minute session. If it takes longer to add the extra minutes, don't worry, there's no rush. It doesn't matter how far you go or how long it takes you to work up to 30 minutes of running.

Safety

You should be able to avoid injury to your muscles if you warm up properly before running, stretch and cool down afterward, and build up gradually to a regular exercise program. However, if you feel pain after running, be sure to have it checked. Other safety factors to consider include not running in traffic or other polluted areas and not running in dark clothes at night. You can avoid these problems by running on an athletic field, golf course, track, or jogging trail rather than on the sidewalk or street.

If you start your running program in the spring, summer, or fall, you may become discouraged when the weather turns bad in the winter months. There is really no reason you shouldn't run in the winter, as long as you dress properly. Running on icy or slippery surfaces is dangerous, so be careful and sensible about running in the winter; a broken leg or sprained ankle will not promote your general conditioning. Running in cold weather may be hard for people with EIA. Two easy steps can make it much easier: Take two puffs of albuterol or other bronchodilator before you go out, and wear a mask or scarf around your nose and mouth, so the air you breathe in will be warm and a bit moist.

SWIMMING

Where to Swim

You will need a pool, lake, river, or ocean. Unless you live in a part of the country where the weather is good and you can swim outside all year round, you will want to swim in a pool that is convenient to get to and affordable to use. A summer swimming program at a beach or lake won't give you any long-term benefit if you only swim for 2 or 3 months out of the year. Additionally, rivers and oceans have currents, waves, and tides that may interfere with a regular, sustained swimming program. If you don't have a pool or ocean in your backyard, there are many places where you should be able to swim free or at a moderate cost. Many high schools and colleges have pools that are open to the public during certain hours. Many people swim at municipal or community pools. Most YMCAs and many health clubs and hotels have swimming pools that can be joined for a reasonable fee.

Equipment

Once you have found a place to swim, the only equipment or special clothing you really need is a bathing suit. For a regular exercise program, a one-piece nylon or Lycra tank suit is best. Both nylon and Lycra suits wear well and dry out quickly. Goggles are useful if you are swimming in a pool or in salt water, because both chlorine and salt can be very irritating to the eyes. If you wear glasses or contact lenses, you can purchase goggles with corrective lenses for very reasonable cost (ask your eye doctor or swim shop for details). If you have long hair, a bathing cap will keep your hair out of your face and out of a pool's filter system. Caps also protect hair and scalp from the drying effects of chlorine.

Safety

NEVER SWIM ALONE! There should always be a lifeguard at the pool or beach. While you are probably less likely to drown in a swimming pool than in a lake, river, or ocean, always make sure that there is a lifeguard present. Failing that, use the "buddy system," swimming with a friend who can pull you out of the water or run for help if you need it. You should also learn some basic water safety techniques. The risk of pulling muscles or tendons while swimming is much less than while running or bicycling. If you are swimming smoothly, your muscles should get an even workout. Most injuries occur from diving into shallow water, swimming into the side of the pool, or sustaining cuts from rocks or trash on the bottom of a river or lake.

Learning to Swim

Swimming is most enjoyable when you have a smooth, comfortable stroke. If you do not know how to swim well or if you want to improve your stroke, swimming lessons will be helpful. This does not mean that you have to start training to make the Olympic team, but you should be able to execute the various strokes properly. As in running and bicycling, the goal is not speed, but rather sustained, even exercise over time. There are many places where you can learn to swim. The Red Cross and the YMCA are probably best known for their swimming programs, but any reputable class will do. Many places offer swimming lessons designed especially for adults.

Starting to Swim

As with running, don't push yourself too hard or too fast at first. A 10-minute session that alternates a strenuous stroke like the crawl (freestyle) with a more restful stroke (breast stroke or side stroke) should get you off to a good start. Try to schedule your swimming sessions three or four times each week for the first few weeks. Gradually work up to longer sessions by adding a few minutes to each session after the first week or two. Your goal should be to swim for at least 30 minutes during each session. Again, remember that you can take as many weeks as you need to reach this goal. It doesn't matter how many laps you swim or how fast you swim them.

BICYCLING

Equipment

If you plan to cycle outdoors, a sturdy bike with three to 12 speeds is your basic piece of equipment. You can get a touring bike, with relatively skinny tires, or a fat-tired bike, which can be used for off-road cycling or for handling rough or wet roads more readily than the skinny tired bikes. If you want to go really fast on a smooth road, the skinny-tired bikes are the ones for you; if you're more into riding on rough surfaces, or feeling more secure, look into fat-tired models. A cycling helmet is also essential to prevent head injuries if you fall or are thrown from your bike. If you plan to cycle indoors, there are many good models of stationary exercise bikes. However, before you buy one, remember that riding a stationary bike can be extremely boring. Some people set the bike up in front of the television and pedal as they watch. Others listen to music or read while they ride. Most people who just cycle in a bare cellar don't stay with it very long.

Preparing Your Bicycle

Your bicycle should be in good condition each time you begin a ride. Make sure that the seat is properly adjusted, because this will increase the efficiency and comfort with which you ride. Raise or lower the saddle so that your leg is fully extended when your heel is placed on the pedal at the bottom of its cycle. This will cause your leg to be slightly bent while pedaling with the ball of your foot on the pedal. Before each ride, briefly inspect the tires, brakes, and wheels of your bike to make sure that they are in good order. If any part is not working properly, have it fixed. Proper maintenance of your bike will help to ensure safe riding.

Safety

Wear a bike helmet! Bike paths and lightly trafficked roads are recommended over city streets and highways. *Wear a bike helmet!* Familiarize yourself with the traffic laws regarding bicycling and obey them. *Wear a bike helmet!* If you plan to ride in the evenings, be sure that you have the proper lights and reflectors on your bike and wear light-colored clothes so that motorists and other riders can see you. There are wonderful little battery-powered blinking lights available to attach to your belt or bike seat that are visible from a long way away. And, did I mention?: *Wear a bike helmet!*

Clothes

The clothes needed for bicycling are similar to those for running, except that you will build up less heat and give off more heat on a bike than on foot, so you'll have to dress more warmly (and with more wind protection) on the bike. Be sure that your pants legs fit snugly so that they won't get caught in the gear sprockets or chain. Be sure that your shoelaces are tucked in so that they don't get caught in the sprockets or chain. And, on your head? *Wear a bike helmet!*

Starting to Cycle

As with running and swimming, start out slowly and build up to longer periods of exercise. A 10- to 15-minute ride three or four times a week is a good way to start out, adding extra minutes to each session after the first week or two. Alternate slow, easy riding with fast, hard riding until you are riding for 30 minutes, three to five times a week. Strive toward a continuous, comfortable ride of increasing duration, rather than a ride that covers a certain distance.

SUMMARY

Patients with CF can and should exercise, at virtually every stage (and age) of life. They reap the same benefits from exercise programs and an active lifestyle that other people do (and perhaps even more): They can become more physically fit, and can do more exercise than if they are sedentary. Exercise helps patients with CF keep their lungs clear of mucus. Exercise helps a lot of people emotionally, too, by reducing stress. Exercise may even enable patients with CF to live longer.

11

Genetics

THE BASICS

1. Cystic fibrosis (CF) is inherited. In order to be born with CF, you have to get two abnormal CF genes (one from each parent).
2. People with just one abnormal CF gene are called "carriers," and do not have CF.
3. Each time two carriers have a baby, the chances are one in four that that baby will have CF, even if the couple has already had one or more babies with CF.
4. It is possible to test during a pregnancy whether the baby will have CF.
5. It is possible to test to see if someone is a CF carrier, but the test will miss some carriers.
6. Gene therapy may some day cure CF.

Cystic fibrosis (CF) is a genetic disorder, which means that it is determined by the genes a person has inherited. There are millions of genes located on the chromosomes within each cell in the body. The genes are made of DNA, the basic determinant of our body makeup. Genes come in pairs, with one gene having come from each parent. As a mother's eggs are formed, each egg has only one set of genes, rather than the double set that exists in all the other cells in her body. Similarly, each of the father's millions of sperm has only one gene for each characteristic. When the sperm and egg unite, the fetus they develop into will have one set of genes from the mother and one from the father. The genes determine all of our physical characteristics, from the shape of our ears to the color of our hair. What makes each of us unique physically is the combination of genes that make up our cells.

Different gene combinations work in different ways. In some cases, a gene is *dominant,* meaning that it is the gene that will be expressed, regardless of what the gene is that accompanies it. A dominant gene completely determines the outcome. An example of this (although it's a bit oversimplified) is the brown-hair gene. If a baby gets one brown-hair gene, he or she will have brown hair, no matter what the other hair-color gene is. In other cases, there is the *recessive* gene, which will not be noticed at all unless it is paired with an identical gene. At a first approximation, red hair is a recessive characteristic, so most redheads have received two red-hair genes—one from each parent. A baby with one red-hair gene and one brown-hair gene will usually have brown hair. Finally, there is the gene interaction where each gene contributes something so that the resulting characteristic is a combination of what each would have determined by itself. An example of this is skin color. When a very dark-skinned person and a very fair person have a baby, the baby's skin is often a color that is in between the parents' skin colors.

We all have two copies of the CF gene—the gene that determines whether or not we have CF—and for most people both copies are normal. CF is a recessive disorder, which means that a baby who gets an altered (abnormal) CF gene from only one parent will not have CF, and will have no sign of CF. CF occurs *only* if a person has received an altered CF gene from each parent. For a parent to pass on an altered CF gene to a child, she or he obviously must have one of those genes. In almost every case, the parent carries one altered CF gene and one normal CF gene in each of his or her cells. Yet there is no evidence at all that they carry the altered CF gene until they have a child with CF. People who have one altered CF gene and one normal CF gene are called *carriers* because they are not affected by the gene but carry it and can pass it along to their children. Whether their children will have CF depends on what gene the other parent contributes. In the unusual case where a parent has CF, he or she has two altered CF genes in each cell, and *must* pass on one of those to each child. As with carriers, whether their children will have CF depends on what gene the other parent contributes.

Figure 11.1 shows the possible combinations if two parents who are each carriers have children. For each parent, half of their eggs or sperm will have the altered CF gene, and half will have the normal CF gene. The chances of a sperm that carries the altered CF gene fertilizing an egg with the CF gene are exactly the same as its fertilizing a normal egg. This means that there are only four possible combinations of genes from these parents, and each is just as likely to occur as the others. *Each time this couple has a child*, the chances are one in four that the baby will get two altered CF genes and will have CF; two in four (a "50 : 50" chance) that the baby will get one altered CF gene, and therefore will not have CF but will be a carrier; and a one in four chance that the baby will not get any altered CF gene at all.

Chance and statistics can be confusing to understand at first. People may assume, mistakenly, that if their chances are one in four that a baby will have CF, and they've already had a baby with CF, then the next three children can't have

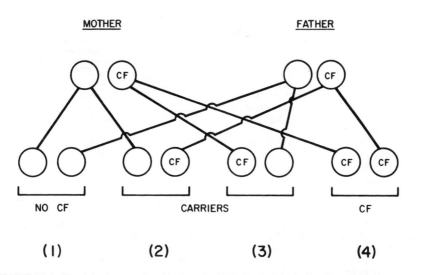

MOTHER FATHER

NO CF CARRIERS CF

(1)   (2)   (3)   (4)

FIGURE 11.1. The inheritance of cystic fibrosis (CF). Each parent of a child with CF has one abnormal CF gene (*circle* labeled "*CF*") (*1*). The abnormal CF gene causes no problems if it is paired with a normal CF gene (*blank circle*). When two parents who each carry an abnormal CF gene have children, each parent passes on either the abnormal or the normal CF gene. The figure shows the possible combinations of genes that children of carriers can have: (*1*) A normal CF gene from both father and mother; (*2*) a normal CF gene from the mother and an abnormal gene from the father; (*3*) an abnormal CF gene from the mother and a normal gene from the father; and (*4*) an abnormal CF gene from each parent. Each of these four combinations is just as likely to occur as the others, meaning that the chances of two carrier parents having a child with CF is one in four each time they have a child.

CF. This is not so—*each* time they have a child, there is one chance in four that the child will have CF. There are families with three children, *all* of whom have CF, and others in which both parents are carriers, yet *none* of their children have CF. With statistical chance, the numbers work out over hundreds or thousands of cases, which doesn't much help the individual family.

Consider the example of a deck of cards. There are four suits: hearts, diamonds, spades, and clubs. If the cards are shuffled well and are not marked, and you try to pick a diamond, your chances will be one in four. Nevertheless, you know very well that you might pick ten cards one time before you get a diamond, and another time you might pick four diamonds in a row. If you picked cards all morning, by the time you'd picked 1,000 cards you'd have come pretty close to 250 diamonds, but those first few might have been almost any pattern.

Thus, although you can know the overall statistics, they won't necessarily be helpful in an individual case. So, in families trying to decide on their family's future, they can consider their statistical chances. If they have had a child with CF, it means the parents are both carriers, and the chances for each pregnancy resulting in a child with CF are one in four. Some people consider one chance in

TABLE 11.1. *Risks for Individuals of North European White Background of Having a Child with Cystic Fibrosis*

One Parent	Other Parent	Risk with Each Pregnancy
No CF history	No CF history	1 in 2,500
No CF history	First cousin has CF	1 in 400
No CF history	Aunt or uncle has CF	1 in 300
No CF history	Nephew or niece has CF	1 in 200
No CF history	Sibling has CF	1 in 150
No CF history	Has CF	1 in 50
Sibling has CF	Sibling has CF	1 in 9
Sibling has CF	Has CF	1 in 3
Sibling has CF	Known carrier	1 in 6
Known carrier	Known carrier	1 in 4
Known carrier	Has CF	1 in 2

CF, cystic fibrosis.

Risks are actually slightly higher than listed because the list assumes that (excluding siblings of patients with CF) someone who is a carrier has one parent who is also a carrier. It is actually possible that both of this person's parents are carriers, and that means that each of this person's siblings has greater than a 50:50 chance of being a carrier. Risks to other ethnic groups will generally be different (see Table 11.2).

four to be great odds, whereas others think they're dreadful. Great chances or dreadful, brothers and sisters of patients with CF should all be tested to see if they have CF, even if they have been perfectly healthy, because each child born to the parents of someone with CF does have a one in four chance of having received the two altered CF genes, and many people with CF can be healthy for a long time before symptoms appear.

What about the chances of having a child with CF if there is CF in the family of one parent (or parent-to-be) or the other? What if you have a nephew, niece, brother, sister, or cousin with CF? Table 11.1 shows the chances in different situations, depending on the parents' family background.

HOW COMMON IS THE CYSTIC FIBROSIS GENE?

Sometimes it can seem to new parents of a child with CF that they were just unbelievably unlucky for two carriers of a disease gene to get together. But, carrying a harmful gene is very common: Geneticists estimate that every healthy person carries between three and five different harmful genes. And the altered CF gene is not unusual. In fact, it is quite common, occurring in about one in every 25 white people in North America. It's less common in other ethnic groups (one in 17,000 black people in Washington, DC; one in 90,000 Asian Americans in Hawaii), but has been reported in individuals on every continent (except, perhaps, Antarctica!), and from virtually every racial background. Table 11.2 shows how common CF is in different countries.

Not only is the CF gene common, it's also old: CF has been with us for somewhere between 3,000 and 53,000 years. People sometimes wonder how an

TABLE 11.2. *Incidence of Cystic Fibrosis in Different Countries*

Country (or Group)	One Baby with CF per Live Births[a]
Alberta (Canada) Hutterites	313
Afrikaners (Southwest Africa)	622
Ireland	2,000
Australia	2,500
United Kingdom (England)	2,500
North America	2,500
France	3,000
The Netherlands	3,500
Germany	4,000
Denmark	4,500
Ashkenazi Jews in Israel	5,000
Sweden	8,000
Italy	15,000
Finland	40,000

[a]Numbers listed are patients with cystic fibrosis per live births (so, for Ireland, of every 2,000 babies born alive, one has CF).

altered gene that causes disease can persist for so long. Getting two copies of the altered gene clearly gives a person big disadvantages. Until very recently, no one with CF lived long enough to have children, so why should the gene still be around? For some other genes that cause recessive disorders (remember, those are problems where you need to get one abnormal gene from each parent), there has been discovered a "carrier advantage," sometimes termed "a heterozygote (see below) advantage." meaning that carriers of the gene have some benefit, some advantage, over those who do not carry the gene. A well-known example is sickle cell disease, a terrible problem that kills many young black people. Carriers of the sickle cell gene are said to have "sickle cell trait," and they have been known for some time to be less susceptible to malaria than people who do not have sickle cell trait. Well, if malaria is killing off whole villages in Africa (as it has done throughout the ages), and you have something that keeps you alive when many others are dying from malaria—and that gene protects you—then you will survive.

Many different guesses have been made about what the "heterozygote advantage" might be for CF carriers. Things like increased fertility of the carriers, less asthma, or increased resistance to intestinal infections have all been suggested, but none has been proven.

Recent advances in molecular genetics enabled researchers to zero in on the CF gene, to determine that CF is caused by a single gene (and not a series of genes), and, in 1989, to discover and analyze the gene itself. That gene is located on the seventh of the 23 human chromosomes. The discovery of the gene has led to a virtual explosion in our knowledge about CF, has made possible the creation of a "CF mouse," has expanded our ability to identify CF carriers, and to diagnose CF in living patients, in unborn fetuses, and even sometimes in patients who have already died. The discovery of the gene has even enabled people to hope that the day may be approaching when CF will be cured with gene therapy.

To understand the importance of this discovery, let's take a little detour, to a crash course in basic genetics. Hold on to your hats!

WHAT IS A GENE?

A gene is a unit of DNA that directs the production of a protein. DNA is considered by scientists to be the basic blueprint of our body's structure and function. DNA in turn is made of pairs of chemicals called *nucleotides*. The chemicals or *bases* that make up these nucleotides are adenine, guanine, thymine, and cytosine (abbreviated A, G, T, and C). These nucleotides form long double chains, wound around each other in a "helix." The strands are held together by specific pairing of the nucleotides. Adenine always pairs with thymine, and cytosine with guanine. These chains of pairs of nucleotides ("base pairs") are the DNA. The incredible array of different information that is contained in these structures seems to be explained entirely by the order in which those four simple chemicals line up with one another.

The average gene is made up of about 30,000 nucleotides or base pairs. All of the human genetic information is stored on 23 paired *chromosomes*; each chromosome stores about 5,000 genes. This dizzying amount of material is all stored within each and every one of the millions of cells that make up our bodies! To get an idea of the dimensions we're dealing with here (Table 11.3), let's look at the genetic information in terms of *distance*: If one nucleotide were 1 inch long, a gene would be 700 yards long, a chromosome 1,900 miles, and all of the human genetic information (called the human *genome*) would stretch twice around the earth's equator! Instead of distance, what if genes were *time* (a kind of crazy idea)? Well, if a nucleotide were 1 second, a gene would be about 8½ hours, a chromosome nearly 4½ years, and the whole genome 1 century! And, all this is packed into each of our body's cells; cells too tiny to see without a microscope.

The way genes dictate what our body's cells do is by directing ("coding") the production of proteins; it's the proteins that really do the work. These proteins are made of *amino acids*, and the various portions of the gene call for various

TABLE 11.3. *The Relative Dimensions of the Components of Human Genetic Material, Expressed as if They Were Time or Distance*

Unit	Time	Distance
Nucleotide	1 s	1 inch
Gene	8½ h	700 yd
Chromosome	4½ y	1,900 miles
Genome	1 century	2 equators

Thanks to Dr. John Mulvihill, formerly of the University of Pittsburgh.

amino acids, with three pairs of nucleotides per amino acid. All together, the particular amino acids and the order in which they are placed determine what the resulting protein looks like and does. It turns out that not all of the gene is involved in coding for protein production; relatively short portions, called *exons*, do the directing of amino acid placement and protein production. These exons are separated along the length of the gene by long stretches of inactive DNA. The inactive stretches are called *introns*.

THE CYSTIC FIBROSIS GENE

The CF gene is very large, containing about 250,000 base pairs (about eight times as many as the average gene). The protein made under the direction of the CF gene contains 1,480 amino acids. (For those of you who've been following the complicated math here, you'll have noted that if it takes three base pairs for one amino acid, 250,000 base pairs could have resulted in over 80,000 amino acids, instead of a measly 1,480; this shows how much of the CF gene—like most genes—is made up of introns, that is, inactive DNA.) This 1,480–amino acid protein has the unwieldy (but accurate) name CFTR, for *c*ystic *f*ibrosis *t*ransmembrane conductance *r*egulator protein. The main function of this protein is to direct traffic across cell membranes, especially traffic of salt (sodium and chloride). Abnormal movement of chloride and sodium (and water) across cells seems to explain many of the problems seen in people with CF, and this abnormality is felt to be the basic defect in CF. It is discussed at length in Chapter 1, *The Basic Defect*. Since the CF gene is responsible for producing the CFTR protein, the gene is sometimes referred to as the *CFTR* gene. To make things even more complicated, *everyone*, not just people with CF, has two *CFTR* genes, and makes CFTR protein. The difference between patients with CF and people without CF is in the structure (and therefore also the function) of the CFTR protein. When the CFTR protein is normal, sodium, chloride, and water all act normally, secretions are not extra thick, and no disease results.

When the CF gene is abnormal, in any of a number of ways, the amino acid composition of the protein it produces will differ from the normal CFTR protein, and it will, therefore, not function normally. If both copies of the CF gene are abnormal, there will be no normal CFTR protein, and this will cause the problems that make up CF. Far and away the most common alteration (*mutation*) in the gene that causes CF occurs in exon 10, and is the loss of three (out of a total of 250,000!) base pairs, leading to production of a protein that is missing one amino acid (out of 1,480). The missing amino acid is phenylalanine, and it is missing from position 508 of the protein structure. By a strange spelling agreement, geneticists abbreviate phenylalanine, "F." Together with the scientific notation "delta," written "Δ," meaning *deleted*, this gives the common CF mutation the name "delta F 508," or "ΔF508." About 70% of CF chromosomes (in North America) have the ΔF508 mutation. About 50% of North American patients with CF have two copies of ΔF508 (one from each parent), whereas 40%

TABLE 11.4. *Some of the More Common Cystic Fibrosis Gene Mutations and their Characteristics*

Mutation	Geographic/Ethnic Incidence	Other
ΔF508[a]	70%–75% in North America	Pancreatic insufficiency
W1282X[a]	50%–60% in Ahskenazi Jews; 2.1% worldwide	Pancreatic insufficiency
G542X[a]	3.4% worldwide	Pancreatic insufficiency; ? more meconium ileus
G551D[a]	2.4% worldwide	Pancreatic insufficiency
3905insT[a]	2.1% worldwide	Pancreatic insufficiency
N1303K[a]	1.8% worldwide	Pancreatic insufficiency
R553X[a]	1.3% worldwide	Pancreatic insufficiency
621 + 1G→ T[a]	1.3% worldwide	Pancreatic insufficiency
1717 − 1G→ A[a]	1.3% worldwide	Pancreatic insufficiency
A455E[a]	3%–7% in The Netherlands 0%–0.2% in North America	Pancreatic sufficiency[b]; mild lung disease
3849 + 10kb C→ T[a]	1.4% worldwide; 4% in Israel	Pancreatic sufficiency,[b] normal sweat chloride; most males not sterile; lung disease varies from mild to severe
R117H[a]	0.8% worldwide	Pancreatic sufficiency[b]; slightly lower sweat chloride; older age at diagnosis
R334W[a]		Pancreatic sufficiency[b]; older age at diagnosis
R347P[a]		Pancreatic sufficiency[b]
P574H[a]		Pancreatic sufficiency[b]
Y563N[a]		Pancreatic sufficiency[b]

[a]"Compound heterozygotes," in most cases, meaning these patients had one copy of the particular mutation noted and one other cystic fibrosis mutation (usually ΔF508).
[b]Pancreatic sufficiency in most, but not all, cases.

have one *ΔF508* gene and one of the other abnormal CF genes. (Someone with two copies of the same gene mutation is called *homozygous* for that mutation, from the Greek "homo," meaning "the same," and "zygote," for yoke, meaning two of the same genes are yoked or linked together. This contrasts with *heterozygous*, meaning two *different* things linked together; "compound heterozygote" is the term used for someone who has two different mutations. A CF carrier, with one normal and one abnormal gene, is also sometimes called a CF heterozygote.)

After ΔF508 was discovered, it was originally thought that there would probably be five or six other mutations that would account for the other 30% of CF mutations. By the time of the writing of this book, 14 years later, more than 1,000 different CF mutations have been identified! Most of these mutations are very rare, occurring in only a very few cases, some in only one case. There are a few that are mutations not so rare, and the frequency of different mutations varies, depending on a population's ethnic and geographic background. For example, "W1282X" is uncommon in non-Jewish people, but found in nearly 50% of the chromosomes of all Jewish patients with CF. "G551D" is relatively

TABLE 11.5. *Ethnic Groups in Which a Few Mutations Account for Most of the Cystic Fibrosis Chromosomes*

Group	Mutations, No.	Cystic Fibrosis Chromosomes, %
Alberta (Canada) Hutterites	2	100
Welsh	29	99.5
Brittany Celts	19	98
Ashkenazi Jews	5	97
Belgian	17	94.3

From Dr. Garry Cutting, Johns Hopkins University, with permission.

common in people of Celtic origin, occurring in 5% of abnormal CF genes in Ireland and England. See Table 11.4 for other examples. Taken all together, the known mutations explain about 98% of all CF chromosomes. In a few specific ethnic groups, a very few of the known mutations account for almost all of the patients with CF (Table 11.5).

DIFFERENT MUTATIONS: DIFFERENT DISEASES?

Whenever several different variations of a gene can cause problems, people wonder if the different variations of the gene cause different problems. Geneticists talk about the *genotype–phenotype relationship*. Genotype just means the combination of genes that one has. "Phenotype" comes from the Greek word that means appearance, and refers to what you see in a person: the outward evidence of various processes. In the case of CF, we know that some people seem to have a worse form of the disease, with severe lung disease and lots of hospital admissions, whereas others are pretty healthy, and some don't even need to take pancreatic enzymes. Whether someone needs to take enzymes, and how healthy his (or her) lungs are, make up his or her phenotype. So when people wonder about the genotype–phenotype relationship in CF, they wonder whether different CF mutations cause any of the variations we see in how CF affects different patients.

As with so many things, the answer seems to be "yes and no." The "yes" part has mostly to do with pancreatic function, and whether someone needs to take enzymes or not. Almost everyone with two copies (one from each parent) of the most common CF mutation, *ΔF508*, needs to take enzymes (they have "pancreatic insufficiency"). There have now been several different CF mutations discovered that are associated with pancreatic sufficiency (that is, you don't need to take enzymes), if you have one of these genes, even if it's paired with one *ΔF508* gene. Table 11.4 lists some of these genes. Unfortunately, some geneticists have referred to the genes associated with pancreatic insufficiency as "severe," while those associated with pancreatic sufficiency are called "mild." The "mild" versus "severe" distinction holds true only for how the pancreas is affected (the need to take enzymes or not). This is confusing, since the pancreas has relatively little to do with the overall health of patients with CF and how long they live.

The more important question is harder to answer: Are variations in the amount of lung disease related to different CF mutations? With few exceptions, the answer seems to be "no." The differences in the severity of lung disease among people with two copies of *ΔF508* seem to be much greater than differences between those with different genes. That is, factors other than the particular brand of CF gene mutation are most important in determining how bad someone's lungs are. These factors could be environmental or genetic.

Factors that are known to influence lung health in patients with CF more than their particular CF mutation include things in the environment, including exposure to cigarette smoke and viruses, and the aggressiveness of treatment. In a way, this is good news, since things over which patients and families have no control (what gene they happen to have) may end up being less important to their survival than some things over which they do have control (treatments, avoiding cigarette smoke).

It is possible that there are genetic factors other than the CF mutation itself that influence someone's CF phenotype. As one example, let's consider a gene that controls the amount of a protein called α_1-antitrypsin. This protein helps protect the lungs against some destructive chemicals that can be released by bacteria and by white blood cells sent to fight those bacteria. If you don't have enough of this α_1-antitrypsin protein, your lungs can be damaged (in fact, extreme deficiencies of this protein can cause emphysema in young nonsmokers similar to the emphysema seen in older people after a lifetime of smoking cigarettes). One small study from Denmark hinted that patients with CF with the gene for lower levels of the protective protein have worse problems with infection in their lungs than those with normal α_1 levels. If someone with CF has another lung-damaging gene, the lungs will likely be worse. Similarly, inherited susceptibility to infection should make CF lung disease worse, because so much of CF lung disease has to do with infection. In real life, there have not yet been other specific genes discovered that have explained differences in the health (or "phenotype") of groups of people with CF.

THE CYSTIC FIBROSIS MOUSE

Until very recently, no animal had CF. Now, with genetic engineering, scientists have been able to alter the genes of a mouse embryo, resulting in mice with two mutations of the CF gene. In some important ways, these mice can be considered to have a mouse form of CF. Study of the so-called "CF mouse" is helping researchers examine the effects of different forms of the CF gene on the functioning of different cells and organs. Scientists hope that this will increase our understanding of CF, and will allow for the speedier testing of new CF treatments. It is important to remember that, some certain Disney characters aside, mice are not people, and it may be difficult to translate some of the findings in the "CF mice" into humans. Two examples: The earliest versions of the CF mouse had no lung problems, but did have severe intestinal blockage, which killed most of the animals within the first 40 days of life. This intestinal blockage may be something like human meconium ileus (see Chapter 4, *The Gastrointestinal Tract*), but it's clearly not identical to what happens in most people with CF. The second example is that the very structure of mouse lungs is quite different from human lungs; mice don't have some of the important mucus-secreting glands that humans have, and these glands are thought to be a source of much of the lung trouble in people with CF.

PRENATAL TESTING

For nearly every couple who already has a child with CF, it is now possible to tell reasonably early in pregnancy (16 to 18 weeks) if an expected child will have CF. To do this testing, a sample of the amniotic fluid (the fluid that surrounds the fetus inside the uterus) must be taken by putting a needle directly through the mother's abdominal wall into the uterus (amniocentesis). This procedure has some risks, but has been used safely for many years for a range of prenatal tests, the best known of which is the test for Down syndrome (performed mainly for women older than 35 years). The fluid includes cells from the fetus, and these cells can be analyzed to see if they contain the CF gene mutations already known to be in this family. If they do, then the fetus would be born with CF. If they have only one abnormal CF gene, the fetus would be a carrier, and if the cells have none of the CF mutations, the fetus would neither have CF nor be a carrier.

Another method of obtaining cells from a fetus to test for CF can be carried out even earlier in pregnancy (at 10 to 13 weeks). This method is called chorionic villus sampling (CVS). In this procedure, a small tube is inserted through the vagina and cervix into the mother's uterus. Once the tube is in the uterus, suction is applied, and a small sample of cells from the placenta is taken for analysis. The analysis and significance of the results are the same as for amniocentesis. Both amniocentesis and CVS have risks to the fetus and to the mother, but the risks are usually quite small. Both tests have been in use for a long time, and—in experienced hands—are quite safe.

Many families have used these new methods to decide to continue a pregnancy if the fetus is shown not to have CF, or to stop the pregnancy (with an abortion) if the fetus has CF. For people who would not consider having an abortion, these tests are less useful. In unusual cases, the family may decide to continue the pregnancy regardless of the result of the testing on the fetus but they believe strongly that they need to know ahead of time for their peace of mind if it turns out that the new baby will not have CF and for planning their lives if the new baby will have CF. In these cases, testing is reasonable because the benefit of knowing ahead of time for the family outweighs the small risks to the fetus and mother.

The main use of these tests is for couples with a child with CF. But there are a few other instances where they might be used. For instance, if the cousin of a patient with CF wants to get pregnant, and she and her husband are found to be carriers, they would be able to use the prenatal testing. In fact, in any couple where both partners are carriers, testing could be done to see if their baby would be born with CF. Of course, if carrier testing (see below) shows that one spouse is not a carrier, then the risk of having a child with CF is very low (but not zero, see below) for the couple.

CARRIERS

If a brother or sister of someone with CF does not have CF, there are two chances in three that this sibling is a carrier. Here's why: As illustrated in Figure 11.1, if both parents are carriers, there are only four possible combinations of CF and non-CF mutations that their children could have. One combination gives CF (two mutated CF genes); two combinations result in carriers; and one combination has no CF mutation. Once you know that a brother or sister does not have CF (and you'll know that after a properly performed sweat test), there are only three possible combinations, two of which result in carriers. Table 11.6 shows the chances of various people being CF carriers. Until very recently there was no carrier test for CF. The only way you knew if someone was a carrier was if he or she had a child with CF. With recent advances in molecular genetics, a genetic test can now tell if a relative of a CF patient is a carrier. The test can also be used in cases where there is no family member with CF.

The way the test is done is to send some of the person's cells to one of the genetic diagnostic laboratories for analysis. The cells can be obtained from a routine small blood sample or by gently swirling a cotton swab inside the person's cheek. The laboratory technologist will then look at the cells' DNA for anywhere between one and 1,000 of the CF mutations. In the case of a close relative of a patient with CF, the important mutations are the ones that the patient has. If a brother or sister of the patient with CF does not have one of the same CF mutations that the patient has, he or she is not a carrier. Period. If cousins, aunts, or uncles are being tested, and they don't have one of their relative's known CF

TABLE 11.6. *Risks of Being a Cystic Fibrosis Carrier*

Relationship to Patient with CF	Risk of Being a Carrier
Parent of a patient with CF	1 in 1 (100%)
Unaffected sibling of a patient with CF	2 in 3
Aunt or uncle of a patient with CF	1 in 2
Nephew or niece of a patient with CF	1 in 3
Cousin of a patient with CF	1 in 4
None known (northern European)	1 in 25

CF, cystic fibrosis.

Risks are actually slightly higher than listed, because the list assumes that (excluding siblings of patients with CF) someone who is a carrier has one parent who is also a carrier. It is actually possible that both of this person's parents are carriers, which means that each of this person's siblings has greater than a 50:50 chance of being a carrier.

mutations, they probably are not carriers either. For someone with no family history of CF, or where the CF relative's mutation was not known, the laboratory technologist will look for all of the most common mutations. Finding one of these mutations confirms that the person is a carrier. Not finding a CF gene makes it less likely that the person is a carrier, but in most populations does not rule it out completely. Just how much less likely you are to be a carrier with a negative carrier test depends a bit on your ethnic background. As Table 11.5 shows, in a few ethnic groups just a few mutations account for virtually all cases of CF, whereas the 2 to 3 dozen most common mutations account for about 85% to 90% of CF chromosomes.

GENETIC DIAGNOSIS OF CYSTIC FIBROSIS

In some cases, gene testing can be used to help make the diagnosis of CF itself. This issue is discussed at greater length in the *Introduction*, in the section called "Making the Diagnosis." The procedure for obtaining cells for testing is the same as for carriers: either a blood sample or a gentle brushing from the inside of the cheek can be used. If two of the known CF gene mutations are found, almost certainly the person has CF. If one or none is found, it is less likely, but not impossible, that the person has CF.

Even though DNA analysis has a gee-whiz, high-tech gloss to it, in most cases, the sweat test remains the "gold standard" for diagnosing CF. This is true in part because there have been rare cases where the genetic testing appeared to confirm two abnormal CF genes, and yet the person did not have CF. This may be particularly true for men who are healthy and are discovered to have two apparent abnormal CF genes as they are being evaluated for infertility: You'll recall from Chapter 5, *Other Systems*, that most men with CF are sterile because they have a complete blockage, or even absence, of both the right and left *vas deferens*, the tubes that normally carry sperm from the testicles to the penis. There is an uncommon form of male infertility not associated with any other evidence of CF, called congenital bilateral absence of the *vas deferens*, usually abbreviated CBAVD (congenital: you're born with it; bilateral: both sides). It turns out that a lot of these men have one abnormal CF gene. Some have two unusual CF genes. One abnormal CF gene that has been associated with this form of infertility is *D1270N*, and another is *R117H-7T*. Men with CBAVD and two copies of *R117H-7T*, or one *D1270N* together with one *ΔF508*, but no other evidence of CF, should not be considered to have CF. In this case, finding two abnormal CF genes does not make the diagnosis of CF.

Three particular cases stand out where gene testing may be very useful in making the diagnosis of CF. The first and most common is in someone who has signs, symptoms, and perhaps even family history that suggest CF, yet the sweat test does not give a definitive answer. This is quite unusual, but the occasional baby does not produce enough sweat to analyze, and the occasional baby or older person has a sweat test result in the "gray zone": not definitely positive, not definitely negative. Finding two CF genes in someone like this will make the diagnosis of CF much more likely.

The second situation in which DNA analysis for the CF gene may be useful in diagnosing someone with CF (or helping to rule it out) is the very unusual one in which there is not an accredited CF center for performing the sweat test. If someone lives 'way out in the boonies, and travel to a laboratory skilled and experienced in performing sweat tests is temporarily impossible, a blood sample could be sent by express mail to a diagnostic laboratory, with results back within a week or two. The cost of the DNA testing is comparable to that of a sweat test (even cheaper in some laboratories!).

The final situation where DNA testing can help make or confirm the diagnosis of CF is in someone who has died. This situation arises more often than you might think: A baby gets very sick and dies before testing can be done (or before CF is considered) or someone has a relative who died a long time ago, and only now has the possibility of CF been considered. If blood or a small piece of tissue is obtained within a few hours after death, the cells will still be enough for testing. Amazingly, if an autopsy was done (even years before), it may be possible to do DNA analysis on any remaining autopsy microscope slides or tiny blocks of tissue that have been preserved embedded in paraffin. Obviously, in these cases, making the diagnosis cannot help the patient who has died, but it can be tremendously helpful for the patient's family.

GENE THERAPY

Gene therapy is discussed at greater length in Chapter 16, *Research and Future Treatments*. Gene therapy is placing a healthy gene into cells affected by an abnormal gene, and having that healthy gene take over the function of those cells. In CF, this would be getting a healthy *CFTR* gene into cells in order to correct the abnormalities in salt (sodium and chloride) and water traffic across the cell membranes. This would be most important in the lungs. Big strides have been made toward developing successful (safe and effective) gene therapy since the discovery of the CF gene in 1989: Gene therapy has worked in the test tube, in individual CF cells, and it seems to have worked in CF mice. But it is a long way from here to having it work in human beings. Nonetheless, work continues, and most CF researchers think the day may come when gene therapy will provide a cure for CF.

12

The Family

THE BASICS

1. Hearing that a child has cystic fibrosis (CF) is very stressful for parents.
2. As parents learn more about CF, and see their children doing better, the stress lessens.
3. CF center staff expects you to have many questions, and want you to ask them. They know that it takes a long time (years) to learn all there is to know about CF.
4. Children with CF should be treated normally: They need to do homework and chores, and should be allowed to participate in all normal childhood activities. Children treated this way grow up healthier emotionally and physically.

As a chronic disease that requires a vigorous schedule of daily treatments, cystic fibrosis (CF) imposes significant stress on the affected child, the parents, and any brothers and sisters (whether or not they also have CF). Understanding the reactions to this stress and learning about effective methods to cope with them are important to the care of the child with CF and to the functioning of the family.

This chapter discusses the variety of reactions that parents have to the diagnosis and management of CF, the methods for dealing with the daily stresses, and suggestions for how the family and the medical team can work together most effectively.

YOUR CHILD HAS CYSTIC FIBROSIS

Parents and other family members experience a variety of emotions when told a child has CF. Family members may say to themselves, "I can't believe this. This can't be happening to *my* child and *my* family. I don't know what to do. What does the future hold? Is there anything I can do for my child? Could I have prevented this?" All of these reactions—anger, denial, shock, grief, helplessness, confusion, despair, sadness, and fear—are very normal responses. These emotions are part of a *grieving* response. Just as a person experiences many of these feelings when a loved one dies, parents feel many of the same emotions when they learn that a child has a serious health problem. The parents "mourn" the loss of the perfect, healthy child that they had expected. Another very common response on learning the diagnosis of CF is one of relief—if a family has taken their child to many doctors over a long period of time, they may be *relieved* finally to have been given a reason for their child's health problems. This sensation of relief may be very puzzling, and the parent may even feel guilty about it.

With more babies being diagnosed through newborn screening (see Chapter 2, *Making the Diagnosis*), the opposite may be true: A baby that seems perfectly healthy baby and a blindside "hit," often in the form of a call from the pediatrician's office, "your baby has CF," or "you need to schedule an appointment at the CF clinic." This can certainly come as a shock.

No matter what the reaction, it's important that each family member has someone to confide in—a trusted, understanding friend or health professional with whom he or she can share feelings. It may be difficult for the parents to talk about CF with one another, especially immediately after the diagnosis is made. Strong emotions may make it too hard to listen and understand another person's pain, grief, or anger—even if it is a spouse. A husband and wife may find that they react very differently to the diagnosis ("how could he feel *that* way?"), making discussion even more difficult. Since they are two individual people, they may experience varying reactions at different times. And it is hard to *give* support and understanding to anyone—even your spouse—when *you* may be hurting badly yourself. This can put a strain on the relationship unless both husband and wife try to remember that it is normal and that the spouse's reaction does not reflect a lack of caring. It is important to try to be open and nonjudgmental about each other's reactions. A third person may be able to help a couple get through this difficult time.

At the time of diagnosis, the family will be given extensive information about CF and its management. The flood of emotions may make it hard to concentrate on what the doctor is saying and to remember this information. Despite an initial lengthy discussion with the doctor, it is not uncommon for parents to retain very little of what they have been told; they may feel that they have a poor understanding of CF and have many unanswered questions.

The team at the CF center is aware that it is difficult to comprehend all this information at such a stressful time. They know that it is important to review the information many times and they plan to spend ample time with the family for this purpose. Learning about CF is a continuous process that goes on over many months and years. The CF center staff *expect* this, view education as a very important part of their jobs, and *want* you to ask your questions, great or small.

Many parents find it helpful to write down their questions and discuss them with the doctor, nurse, or social worker, in person or by phone. Typical questions that many parents ask are the following:

- Will CF affect my child's brain function?
- Will my child look any different from other children?
- How will CF affect my child's daily life?
- How long will my child live?
- Is there something I did during the pregnancy to cause my child to have CF?
- Could I have prevented this?
- Should I limit my child's activity?
- Can my child go to daycare and school?
- Do my other children have CF?

Some families are reluctant to ask these questions out of fear of what the answers might be or fear that they may appear insignificant or too simple. Your physician and the team members at the CF center understand and encourage the families to ask all their questions—no question is too insignificant to be considered, and even answers that are hard to hear are seldom as horrible as people's imaginations.

Because manifestations of CF are so different in each child, it is often difficult for the doctor to be specific in answering many of the parents' questions. No one can predict the exact effect of CF on a child's lung function, growth, activity, or life span. The uncertainty is very frustrating and frightening, for it means that the family must live with the unknown from day to day. Even though the doctor cannot make any predictions for a specific child, he or she can explain to the parents the range of disease in CF and perhaps where the child falls in this range. On the whole, most children with CF should be expected to attend school regularly, to be able to participate in sports, and to play with other children without restriction, that is, in general to carry out the work and play of normal children.

It can be very helpful if you are aware of the different stages of development that your child will go through and how these might influence CF care. For example, it helps to be prepared for the wonderfully challenging time when a toddler begins to express her or his own preferences ("NO!!"), which you'll notice I didn't call "the terrible twos." Social workers and others in your CF center can help you anticipate these times and how to work in important treatments *and* enjoy your toddler. Similarly, teen years can bring their own challenges, and anticipating them can help both you and your child.

BEGINNING HOME CARE

In addition to obtaining information about CF, it is important that parents learn techniques in caring for their child with CF—particularly the methods for respiratory treatments and enzyme administration. In the past, many physicians recommended that the newly diagnosed infant or child be admitted to the hospital for thorough evaluation of respiratory function and growth and for education of the parents. While this idea was frightening to the family (and disapproved by short-sighted "bottom-line" oriented insurance clerks), it often helps if they realize that an admission to the hospital provides the valuable opportunity for the parents to have daily contact with the CF team, and lays the groundwork for a lifetime of successful health care—perhaps preventing or minimizing the need for future hospitalizations. The doctors, nurses, social worker, respiratory therapists, and dietitians used this time to teach the family about home management of CF and begin to develop an important working relationship with the family.

In recent years, hospital admission for initial CF education has become much less common. Instead, many centers schedule several clinic visits back-to-back (e.g., every week for several weeks in a row) to try to accomplish the same goals of initiating the learning process, and helping families through the difficult time that follows their hearing the diagnosis. Families may be invited to bring other important people (most often grandparents; sometimes older siblings, aunts or uncles, etc.) to these sessions.

No matter how thorough the instructions and how skillful the parents, most families are nervous about beginning therapy at home. At the same time they are beginning enzyme administration and respiratory treatments, they may be facing an already busy child-care schedule, work schedule, or both. With the help of a nurse or social worker, the parents may benefit from sketching out a daily schedule, which takes into consideration *their* family's needs. The doctor, nurse, or social worker may be able to arrange for a meeting with a family more experienced with CF who can serve as an important source of information and support.

In addition to the confusion of a new schedule and nervousness about new treatments, parents may find themselves faced with a cranky baby who is hard to comfort. Some babies with CF are fussy eaters, and before diagnosis have been irritable because of lung infection, hunger or chronic abdominal discomfort, and diarrhea. Because they have been hard to feed, hard to soothe, and haven't grown well, their parents may feel helpless and incapable.

Many parents say that although they *love* their infant, they find it difficult to *like* him (or her) because he or she is so irritable and is frustrating to care for—and they feel guilty about resenting their own child. It may be hard for the parents to talk about these feelings or even for parents to admit them to themselves. These feelings, while very troublesome to the mother and father, are very common, normal reactions.

Gradually, as babies become accustomed to their new medications and treatments, the chronic digestive symptoms will be relieved and they will begin to gain weight. As babies feel better, they become more contented, and their parents can draw much satisfaction from their daily efforts and the successful "settling in" at home.

EXPLAINING CYSTIC FIBROSIS TO OTHERS

Once the diagnosis of CF has been confirmed and the parents have begun to learn about CF, they must begin to explain CF to grandparents, other family members, and friends. This may be difficult to do. However, an honest, simple explanation is essential—it will set the tone for how others react to their child for many years to come. Although CF is a chronic progressive disease that may result in shortened life span, many patients live to middle age, or even beyond. As the prognosis for CF improves, it is important that children and teenagers be raised with the idea that they should look forward to being active, productive adults. In order to promote independence and goals for the child with CF, the parents and others with whom the child lives and works must share an outlook of hope and encouragement for the child. Many questions are difficult to answer, but each successful encounter makes the next one easier to handle.

Following are some of the important points that parents may want to share with others:

- CF does not affect the brain or intelligence.
- No part of CF, including the cough and loose stools, is contagious.
- CF is a genetic disease caused by inheriting a gene mutation from each parent; it could not have been prevented and it is no one's *fault* (some grandparents have difficulty accepting the idea that an abnormal gene came from *their* side of the family).
- CF is not curable, but it is treatable.
- The treatment for CF must be carried out each day and consists primarily of respiratory care and enzyme administration, both of which must be made non-negotiable and normal parts of every day.

YOU AND YOUR CHILD

One of the most valuable gifts you can give your child with CF (and yourself) is to treat him or her as a *normal* child *who happens to have CF*, and not as a case of CF, nor as a poor, sickly weakling who should not be expected to do normal things. First, most children and adolescents with CF are not limited in their physical or mental capacities by their disease. Many play sports, some even excel at sports; many excel in school. But, as surely as day turns into night, children whose parents expect them to fail and to be unable to take care of themselves will fail and will grow up thinking poorly of themselves. Children should know that they have CF, and that having CF means certain things are different from other kids (need to do chest treatments, need to take enzymes with meals). Many children who feel unfairly singled out because of having to do special things because of their CF take some comfort in knowing that many kids have to do different things: Some children may have diet restrictions that the CF child doesn't;

some may need a wheelchair, as the child with CF doesn't; some may need braces, and so forth.

But, they should also know that they have the same rights, privileges, and responsibilities as anyone else in the family or school. They go to school, have friends over, play sports, and so on. They need to do homework, help with the dishes, and so on. Treated normally, they will think of themselves as normal, and will *be* normal. In reviewing this book, several teenagers and young adults with CF urged me to stress that children with CF should never be allowed to use CF as an excuse for getting out of unappealing chores or responsibilities.

In fact, most parents and children with CF are able to adopt this very positive outlook, which in turn not only makes the children wonderful to be around, but also has a very positive influence on their health.

YOU AND YOUR OTHER CHILDREN

In many ways, having two children is more than twice as hard as having one. Although the bond between siblings in most cases ends up being among the strongest on earth, sibling rivalries and jealousies exist at one level or another in most families. Most parents are able to keep these rivalries and jealousies from erupting into outright armed conflict, but at times the peacekeeping role can be challenging. If one child has CF, this can add a dimension to the challenge. The child with CF may resent the other child for *not* having it ("Why me? It's not fair!"), while the child without CF may resent the extra attention the child with CF gets (treatments, trips to the clinic, perhaps even visits and gifts in the hospital). It's a balancing act—that most parents end up doing very well—to make absolutely certain that the child or children with CF get all the needed treatments, while the other child or children realize that they too are cherished.

YOU AND YOUR SPOUSE

In conjunction with the treatment of CF, parents find themselves faced with new stresses on their marriage: Care of the child takes up more time—how should they divide the responsibilities? Medicines and doctor visits are expensive—how can their budget accommodate this? There is a risk of subsequent children having CF—how can they work out their sexual relationship and family planning? The child with CF needs discipline as any other child—how should they handle discipline for a "sick" child? The other children need attention or one parent's job may be in jeopardy—how can they cope with preexisting family problems in the midst of this new stress?

An important starting point for handling each of these stresses is for the couple to be open and honest in sharing their feelings with one another. Good communication will help to define the problems from each partner's perspective, starting both partners on the path to developing mutually acceptable solutions. As the husband and wife work *together* to resolve conflict, many couples report that their relationship is strengthened and they are better prepared to face future challenges together. Many experts in family relationships stress the need for couples to make some time alone with each other, whether it's an evening out to dinner and a movie or just a walk together in a local park. These times can reinforce the couple's relationship with each other and make it easier for them to face any stresses, including those brought by CF. (The child benefits from parents' having some time to themselves, too: Parents leaving a child with a trusted babysitter, be that a relative, friend, or professional, give the child an important lesson in security, and teach the child that (a) the parents *will* return and (b) the world is safe place, even without the constant presence of the parents.)

If one spouse is employed outside the home and the other is responsible for child care, the employed spouse will probably have a limited amount of time to administer treatment. However, it is important that parents share responsibility for the child's care, even if it can only be to a limited extent. This shared responsibility demonstrates to children that their parents are unified in their approach to their care; it also may help to avoid resentment that can arise when one spouse is solely responsible for treatments.

Financial worries can cause much strain within a family. Insurance coverage may be inadequate or nonexistent. State-aid programs may be helpful in some situations. Many clinics have a "patient representative" or a social worker who can put parents in contact with appropriate financial resources.

As the husband and wife cope differently with their reactions to the diagnosis of CF, their desire for sexual intimacy may be altered. These differing needs may serve to create further conflict and misunderstanding. Overshadowing these differences may be fear of another pregnancy and the birth of another child with CF. An atmosphere of open, honest communication is essential for the resolution of these differences.

Sometimes the stresses associated with a diagnosis of CF are too much for a couple to handle without outside help and guidance. The CF center team can be a valuable resource in assisting the family; they may recommend further assistance from a psychologist, counselor, or clergy. The family's pediatrician or family doctor may also be of great assistance. Although these professionals are not CF experts, they may have known the family for a long time and often are very willing to provide support. It is essential that a family seek help promptly if difficulties arise in coping with the diagnosis of CF or with related issues. Such problems do not "just go away" and must be handled directly and aggressively. Unless properly managed, problems with stress and communication within the family may persist, having an impact on CF management and adversely affecting the child's health.

GOING TO THE CYSTIC FIBROSIS CLINIC

Most patients with CF will have clinic visits scheduled for between four and eight times a year, more just after diagnosis and when someone is sick. These visits are very important to maintaining the patient's good health, but for many people they are not easy. Depending on the distance you live from the center, the number of tests to be done, and how busy or organized the clinic happens to be that day, a variable amount of time (often a whole day) is lost to other activities. This may mean losing a day's work (and wages), spoiling a perfect school attendance record, missing a team or chorus practice, and so on. It may be expensive to drive and park.

Beyond the financial and logistical nuisance of clinic visits, they may be difficult emotionally, too. For some young patients, there is the fear of shots (despite experience and assurances that there are unlikely to *be* shots, except for a yearly "flu" shot, and yearly blood work) or the fear of hospital admission. For some patients and families, it may be less focused, but scarier than that: Going to CF clinic is a rude reminder that the child *has* CF. Many families—including many who do absolutely every treatment, every day—are able to put CF aside and not think of it or its long-term implications most of the time. But, a clinic appointment brings CF back into the center of the family's existence for a brief time.

There are some things that may help ease the emotional burden of a trip to clinic. The first is the realization that most clinic visits are actually quite pleasant, with a number of people who are truly glad to see you and your child and with a minimum of unpleasant tests or treatments. At most visits, there's a positive report from the physician, or an optimistic and realistic plan arrived at to attack a problem you knew about before you came. It's relatively unusual for a bad problem that is a big surprise to be discovered at the clinic visit. Parents can help nervous children prepare by stressing the positives: "You'll get to see_____" (fill in the blank with a favorite nurse or doctor or waiting room toy), and we'll go out to eat afterward (or to the museum, zoo, mall, etc.). It is *not* helpful to say over and over to a frightened toddler, "They're not going to *HURT* you; I won't let them *HURT* you," because that can even plant the idea of hurting in the child's mind.

GOING TO THE HOSPITAL

Occasionally, hospitalization may be necessary. Admission to the hospital upsets the daily routine of a family, and, in effect, creates a crisis. This topic is dealt with at length in Chapter 7.

SUMMARY

Having a child with CF adds stress to a family, particularly when the diagnosis is made. With time and education, if parents make an effort to work together, the stress eases, and the family can even be made stronger by this stress. Parents can work together with CF center staff to learn about CF. CF center staff expect (and want) parents to ask many questions, because learning about CF is very important and takes years. Children with CF should be brought up normally, with the same plans, expectations, and responsibilities as other children. Most children with CF grow up with healthy positive attitudes they've gotten from their parents, and this positive outlook helps their physical health as well.

13

The Teenage Years

THE BASICS

1. The teenage years can be wonderful and healthy for people with cystic fibrosis (CF).
2. The teen years are a crucial time for CF patients' health. If the lungs are neglected, they can easily be damaged irreparably; with good care, they can often remain very healthy.
3. Teens with CF can do virtually everything that their friends without CF do: school, college, date, plan careers, and so forth.

HOW DO TEENAGERS RATE THEIR OWN CHAPTER?

If you read the *Preface* to this book, you saw that teenagers with cystic fibrosis (CF) are one of the main reasons for this book's having been written. There are a few reasons for that, and a few reasons why you deserve your own special chapter. Teenagers are caught between two extremes: adults—out on their own, totally *independent*, and with their own chapter in this book—and children—totally *dependent* on parents for everything, and with a lot of the rest of the book focused on their needs. There are special questions that are of more concern to teenagers than other people (education, deciding on a career direction, establishing relationships—including intimate relationships with people of the other sex, and even deciding who you are and who you are going to be). And, there are a lot of you: In 2001, there were 22,732 patients with CF aged 0 to 74 years (that's right, 74!) seen in CF centers in the United States, and 4,832 of them were aged 13 to 18 years. That means about 21% of all patients with CF are teenagers. Finally, perhaps more than any other 7-year period, the teenage years determine what will happen to your health for the rest of your life, based in large part on what you yourself decide to do about it. Unfortunately, many teens with CF have made what they later realize have been *bad* decisions about their health, and have paid a big price for those decisions, for the rest of their lives. I want to help convince you to make *good* decisions and to be able to reap the benefits of them, for the rest of your longer, healthier lives. In addition to the problems that everyone always talks about with the teen years, these years can be wonderful, and your CF does not need to change that.

You will find some of the information in this chapter other places in the book, as well, particularly Chapter 14, *Cystic Fibrosis and Adulthood*.

MEDICAL ISSUES

In this section, I'll address the various organ systems of the body that are affected by CF, and how either the effects or the treatment might be different for teenagers. You'll find more details about each organ system in its own chapter (for example, lungs are discussed at great length in Chapter 3, *The Respiratory System*). You probably know a lot of this stuff already, since you've had CF all your life, but most likely you haven't had the opportunity just to sit down and learn about CF; rather—if you're like 99% of teenagers with CF, it's been a matter of picking up a bit here and a bit there as you go to clinic, get your treatments, have arguments with your parents, and so forth.

Lungs

Far more than any other part of the body, it's the lungs that determine the health of people with CF and how long they live. The lungs account for 95% of the deaths from CF. Fortunately, there's a lot you can do to influence the health of your lungs.

First, you need to know what happens in the lungs of people with CF. For the full story, you can go back to Chapter 3, *The Respiratory System*, but for the brief version, here we go: Thick mucus blocks the bronchi (air tubes, sometimes called *airways*) of people with CF. It doesn't *totally* block them, but it blocks them enough that infection and inflammation can take hold. Infection you understand: Germs (mostly bacteria, but also viruses, and occasionally fungi) can grow in the bronchi and cause damage. *Inflammation* is what happens when the body responds to these invading germs: White blood cells are sent to fight the infection, and—in a kind of chemical warfare—they release toxic chemicals that attack the bacteria. Unfortunately, these chemicals can also damage the cells that line the airways, causing swelling and cell damage. Some of the bacteria themselves release the same kinds of chemicals and cause the same kind of damage. If the infection and inflammation go on too long or too often (and nobody knows exactly how long "too long" is, or how often "too often" is), airway cells are killed, and scar tissue is formed. For each little infection, it's probably only a little bit of scar tissue that's formed, but once scar tissue forms, it can never become normal, and over months and years that "little bit" of scar tissue for each little infection adds up, so that eventually virtually the whole lung becomes a mass of infected *cysts* (fluid-filled sacs) and scar tissue. In fact, since scar tissue is called *fibrosis*, you can see where the name *cystic fibrosis* comes from.

So, the idea in treating the lungs of someone with CF is to prevent this progression of airway blockage, infection, inflammation, and scar tissue formation. Since there are three ingredients in the recipe for scar formation, there are three targets for treatment, namely, (a) reducing or preventing airway obstruction, (b) treating or preventing infection, and (c) treating or preventing inflammation.

Minimizing Bronchial Blockage

Airway-clearance techniques are used to minimize bronchial blockage. These techniques include CPT (for *chest physical therapy*), the Flutter, percussion vests, *huffing, autogenic drainage, PEP* (positive expiratory pressure) masks, and several others. You've probably heard of one or more of these, and have probably had countless treatments with at least one of these techniques. You *may* even have realized how effective they can be in keeping your airways unblocked, and you never miss a one. But, there's a reasonable chance that you've thought they don't make any difference, or perhaps part of you realizes they help, but you skip a lot of treatments because they're a bother.

The thing is, they *do work*. Studies have shown a significant deterioration in lung function after 3 weeks of missed treatments, even in people whose lungs are in pretty good shape. But a big catch is that if your lungs are in pretty good shape, you will probably not *feel* a difference after getting (or missing) an individual treatment. Our lungs—all of us, CF or no—are notoriously insensitive. By that, I mean that we cannot tell when our bronchi are blocked. In a famous experiment, people breathe through a small plastic tube, with their eyes closed. Then the doctor conducting the experiment gradually blocks the end of the tube until the person doing the breathing feels a blockage. Most people can't tell those tubes are blocked until they're more than 50% blocked! The same is true if the breathing tube is your own airways, and not a plastic tube you hold in your lips. So, you can't go only on the basis of how you feel: "My breathing feels good, so there must not be any blockage." There can be substantial blockage before you feel it. This is true if the blockage happens quickly (as you just saw, with that tube-blocking experiment); it's ten times truer if the blockage develops slowly. As with so many other things, gradual changes are very hard to notice: You don't see a kid brother or sister (or the grass) grow taller from day to day, but let a few months go by and they don't fit their jeans anymore (and the grass now looks like a wild field). The difference between those examples and the lungs is that it's never too late to buy a new pair of jeans for your kid sister; and the lawn can be mowed when it's tall—it'll be harder, but it can be done. If the lungs are let go for too long, it may be impossible to get them back in shape again. You may be able to gain some control over infection and inflammation, but the parts that have been replaced by scar tissue can never be made into healthy lung tissue again.

One big problem with the older (and still useful) ways of clearing mucus from the lungs, like CPT, was (and is) that for these to be done well, you had to have someone else do them to you. That "someone else" was almost always a parent. That's fine when you're a baby or young child, but gets harder when you and your folks may not see eye-to-eye on everything, including exactly *when* something is supposed to be done. You have your schedule of activities, friends, and so on, your parents have their own schedules, and the two might not coincide. This can be an area of conflict between teenagers and parents (ever notice how a *lot* of things can be an area of conflict between teenagers and parents?). If this has been a problem for you, there's very good news. There are some treatments that are as effective as (maybe even *more* effective than) the old CPT. You can read more about these in Chapter 3, *The Respiratory System*, and in Appendix C, *Airway Clearance Techniques*. Here's exactly what Chapter 3 says about one of these techniques, namely, the Flutter valve.

> This is a hand-held device, small enough to carry around in your pocket, that looks a little like a kazoo. It has a stainless steel ball in it that vibrates up and down (flutters, you might say) as you blow into the tube. The vibrations are transmitted backward down through the patient's mouth into the trachea and bronchi, where they shake mucus free from the bronchial walls. Many teenagers and adults who had done traditional chest PT for years have become "Flutter converts," saying that the Flutter is more effective in helping them bring up mucus, letting them feel when there's excess mucus there, and to know when they've cleared their airways. The Flutter has the advantage of enabling patients to work on airway clearance without help.

Much the same kind of thing can also be said about a newer device, the vibrating vest—although it's much harder to move from one place to another than the Flutter, and is very expensive ($17,500!), it too can give very effective airway clearance for teenagers, without help or interference from parents.

Autogenic drainage, the PEP mask, and the active cycle of breathing are all airway-clearance techniques that also can be done independently. These last three techniques are used more in Europe than they are in the United States and Canada. They seem to work well, but you need to be taught how to do them by someone with a lot of experience in using them.

Exercise

Exercise is another thing that also helps to clear mucus. Many of you have no doubt noticed that you cough and bring up mucus when you exercise hard. Right now, most CF doctors recommend that exercise be used *in addition to* one of the other airway-clearance techniques (and not instead of them) but it is clearly helpful.

Mucus-thinning Drugs

CF mucus is hard to clear because it's so thick and sticky. Thinner mucus should be easier to move up out of the lungs. There are a couple of drugs available (and some others that might be available before too long) that make CF mucus thinner. These drugs work extremely well, in a test tube. It's hard to know ahead of time which actual patients these drugs will help, but for *some* people they *do* seem to be very good. The main drug in this family is DNase (Pulmozyme). DNase is breathed in once a day, in an aerosol. One study with 900 patients (!) showed an overall small improvement in lung function in patients with CF who took DNase once a day for 6 months, compared with no change in lung function in those who took a *placebo* (a drug that looked and tasted like DNase, but had no effect). Some patients definitely feel better when they take DNase, and some say they breathe easier. Almost no one is hurt by the drug (except financially, since it costs about $12,000 a year). A very few patients who have more severe lung problems and lots of thick mucus stuck in their lungs have had trouble when the DNase has freed huge amounts of newly thinned mucus all at once. For these few patients, it's been too much fluid in their airways for them to handle comfortably. One surprise about DNase is that it helps improve pulmonary function tests (PFTs) even in patients who do not seem to have a lot of thick sticky mucus in their airways. We're not sure why it helps those people, but it might have other effects in addition to thinning mucus.

Mucomyst is an older drug that does the same thing as DNase: It breaks down mucus, and makes it thinner, in the test tube. Some patients have benefited from Mucomyst, but many have had worsened inflammation within their airways, or even had asthma attacks after taking Mucomyst.

Treating Bronchial Infection

Antibiotics are the main tools for fighting infections, including bronchial infections, that people with CF get. (We often call these times of bronchial infections *pulmonary exacerbations*, which just means times when the lungs are worse than usual.) Antibiotics kill bacteria. They don't kill viruses, but they are often prescribed when someone with CF has a viral infection (like a cold), too, because the viruses can throw off the lung defenses enough that bacteria can take hold there more easily. Antibiotics come in different preparations, including oral, aerosol, and intravenous (IV). Usually, with a new infection, oral antibiotics are used. Antibiotics are prescribed to go in your aerosol if the oral antibiotics aren't working well enough, and if the aerosol and oral antibiotics aren't controlling the infection, then IVs may be needed. IV antibiotics are usually given in the hospital, for at least 2 weeks, and sometimes as long as 3 or 4 weeks, depending on how long it takes to get you back to normal (back to your "baseline" is what we often say, meaning back to where you were before this particular *exacerbation* started).

The steps here are pretty easy to understand. It's *not* always easy to know when to start treatment at any of the steps, when to move on to the next step, or even when you've gotten back to your baseline. The reasons for this are a bit like what I just said about bronchial obstruction: You can't always tell when you've got worsened infection in your lungs or when it's improved as much as it can. Physicians can't always tell that easily, either.

How to Tell If You Need More Treatment

The amount of cough you have is the main clue for most pulmonary exacerbations. Someone who usually has no cough may start with a morning cough, while someone who usually does have some cough may have more cough. Your parents or brother or sister may tell you that they heard you coughing during the night (or the cough may actually awaken you during the night). Your mucus is the next clue. Someone who doesn't usually feel like there's extra mucus inside the chest might start to feel some or start to bring it up. People who are used to bringing up mucus may have more, or it may be darker, thicker, or harder to bring up. Some people may have some trouble catching their breath (they are short of breath) when they go up stairs or run or even just sitting there. There are some signs that aren't obviously connected to your lungs that often go along with a pulmonary exacerbation, including being tired, losing weight, and having a crummy appetite. You might find that you're feeling irritable. All of these changes can signal worsened lung infection (and inflammation). But it may be hard for you to detect any small changes from your baseline, particularly if the changes have developed gradually.

That's where your doctor can help. He or she may be able to tell some things by examining you. Listening with a stethoscope can help. If your lungs are usually clear, but now have *crackles* when your doctor listens, or perhaps more crackles than usual, that suggests extra mucus and infection. (If you're wondering what crackles sound like to the physician, reach up to next to your ear, take a few strands of your hair, and roll them back and forth between your fingers. The sound the hairs make rolling over each other is what crackles sound like: Now you're a doctor! Well, maybe not, but now you know what we hear when we say we hear crackles.) But if you have no crackles, or only in the same places you always have them, the listening might not have told the whole story. Your weight will be important: If it's down, without another explanation, the most likely cause is your lungs (lung infections make you lose weight several ways; if you're breathing harder, your breathing muscles use up energy and calories, just as any other prolonged muscular exercise can do—your body also uses calories to fight infection; and finally, having a lung infection can often make you lose your appetite, so you won't feel like eating as much as usual).

Finally, PFTs (breathing tests) can be a big help. You've probably had these a bunch of times: You blow into a tube, and a machine records numbers. These numbers mostly tell how quickly you've been able to blow air out of your lungs and that tells how much blockage there is: the more blockage, the slower the air comes out. If the larger bronchi are blocked, that will affect the first part of the breath, and if the small bronchi (the ones further out in your lungs) are blocked, that will have more of an effect on the last part of the breath. The PFTs are a much more sensitive tool than your doctor's stethoscope, or your ability to feel how hard it is to exhale, for telling just exactly how much obstruction you have in your lungs.

Since the physician (with or without the PFTs) can often detect changes that you hadn't been aware of, it's usual for regular checkups to be scheduled somewhere around four to six times a year. If an unexpected problem shows up at one of the regularly scheduled clinic visits, it's usually possible to start effective treatment before irreversible lung damage has set in. If you waited a year between appointments, it is certainly possible to have some lung damage that's gone beyond the stage of recoverability, *even if you feel pretty good*. That's why it's important to keep those clinic appointments. A lot of people think of doctors' appointments as what you do when you're sick, but there is now good evidence that patients with CF who are seen more frequently—even when they're well—stay healthy longer than those seen less frequently.

Fighting Inflammation

The main way to fight inflammation is to fight infection. For most people, controlling infection with antibiotics will also control inflammation. But some people with CF (and lots of people with asthma) do better if they also get specific *antiinflammatory* treatment. There are a couple of different kinds of antiinflammatory medications. *Steroids* are the first kind, and *prednisone* is the most common form of steroids used for people with CF. These drugs are very powerful and control inflammation very well: There are many people whose breathing is a lot more comfortable when they take prednisone. Unfortunately, prednisone (and all other steroids, too) has some side effects that are unpleasant or even dangerous. The two side effects that probably bother teenagers the most are that they can cause acne and they can cause some puffiness, particularly of the face ("chipmunk cheeks"). Another antiinflammatory medication that's being used a lot recently is *ibuprofen*. You've probably used ibuprofen on occasion for headache or other minor ache or pain. A study has shown that ibuprofen taken in fairly high doses over a 4-year period seemed to slow the deterioration in lung function in patients with CF. You'll note I didn't say that it *improved* lung function, but it slowed how quickly lung function got worse. So, this is not a medicine that is going to make you feel better after you've been on it for a day or so. Even if it helps, you won't be able to tell. There are some other problems with the drug, too. Ibuprofen can cause kidney problems and can cause stomach ulcers. It's possible that your CF doctor will want you to take this drug, and it might be good for you, but be sure you understand the possible side effects, and also understand that—even if it's helping—you probably won't *feel* any better on it.

There are a couple of antiinflammatory inhalers that are very effective for people with asthma, and might also help in CF. One family of these drugs is inhaled steroids, including budesonide (Pulmicort), fluticasone (Flovent), and Advair [a combination of budesonide and salmeterol (Serevent)—which is a long-acting bronchodilator, like albuterol, but longer lasting]. One of the differences between these steroids and prednisone is that these are not absorbed into the bloodstream (or absorbed in tiny amounts), so as a rule they don't cause side effects (no acne, no chipmunk cheeks). Another difference is that they are not as powerful, and don't do very much to make you feel better *right away* (even in people with asthma for whom they work extremely well, they *prevent* problems, and don't cure problems once they've started). Another inflammation-preventing inhaler is cromolyn sodium (Intal), and its brother, nedocromil sodium (Tilade). Like the steroid inhalers, these are effective for people with asthma, have no side effects, and will not make you feel better, but *might* prevent you from developing more inflammation in your bronchi.

Complications of Lung Disease

Problems that are the indirect result of CF include *pneumothorax* and *hemoptysis*, and both are discussed in Chapter 3, *The Respiratory System,* and in Chapter 14, *Cystic Fibrosis and Adulthood.* Very briefly, *pneumothorax* is a collapsed lung, and can be serious, but is quite uncommon. Anyone who develops a very sudden sharp pain on one side of the chest, along with being short of breath, should call the CF center because this might be a pneumothorax and need quick treatment. Another problem is *hemoptysis*, or coughing up blood. It's not uncommon to have some blood streaks in the mucus, and a few people have pure blood. This is very scary, but usually not nearly as dangerous as it might first appear. See Chapter 3 for more details.

Gastrointestinal System

There's not very much different for teenagers in the gastrointestinal (digestive) system. The main thing is the need for enzymes with all meals and most snacks (all the ones with fat or protein in them; see Chapter 6, *Nutrition,* for details). About 90% of all patients with CF need to take enzymes for full digestion of their food. You're probably already familiar with what happens if you miss your enzymes, or don't take enough: abdominal pain, loose, greasy, smelly stools, and maybe more gas. Surprisingly, some teenagers may need slightly fewer enzymes than they needed as children. Intestinal blockage, called DIOS (distal intestinal obstruction syndrome), is more common in teenagers than in children, and can be extremely uncomfortable (abdominal pain, no stools). This kind of intestinal obstruction can often be treated by drinking a glass of water or juice with a powder called Miralax, but some people may need a special enema (in the radiology department of the hospital) or even surgery. If the problem is caught and treated early, it's easier to avoid the more invasive treatments. So, if you're having "stomachaches" and fewer bowel movements than normal, let someone know.

Diabetes

About 10% to 15% of teenagers with CF develop diabetes, a condition where the pancreas does not make enough insulin, and therefore the amount of glucose (sugar) in the bloodstream increases, and some glucose is lost in the urine. Losing sugar in the urine means several things: You lose calories, so you might well lose weight and energy (before diabetes is diagnosed and treated, people often feel drained and dragged out without knowing why). In addition, sugar in the urine makes you lose a lot of urine, and you're likely to notice that you're getting up in the middle of the night to pee, and you're thirsty all the time. If you have these symptoms, you should be checked for diabetes. Diabetes is usually treated with a special diet (mostly cutting down on soda pop, candy, and other "concentrated sweets"). Most people with CF diabetes end up getting insulin shots one to three times a day. These shots are surprisingly easy to get used to and make an amazing difference in how good someone feels. Developing CF diabetes is often a case of "good news disguised as bad news." Hearing that you have *another* problem—and one that needs several shots a day!—certainly at first seems like bad news. But it's good news in a couple of ways: First, diabetes in people with CF is usually less severe than diabetes in young people without CF. Second, studies from Scandinavia have shown that people with CF who start insulin shots often improve their nutritional status *and* their pulmonary function, back to where it had been as long as 2 years before the diabetes was discovered!

Liver

Some patients also have liver problems, and these are discussed more in Chapter 4, *The Gastrointestinal Tract*).

Other Systems

Sweat Glands

You probably know that people with CF have extra salty sweat. That's what makes the sweat test such a good test for CF (analyze sweat, and if there's a lot of salt in it, that means the person has CF). It also means that people with CF lose more salt than normal when they sweat, and will have to take in more salt in their diet than others, especially during hot weather, and particularly if they're exercising a lot. This is something that your taste buds are pretty good at telling you: In most cases if you *need* more salt, you'll *want* more, and you'll find yourself heading for the chips or pretzels or pickles, or just using the salt shaker more at meals. It's not necessary or useful to take salt pills.

Reproductive System
General

Both boys and girls with CF may be delayed in going through puberty (growing and developing). This can be a big worry for young teenagers when their friends (or not-friends) are bigger and look more mature. Locker rooms make the differences and delays in development embarrassingly obvious. It's good to keep in mind that almost everybody with CF will catch up, even if it's a year or so later.

Males

Everything about the reproductive system in men with CF is normal, except one little tube. That tube, the *vas deferens*, is the tube that takes sperm from where they're made (the testicles) to the penis, and in 98% of men with CF it's blocked or even absent. That means that men with CF can and do have a completely normal sex life, but there are no sperm in the semen when they ejaculate. In almost every case this means that men with CF are *sterile*, that is, they cannot get a woman pregnant. You can have your semen analyzed to see if there are sperm present (as there will be in 2% of patients). There's more about this in Chapter 14, *Cystic Fibrosis and Adulthood.*

Females

Everything about the reproductive system in women with CF is normal, except for thick mucus in the cervix (the opening to the uterus). This makes it harder for women with CF to get pregnant. Yet, hundreds of women with CF have gotten pregnant. Some women with CF have irregular menstrual periods. These can be regulated with birth control pills. Many young women have vaginal yeast infections (with itching and burning, especially during urination). Women with CF may be somewhat more likely to develop these infections than women without CF, probably because taking antibiotics makes it easier for the yeast to take hold. These infections can be treated, but only if your doctor knows and gives you a prescription. Some women also have the nuisance problem called "stress incontinence"—leaking a little urine with a cough, sneeze, or laughing. See Chapter 14, *Cystic Fibrosis and Adulthood* for more details.

YOUR MEDICAL CARE: WHO'S IN CHARGE?

Your medical care is like so many other aspects of your life where you're between childhood (where your parents take care of everything for you) and adulthood (where you take care of everything yourself). Ideally, during the teenaged years (actually, *early* in the teen years), you should be starting to take charge. That means knowing your medications (names, doses, times, side effects you've had, and so on), being able to report your symptoms correctly (being honest with your doctor and—a necessary first step—yourself about new or worsened symptoms). That means making a call (yourself) to your doctor to report new symptoms, get a new prescription, or arrange for a new appointment. It's extremely common for a teenager to tell the doctor, "I'm fine," leaving it to the parents to point out that the teenager has been coughing a lot more in the past week or two and needing a nap in the afternoon. This inaccuracy on the part of the teenaged patient is almost never *lying*, but rather a kind of *optimism* that sometimes is called "*denial*" by physicians. The kind of optimism and positive outlook on life that so many people with CF have is very important and healthy, *if it doesn't blind them to symptoms that need attention*. We'll talk a little more about denial and optimism later in the chapter.

Your medical care team is going to include you, your parents, and your physician (as well as other folks at the CF center), and needs to be a cooperative venture. You may not always know when you need more care, more antibiotics, or a clinic visit. Your parents won't always know for sure, and in fact, your doctor can't know either, without good information from you. It's very common for parents to have a hard time giving up their control over their child's medical care. And it's not uncommon for their teenagers to resent this refusal to turn over responsibility. If the resentment is great (as it often is), there are two different ways teenagers express it. One is just to tune out, be sulky, and *let their parents and doctors get away with doing all the talking and making all the decisions for them*. The other is to refuse to have anything to do with treatments, medications, and so forth. By refusing to do treatments, some patients feel that they are taking over control of a part of their lives ("They can't make me do this!"). But it's an unfortunate mistake that ends up almost being: "I'll show you, I'll get sick!" And this approach actually hands control over to *the disease*. A way a patient can really take control of this important part of his or her life is to learn about CF, and say, "*I'll do the front-line monitoring of how I'm doing; I'll call when I'm doing worse; I'll make sure I get more treatments to keep myself healthy*." You can't get rid of CF, but there's lots you can do with your life, including getting as good control as possible of your CF.

PSYCHOLOGICAL AND FAMILY ISSUES

You and Your Parents and Cystic Fibrosis

Although most parents and teenagers get along reasonably well, some are constantly at each other's throats. Even the families that get on well together have times when they get on each other's nerves. The teenagers are embarrassed by and feel nagged and harassed by their parents, while the parents feel exasperated that the teenagers don't listen and don't have a sense of responsibility. These occasional or constant irritations and disagreements can affect CF care. Some teenagers feel that their parents restrict their activities because of CF and are always "on their case" about their diet or doing their treatments.

It's worth keeping in mind that parents who don't care about their children don't nag them about medications or treatments. So, most nagging parents nag because they care (not that that's the best way to show it, and not that nagging is easy to put up with, but it's worth checking back in with that fact now and then). One way a lot of teens with CF have found to get their parents off their case is to grab control of treatments and CF in general away from their parents: Show that you can be more attentive and reliable about your treatments than they ever were. Show that there is no need or point to nagging you, and you've won! They leave you alone, you've gotten control, and your health improves, all in one.

Your Parents, Prenatal Testing for Cystic Fibrosis, and Abortion

A very few teenagers will have the experience that their mother has gotten pregnant, had prenatal testing for CF, and decided to have an abortion because the test showed that the baby would have been born with CF. Others will have heard their parents discuss this question. Sometimes when this happens, the person who's already alive with CF gets the feeling, "Do they wish *I'd* never been born? Do they hate me *that* much?" Of course, this is seldom the case. Almost always when parents make the decision not to have another child with CF (either by not taking the chance and deciding not to have *any* more kids at all, or by using prenatal testing and having an abortion if the prenatal tests show positive for CF), it's not because they regret having had the child or children they already have, but because they want to spare future children the hardships (and there are some, as you know) that come along with having CF.

You and Your Siblings and Cystic Fibrosis

Sometimes CF can seem to cause tension between siblings. Every single person on earth occasionally gets into a "poor me" mood. People with CF are no exception, and you may on occasion think of the unfairness of CF: Why did you get it, and not someone else? If you have a healthy brother or sister, they are obvious examples of the "someone else" who could have gotten CF instead of you. Try to keep in mind that just as it wasn't *your* fault that you ended up with CF, it wasn't *their* fault that you did, either—or that they didn't. Many brothers and sisters of patients with CF also feel (particularly when they're in their own "poor me" moods) that they've been dealt an unfair hand too. It may seem to them that you get all your parents' love and attention, since your parents spend a lot of time giving you treatments, going to the doctor's with you, and perhaps visiting you in the hospital. If you've been in the hospital, you may have gotten gifts from friends and relatives, too, that siblings didn't get. All this might seem to confirm that you're luckier or more loved than they are. You can reduce these feelings by trying to include them in your life and making it clear to them that they are important to you. Of course, this isn't always easy, because younger siblings *can* be a royal pain sometimes.

You and Your Own Attitude Toward Cystic Fibrosis

There are almost as many different approaches to one's own CF as there are people who have CF. Most people have a very strong healthy positive outlook that serves them well. Psychologists who have studied groups of patients with CF are always impressed with what an emotionally healthy group of people they are. In practically all areas of life, a positive outlook brings positive results. You might have heard of "self-fulfilling prophecies." This means that if someone is convinced they'll succeed at something, it makes their success that much more likely. (Certainly, the reverse is true: If you go into something convinced you'll fail, you will.) So, someone with CF who approaches life with optimism and determination (as most people do) ends up doing better and being happier than those who have a more pessimistic approach. (If you find that you just can't seem to get that optimistic attitude, and are sad or depressed a lot of the time, you should let your doctor know, because you can be helped, by talking with someone—social worker or psychologist or psychiatrist—or by some very effective medications.)

Most teenagers with CF are able to go on about their lives without paying undue attention to CF. In fact, when CF rears its ugly head, for example, with an article in the newspaper about CF being a "fatal disease," or with a friend dying, or even with a parent nagging you about taking your aerosols, most people are able to push aside the darker thoughts about dying and go on with their lives. By thinking, "this person who died isn't me," you are able to go on about your business. Some professionals call this "denial," meaning that somebody is denying that they have a disease, or refusing to face reality. Actually, though, I prefer to think of this approach as *optimism*, and I find it a very healthy, positive way to live your life, with one qualification (see below). People who don't push away negative thoughts and who dwell only on the depressing parts of life (CF or other), get stuck in a quagmire and will not have a very rewarding life.

The only qualification about this approach is that you can't be so unrealistically optimistic about life that you ignore (or deny the importance of) signs that you might need more treatment to maintain or improve your health. Don't dwell on them, don't let them run your life, but face them, deal with them, and move on. If you've got more cough, don't pretend you don't, but increase your treatments, contact your doctor for an antibiotic, and get on top of the problem. If your parents nag you about treatments, don't react to the nagging by skipping health-maintaining treatment.

Your Body Image

Body image means how you feel about your body. This is a problem for some teenagers with CF, which shouldn't be terribly surprising because it's a problem for lots of teenagers without CF, too. Many people think they're too short or fat or whatever. In addition to the doubts about their bodies that many, many teenagers have, the teenager with CF may have some specifics to focus on: finger clubbing that might seem ugly to him or her (and likely not very much noticed by others); big chest because of overinflated lungs; skinny, or perhaps puffy chipmunk cheeks from prednisone. For many of these things, nothing can be done other than to try your best to accept them as part of who you are and what you look like, remembering the dedication at the front of this book ("it's not just what you're given, but what you do with what you've got"). For some things, you may be in a position to do something [for example, a number of teenagers with CF were upset enough about being short and skinny that they agreed to have a gastrostomy tube placed (see Chapter 6, *Nutrition*) for overnight feeds]. Many of these people have liked the results of their taking some control over their bodies.

Friends

Friends Who Do Not Have Cystic Fibrosis

Most of your friends don't have CF. You should be able to do everything with your friends that they do. There are just a few qualifications to that last statement: If your friends are smoking and drinking, you shouldn't. It's not a great idea for *anyone* to smoke at all or drink heavily, but these can be more trouble for people with CF than for people without CF. Cigarette smoke is clearly very harmful to the lungs of people with CF, whether they are holding and sucking on the cigarette themselves or whether they're breathing in the *sidestream* or *secondhand* smoke from someone else's cigarettes (sidestream smoke is the smoke that comes from the lighted end of a cigarette that's just sitting there; secondhand smoke is what's exhaled from a smoker's lungs). Too much alcohol can depress your breathing and even a small amount of alcohol can react badly with certain antibiotics and make you feel very sick. If you're old enough to drink, and plan to have a glass of wine or a beer, ask your doctor if that will be a problem with any of your medications.

Late nights, meals out, even trips away, shouldn't be a problem *if you continue to take your enzymes, antibiotics, and other medications, and get in your airway-clearance treatments.*

Whom Should You Tell that You Have Cystic Fibrosis?

This is a hard question that everyone with CF has to decide for him- or herself. People worry that if others know they have CF, they'll be treated as "a case of CF," or a freak, and not be treated for who they really are. And there certainly are horror stories of kids asking, "why aren't you dead if you have CF?" or teachers announcing on a school-wide announcement system that someone has CF and asking the whole school to pray for them (these are true stories). Most CF physicians, social workers, and psychologists believe that if you are just open and matter-of-fact about your CF, you will do much better overall, including dealing with the occasional jerk who does or says something stupid. It's a lot easier just to go about living your life, not carrying around a deep dark secret. Keeping a secret is very difficult, anyway. If you tell *some* people, like your very best friends (and you *should*), it'll be hard for you to know who knows and who doesn't. Instead of going around scared that someone who knows might spill the beans around someone who's not supposed to know, if everyone knows (or at least if you don't care if they know), your life is a lot easier. This doesn't mean defining yourself as *a case of CF*, (you're *not*; you're a person who happens to have CF). And it doesn't mean going up to strangers on the street and saying, "Hi, I'm Arthur (or Anna); I have cystic fibrosis." It just means not hiding the fact, and being comfortable with discussing it. For example, you might meet somebody who complains about needing to take an inhaler for asthma. You can say, "Yeah, I know what you mean. I have cystic fibrosis, and I have to take inhalers too."

Friends with Cystic Fibrosis

Often people with a lot in common can support each other. We tend to seek out people with similar interests and experiences. CF is no exception, and many people with CF get comfort from knowing others with CF—people who can understand what it's like to have a hard coughing spell in the middle of class, or what it's like to have to swallow capsules with a pizza, and so on. (Some people choose *not* to associate with a lot of people with CF, because they don't want to define themselves too much as Someone With CF, and that's fine, too.) A recent change has occurred to make this a little more difficult for people with CF: Physicians and families worry that patients with CF can give each other possibly dangerous bacteria (the most notorious of which is *Burkholderia cepacia*, or just *cepacia;* see Chapter 3, *The Respiratory System*). Because of this concern, there is less opportunity to meet and mingle closely with other people with CF. This limited contact is a bother (and the reason for it can feel scary), but it has probably saved some people from getting sicker. Limiting contact does not mean eliminating it completely, so you still should be able to have friends, perhaps e-mail correspondents, with CF.

Seeing Other Patients with Cystic Fibrosis Get Sicker

This can certainly be hard. Some of your friends with CF will undoubtedly be sicker than you, and you might see some get sicker who you know didn't need to because they didn't take care of themselves. Some others might do every single treatment and still get sicker. Your job is to be as supportive as you can, and to keep in mind for yourself that CF affects different people very differently. Let your friends talk to you if they want, about anything, including their fears and wishes. Sometimes people who are worried about their health—perhaps even worried that they might die—have trouble finding people to talk to about their fears. It might be hard for their parents, who might tell them, "nonsense, you're fine, don't even think about it," and their friends can do them a big service by letting them talk and being supportive and understanding. It can be sad for you to see someone you care about get sicker, and especially sad if he or she dies. You may find a lot of different feelings arising, including sympathy, guilt that you're healthier than your friend, fear that you might get sicker, and so forth. You yourself may need someone to talk to about the feelings their sickness brings up for you. Parents sometimes *are* good people to talk with about this. Other friends may be able to help by listening to you. Your physician or CF social worker has a lot of experience with people going through exactly what you're going through, and they may be able to help.

Seeing Yourself Get Sicker than Your Friends

This too can be hard and sad, and can raise the "it's not fair" feelings that we talked about a little bit ago. It is almost never too late for increased attention to your health to make some difference, so if you've not been taking good care of yourself and you realize that you're sicker, start taking care of yourself *now*. You won't be able to heal scar tissue, but you can slow deterioration, and you will probably make yourself feel better. There is an excellent chance that you'll be able to feel better *about* yourself if you've adopted a positive "I'm going to take control now" attitude.

DATING, MARRIAGE, AND FAMILY

Some of these topics are also discussed in Chapter 14, *Cystic Fibrosis and Adulthood*. When I said that CF should not keep you from having friends, that included boyfriends or girlfriends. People with CF have the same wishes as everyone else, and dating and forming intimate relationships with others are important parts of life for many people. There is nothing about CF to prevent this, although there are a few little points to keep in mind.

If You're Dating, Should You Tell Him (Her) that You have Cystic Fibrosis?

As you have seen, most people think it's a whole lot easier if you are open about having CF. There certainly are cases where a possible boyfriend or girlfriend has hit the road as soon as he or she found out that the person they were dating had CF. Clearly, if that is the way someone will react to hearing about CF, it's better to find that out sooner rather than later in a relationship. If you are close to someone, they need to know. If they are close to you and care about you, they will *want* to know. Their knowing about CF will help avoid a lot of otherwise awkward times and explanations: Why you might have to excuse yourself more often to go to the bathroom; why you take those pills with your meals; what was that embarrassing explosive coughing spell just as you were getting ready for (or worse, in the middle of) a good-night kiss?

Sex

Most of the same things that are true about sex for all teenagers are true for teenagers with CF. In addition, there are a few special considerations. Some of the things that apply to *anybody* include being sure not to get pressured into having sex. Being physically close to someone else can be very special, and many teenagers feel, correctly, that that closeness (whether it's actual sexual intercourse or holding, hugging, and kissing), shouldn't be entered into lightly, and certainly not done without a full understanding of the possible consequences. In addition to the tremendous emotional commitment that having sex with someone entails, there are definite medical consequences as well. The risk of pregnancy is the first that should be considered. You've already learned that *most* young men with CF cannot get someone pregnant, although they can have sex just the same as any other man, and that women with CF are less likely than other women to get pregnant. You absolutely must be clear that some men with CF *can and have* gotten women pregnant, and many women with CF have become pregnant. *Having CF is not adequate birth control*. For young women with CF, it also is essential to keep in mind that there are reasons not to get pregnant in addition to the huge responsibility that anyone would have if they got pregnant. Those additional reasons include the fact that pregnancy can in some cases be very harmful to a young woman's health. (Don't despair; if your lungs are in good shape, you may well be able to have a baby later, when your living situation is stable and you're able to take care of one; this is discussed in the next chapter.) Men can have a semen analysis done to see if they have sperm. If they do not have sperm, they might not need other birth control, **BUT** anyone having sex should be practicing safe sex. Using a condom can protect against STDs (sexually transmitted diseases), including acquired immunodeficiency syndrome (AIDS), as well as protecting against pregnancy.

EDUCATION

Many young people with CF decide to further their education after high school. Many have gone away to college, and lots have even earned graduate degrees. Your CF certainly doesn't interfere with your ability to think, and many patients with CF are outstanding academic successes. Plan your education so that it fits your lifestyle, and so that your health doesn't suffer.

Home or Away?

The decision to go away to college is a big one, especially for someone with CF. For many people—with or without CF—it's not something they want to do, and it certainly is not something that *needs* to be done. But, if you want to attend college away from home, it can be a wonderful experience and an opportunity to establish your independence and, in certain ways, even to define anew who you are. If you decide to take the plunge, you must be certain that your CF care doesn't suffer. You will be in a place where your parents won't be reminding you to eat properly (and providing the food), to take your enzymes, to do your treatments, to insist that you go to (or call) the doctor if you have new symptoms. They won't be there to do your CPT. All of these things must be done, though. One of the saddest things any CF doctor sees is his or her favorite patients going off to school full of enthusiasm and coming back with irreversible lung damage because they neglected their health while they were away. One of the *nicest* things I see is our patients going off, full of enthusiasm, and coming back grown up *and healthy*, because they took care of their health as well as their education! It can be done.

CAREER DIRECTION

CF does not need to dictate your career choice. People with CF have successfully held a broad range of jobs: doctors, lawyers, businessmen and businesswomen, secretaries, school teachers, coaches, construction workers, grave diggers, housewives, husbands, computer repair technicians, and so on. So if you really want a particular career, you can probably have it. It is worth keeping a few things in mind. It's not a great idea to have a job with heavy exposure to airborne pollution, smoke, dust, chemical fumes, and so forth. You should also keep in mind that very heavy physical labor might be difficult to sustain over a period of many years. There are people available who can help you make career decisions. Some of these people include CF social workers, and people connected with your state's Office (or Bureau) of Vocational Rehabilitation. (There's a lot more about careers and employment in the next chapter.)

SUMMARY

The teenage years are full of challenge for people with CF, just as for people without CF. However, for those with CF, the stakes are higher—if they neglect their health during these important years, they might never regain it. If teenagers with CF take good care of themselves, these years can be wonderfully happy, healthy, productive, and fun.

14

Cystic Fibrosis and Adulthood

THE BASICS

1. Most patients with cystic fibrosis (CF) live well into adulthood.
2. Most adults with CF are able to study, work, marry, and do most of the other things that adults do.
3. Adults may have more health problems than younger patients with CF.
4. Adults have to deal with some difficult questions, including what kind of work they can do, whether they can or should have children, and how long they will live.

Until fairly recently, adults didn't have cystic fibrosis (CF); children had it, and they died. Today, most patients with CF can plan to live well into adulthood, with the pleasures and responsibilities that come with adulthood. In fact, nearly 40% of all patients with CF today are 18 years or older, compared with only 8% in 1969. In 2001, there were 9,093 patients with CF 18 years or older followed in CF centers in the United States, compared with only 624 in 1969. Patients now live to an average age of about 33 years, and some experts have predicted that survival will increase to 40 years for someone born today (even without any of the many new treatments that are on the verge of becoming available).

Adults with CF are living fulfilling lives. In 2001, 62% of patients with CF 21 years and older had graduated from high school; this compares with the national rate of 70%. Many of those CF high school graduates went on to college and some to graduate school. Only 22% of patients with CF over 18 years old listed themselves as unemployed or disabled, whereas 25% were students, 37% were working full-time, and 12% were working part-time; 36% of these adults were married or living with a partner.

Upon reaching adulthood, people with CF must contend with some special issues, in addition to those faced by all people as they approach adulthood and in addition to the CF issues facing younger patients and their families. Since the lung problems with CF are progressive (that is, they tend to get worse, slowly, as time goes by), many adults with CF have more symptoms and limitations than they had as children and teenagers. What is true of the lungs is also true to some degree for the other body systems affected by CF: More CF-related problems happen in adults than in children. For this reason, we will have a brief discussion in this chapter of the different organ systems and how they may be affected differently for adults than for younger patients with CF. We'll also discuss some other issues, including medical care, health insurance, employment, marriage and family, disability, and psychological issues.

Newspapers, television, and "the public" (whoever *they* are) often refer to CF as "a fatal disease," which forces even healthy adults to consider the issue of death and dying, which we will address with a brief discussion of death and the adult with CF. More complete discussions of each of these topics can also be found in other chapters. Patients' attitudes and outlook on life have a tremendous influence on what they are able to do, and indeed, on how long they live. Patients with CF typically have a strong, positive outlook, and therefore are able to accomplish many of the normal tasks and enjoy many of the normal pleasures of adulthood, despite having to contend with some difficulties.

DIFFERENT ORGAN SYSTEMS

Respiratory System

Upper Airway: Nose and Sinuses

There is little different about the involvement of the nose and sinuses in adults with CF compared with CF children and adolescents. In all ages, the sinuses will look abnormal on radiographs (x-ray films), and patients may develop nasal polyps, which may or may not respond to nasal sprays, and which may need to be removed surgically. The sinus abnormality is more apt to bother an adult with CF than a child with CF, and some adults will have problems with chronic (long lasting) sinusitis. Headache, constantly stuffed nose, and even increased cough may signal infection of the sinuses, which will usually improve with antibiotic treatment. If sinus problems persist despite antibiotics, sinus surgery (to open up the sinuses and make it easier for them to drain) may be helpful in some cases.

Lower Airways: Lungs and Bronchial Tubes

The lungs, especially the bronchial tubes, are the main source of problems for anyone with CF, with buildup of secretions, infection, and inflammation that if unchecked can lead to permanent damage of the lungs. The lung problems are more likely to occur, and be more difficult to manage, in adults. By age 15 years, about one half of all patients with CF cough up mucus each day, and 85% bring up mucus from their lungs occasionally. Adults have more episodes of infection for which they need to be treated with intravenous (IV) antibiotics, either in the hospital or at home. While pulmonary function tests (PFTs) do not tell the whole story, they can help give a general picture of this situation: You may recall from Chapter 3, *The Respiratory System*, that the forced expiratory volume in 1 second (FEV_1) is the amount of air that can be blown out of the lungs in 1 second, and is a measure of how much bronchial blockage there is (the higher the FEV_1, the higher the airflow, and the less blockage there is). The average FEV_1 for 7-year-olds with CF is 95% of normal (meaning that the average 7-year-old with CF can blow out 95% as much air in 1 second as a healthy 7-year-old), the average FEV_1 for 18-year-olds is 72% of normal, and for 30-year-olds it is 50% of normal. What this shows is that adult patients are more likely than younger patients to have considerable bronchial blockage and generally serious lung disease. Adults are more likely than children to have difficulty exercising. Adults are more likely than children to need to use oxygen (although most will not). Adults are more likely than children to be referred to a lung transplant program for possible lung transplantation (see Chapter 8, *Transplantation*). But, not everyone continues to get worse and worse after they reach adulthood. Some patients remain quite healthy, and even those who have gotten sicker as they have become adults may be relatively stable for a long time. Some adult patients tell us that they don't get sicker each year, but feel that they have to work harder to stay the same.

Of specific *complications* of lung disease (see Chapter 3, *The Respiratory System*), adults are more likely than youngsters to have hemoptysis (coughing up blood) and pneumothorax (collapsed lung caused by a hole in the lung). It is fairly common for an adult with CF to have blood streaking of the mucus that they cough up and spit out, but bringing up a large amount (enough to require hospitalization, for example) is much less common: about 2.5% of patients older than 21 do so (this compares with fewer than 0.4% of children under 15 years old). Although pneumothorax is three times more common after the age of 15 years than before, only about 1% of older patients suffer this problem in a given year. So, even though both of these problems are more common in adults than in children, neither one is a major problem for most adults with CF.

Gastrointestinal System

The symptoms and signs from the gastrointestinal system vary in their effects on adults. Most patients, young and old alike, need to take pancreatic enzymes for the digestion of their food. For some strange reason, it seems that many adults have less abdominal discomfort from their pancreatic problem (and may need fewer enzymes with meals) than children with CF. We don't know why this is so; it may be simply that by the time they are adults, patients have learned how to take their enzymes better, or they've learned to avoid problem foods. It may also be that with age there is a change in their pancreas, stomach, or intestines that we haven't identified. There may be another explanation, too: It may be that some patients are just *used* to the discomfort, so they notice it less.

Distal Intestinal Obstruction Syndrome

Intestinal blockage (DIOS, standing for distal intestinal obstruction syndrome) occurs in as many as 20% of adults sometime during their adult lives. It's not known what causes DIOS, but one factor that has been blamed in many cases is not taking adequate enzymes. DIOS can cause symptoms ranging from mild cramping to severe abdominal pain—that seems a lot like appendicitis—and lack of bowel movements. It can be very serious and occasionally may even require surgery. Because of the possible consequences, changes in bowel habits—especially having no bowel movements for a day—should make you call your CF physician right away. DIOS can usually be treated by drinking large amounts of special liquids (the best known is GoLytely), or if that fails, by special enemas. Patients with CF should never undergo surgery for "appendicitis" without communicating with their CF physician, because DIOS can sometimes mimic appendicitis but can be treated without surgery. Only very rarely is surgery necessary.

Gallstones

Gallstones appear in about 10% to 15% of patients with CF at some time in their lives. This is more likely to happen in adulthood. Gallstones can be completely innocent or can cause pain or block drainage of liver secretions. If they do cause pain, they are usually removed by surgery (taking out the whole gallbladder).

Diabetes

As you saw in Chapter 4, *The Gastrointestinal Tract*, diabetes is much more common in adults with CF than in children, with about 10% (or more) of patients with CF developing diabetes each decade after age 10 years: Almost no one with CF gets diabetes before age 10; about 10% of patients between 10 and 20 years old develop it; by age 30 years, about 20% of patients have developed it. Diabetes is well managed with diet and insulin injections (and in unusual cases, with diet alone). In some centers, oral medications are used to help control the blood sugar level. Other than the bother of watching the diet a little more carefully than before, and of taking extra oral medications or giving oneself injections, it is unclear what impact diabetes has on the health of the patient with CF. One report suggests that it has a negative impact, with diabetic CF patients dying earlier than nondiabetic patients, whereas most studies have found no effect on how long someone will live. Probably, patients who work hard to control their blood sugar levels do better than those whose sugars are poorly controlled.

Liver Disease

Liver disease, including cirrhosis, used to be the second leading cause of death in patients with CF (after lung disease), accounting for about 2% of the deaths among people with CF. Experts predicted that as treatment for the lungs improved, and patients lived longer, more patients with CF would develop liver disease; that is, as there were more adults, there would be more liver disease in patients with CF. This has turned out not to be the case. It seems that most patients who will develop liver disease do so by their teens.

Bone Health

The density of bones of patients with CF tends to fall as patients age. The worse the patient's pulmonary and nutritional health, the lower the density of bone and the greater the risk of bone fracture. The problem is especially pronounced in patients treated with steroids and those who have undergone lung transplantations. Patients need to pay special attention to factors that help bone health, including overall nutrition (including taking pancreatic enzymes), vitamin D and calcium supplements, weight-bearing exercise, and adequate exposure to sunlight. Some patients may need special supplements of bone-building drugs, including alendronate sodium, pamidronate disodium, or calcitonin. This problem is discussed at greater length in Chapter 6, *Nutrition*.

Reproductive System

The reproductive system is more of a concern to teenagers and adults as compared to children.

Men

Some 98% of men with CF are sterile because of a blockage or incomplete formation of the *vas deferens*, the tube that takes sperm from the testicles to the penis. All other aspects of the sex life of adult men with CF are normal, but they cannot deliver sperm to their partners. This means that most men with CF are very similar to men who have had a vasectomy, where the *vas deferens* is cut and blocked for male birth control. Two percent of men with CF do not have this blockage, so you cannot assume that intercourse will not result in pregnancy. This may be good news for someone who wants to father children, or bad news for someone who thinks that CF alone is adequate male birth control. A semen analysis can be done to see if sperm are present. Men with CF have wondered if there was a way to get around the blockage of the *vas deferens*, since the sperm are made normally in the testicles but just can't get out. Recently, a new high-tech microsurgical technique has been developed for *in vitro* fertilization, which has enabled a few men with CF to father children. This technique is called

MESA, for microsurgical epididymal sperm aspiration. Here's how it works: Using a special surgical operating microscope and tiny needle (because the structures are so small) a urologist aspirates (uses suction to pull out) some sperm from the man's epididymis (a crescent-shaped structure attached to the testicle). These sperm are then injected into one of the woman's eggs, which had previously been removed from her ovary and placed in a test tube. The injection technique is different from the usual *in vitro* fertilization procedures (not that any way of fertilizing a human egg outside the body can really be called "usual"). When *in vitro* fertilization is performed, most often the egg and sperm are just put together, with the hope that they'll hit it off and the sperm will enter the egg to fertilize it. But the sperm collected via MESA are generally not mature enough to fertilize an egg on their own, since they are removed before they have had a chance to take their normal maturing trip all the way through the epididymis. Since these somewhat immature sperm would not have much success at fertilizing an egg on their own, they are helped by being injected directly into the egg. The pregnancy rate with this technique may be as high as 50% per attempt. If the procedure works, and the egg is fertilized, the tiny several-cell embryo can be analyzed to see if it carries abnormal CF genes before it is implanted into the mother's uterus to grow and develop (the chances of the baby's having CF are shown in Table 11.1). The procedure is expensive (somewhere around $10,000), is not widely available, and is not covered by most insurance policies. Whether a couple in which the husband has CF wants to attempt this will depend on a number of factors, including (a) who will pay for it, (b) what will the couple do if the embryo is found to have two abnormal CF genes (most couples contemplating this procedure will decide to have the mother-to-be screened for the most common CF gene mutations beforehand), and (c) is the father healthy enough to be able to help raise the child?

Women

The reproductive tract is fairly normal in most women with CF, although a fair proportion of women with CF may have irregular menstrual periods. Women with CF are able to get pregnant, and several hundred have carried their pregnancies to term and had babies, most of whom have been healthy. It is probably a bit more difficult for a woman with CF to get pregnant than it is for one without CF, for a couple of reasons. The first factor that makes women with CF less fertile than normal is that the mucus in their cervix (the opening to the uterus) is—like most mucus in people with CF—extra thick and sticky, making it tough slogging for a sperm trying to swim from the vagina through that cervical mucus to get to the uterus (womb) to unite with an egg. In addition, if a woman's nutrition is poor, or if she is in poor health otherwise (as, for example, from severe lung disease), her periods may not be regular, and the periods may be anovulatory (meaning that no eggs are released). In one recent year, in the United States, 58 women with CF delivered live babies, 14 had a therapeutic abortion, and 11 had spontaneous abortions (miscarriage or stillbirth).

As we discuss a little later in this chapter, the decision to have or not to have children is extremely important for any woman, particularly so for a woman with CF. Pregnancy can have a detrimental effect on the mother's health if her lungs were not in good condition at the onset of the pregnancy. (For most women whose lungs are in good shape, pregnancy does not usually seem to make the lungs worse than they would have been otherwise.)

Birth Control

For many excellent reasons (some discussed later in this chapter), women with CF often decide they do not wish to become pregnant. They certainly should not become pregnant unless and until their ability to take care of themselves (particularly their lungs) and their baby is solidly established. This means that birth control is essential for many women with CF. Not counting abstention (not having sex at all), the most effective birth control method is surgical: tubal ligation. Practically the only disadvantage is that if you change your mind, it will be difficult or even impossible to undo a tubal ligation. The pill is another reliable method of birth control that many women with CF have chosen, and have used safely and effectively. The pill has the further advantage of regulating menstrual periods—a relief to those many women with CF who had had irregular periods. It is theoretically possible that the pill may not work quite as well in women taking antibiotics. This possibility can be avoided by talking with your CF doctor or gynecologist and arranging a special schedule of only 3 or 4 days (instead of the usual 7) each month taking a "placebo" pill. "Barrier" methods (diaphragms and condoms) are somewhat less effective than the other methods; mostly because they must be thought of and used each time a couple has intercourse. Condoms have the important advantage of providing excellent protection from sexually transmitted diseases, including acquired immunodeficiency syndrome (AIDS). You should discuss the pros and cons of the various methods with your physician.

Vaginal Yeast Infections

Somewhere around 75% of all women will have a vaginal yeast infection at some time in their lives. Women with CF are no exception, and probably have more of them than other women because of CF women's frequent use of antibiotics. Women with CF would be expected to have more than their share of vaginal yeast infections (often referred to in the medical literature as thrush or vulvovaginal candidiasis—*Candida* species being the most common yeast causing this infection). This is because being on antibiotics increases anyone's chances of getting this infection because antibiotics kill bacteria, which allows the yeast to multiply. One study from Australia showed this problem to be much more common in women with CF than women without CF, and for episodes of thrush to correspond to times they were taking oral antibiotics.

Furthermore, diabetes also may make a woman more likely to develop a yeast infection, and more women with CF have diabetes. These infections are not dangerous, but can be extremely uncomfortable, causing terrible itching and sometimes burning. These infections can usually be treated successfully with antiyeast cream placed in the vagina. Occasionally, an oral medication might also be needed. Women with CF who get these infections whenever they go on antibiotics can be helped tremendously by starting treatment with vaginal antiyeast medications as soon as they start their antibiotics.

Urinary Stress Incontinence

Urinary incontinence (leakage of urine) is common in healthy women and is even more common is women with CF. As many as half the adult females with CF may have urinary incontinence, usually associated with hard coughing and laughing. Some women with CF say that this problem sometimes interferes with their social life and often interferes with effective airway clearance. The problem with airway clearance is minimized by a trip to the bathroom before airway clearance sessions. Pelvic floor muscle exercises are sometimes helpful for women with urinary incontinence. You should discuss this problem with your physician.

OVERALL HEALTH

Many adults with CF find that they are able to do less and less as time goes on, mostly because of the worsening health of their lungs. This can be very difficult, particularly for people who used to be very active. Recurrent courses of IV antibiotics may be needed, and if they are carried out in the hospital, these courses can have a huge impact on an adult's ability to continue to carry out a normal work and home life. Permanent IVs like Porta-caths and Mediports (discussed in Chapter 7) can enable many adults to get their IV antibiotics at home, thus helping them to continue a relatively normal life.

One of the hardest parts for many people is getting used to using oxygen, something that was necessary for about 7% of all patients with CF in 2001, most of them adults. People—especially children—may stare at you if have this greenish tubing wrapped around your ears and plugged into your nose. Different patients have handled this discomfort in different ways, from ignoring it to answering questions with a gentle explanation of what the oxygen tubing is for ("it's oxygen to help me breathe better because I have a lung problem"). Oxygen is discussed more in the Appendix B, *Medications*.

You may have less energy, find you need to take more time to do things, and schedule more time for rest. Some people may be helped by getting a handicapped parking placard and license plates. If you belong to American Automobile Association (AAA), they can help get you the necessary forms; otherwise, contact your local driver's license bureau.

MEDICAL CARE

The training of physicians in the care of adult patients with CF is just now catching up with the tremendous improvement in longevity. Until very recently, CF was a disease of childhood, and physicians who were trained to care for adults were not taught about CF. Today, there are still too few internal medicine physicians (general medical specialists for adults) who have had training and experience in the problems and care of people with CF. Fortunately, however, there are more and more adult pulmonologists who have taken it upon themselves to become knowledgeable in the care of adults with CF, and medical training programs are beginning to pay more attention to the treatment of this important population. There has been a large effort over the past 5 years for CF centers to develop adult programs, now most CF centers (more than 100) have a program for their adult patients, including physicians who are interested and knowledgeable in the care of adults with CF.

Care at an approved CF center, with its team of experts, is very important. Studies in Europe, Australia, and North America have shown clearly that *patients who receive their care at CF centers live longer than those whose care is not in centers; it's that simple.* This is not to say that the general internist or family doctor isn't capable of participating in the care of adults with CF. Quite the contrary: The primary care physician can be a wonderful ally in maintenance of the health of people with CF just as with people without CF. But the CF care should be coordinated between the primary care doctors and the CF center and not done to the exclusion of the CF center. It is quite important to insist that you have access to center care, particularly in this era when costs may be more important than patient health to some health care plans.

HEALTH AND DISABILITY INSURANCE

Health insurance is a very important issue, because medical care for any chronic illness, including CF, is so expensive. Once a person reaches adulthood, he or she is usually excluded from his or her parents' family insurance coverage. Some states have "over 21" laws, which extend health insurance and/or state programs to adults with certain chronic illness, including CF. Some employers have excellent employee health insurance, but some plans exclude anyone with a "pre-existing condition," meaning that they don't pay any expenses related to a problem that you had before you joined the company, which of course would include CF. Some policies limit how much they pay for a particular illness; many have a lifetime limit to how much they will pay. You should find out if a hospitalization for CF at one time will count as the same "illness" as a previous hospitalization that was also due to CF. Some policies or certifiers are liberal in their interpretation, and might consider one pulmonary exacerbation (see Chapter 3, *The Respiratory System*) a separate episode of "bronchitis," "lung infection," or "pneumonia," and therefore pay for each of them, whereas others will be very strict and consider every episode to be part of CF and be less willing to pay for multiple admissions.

Health Insurance When Changing or Leaving Jobs

If you want to change jobs, for any reason, you may be scared off by the new company's having a "preexisting condition" exclusion in its health insurance that won't pay for medical expenses associated with a preexisting condition for the first 12 months the person is working for the company and is covered by the new company's insurance. Don't let that stop you. There is a federal law, referred to as COBRA (standing for Comprehensive Omnibus Budget Reconciliation Act), that requires that employees be allowed keep their medical insurance for 18 months after they stop working for an employer (unless they were fired for gross misconduct). That means you can start your new job, with the new insurance coverage, but retain your old insurance for the first 12 months. That way, if you have CF-related medical expenses within those first 12 months, the old company's policy will pay for them; then, once you've put in your 12 months, the new policy no longer excludes the preexisting condition. (There are some preexisting condition clauses that have a different 12-month exclusion: They won't pick up coverage of a condition until you've gone 12 months without any medical expenses related to that condition; those are very difficult to get around.)

That's the good news about COBRA and preexisting conditions. The bad news is that to continue your old insurance policy for the 12-month waiting time until the new one kicks in, you have to make the insurance payments yourself. This can amount to several hundred dollars a month, depending on the policy, and may be more than many patients can afford.

It is very important to look very carefully at insurance plans and possible exclusions before making decisions about employment. As we mentioned above, it is crucial to insist on being able to have access to a CF center for your care. Be certain that you will not be prevented from this specialized care. Health care reform bills are being considered in the U.S. Congress. If any of this legislation passes, it may well change what insurance companies are allowed to do in terms of excluding preexisting conditions, and so forth. Stay tuned, and check with your CF center. The center personnel are likely to be up to date on these regulations.

UNEMPLOYMENT

If you must stop working because of your health, there are some programs that can help with income and some help specifically for medical bills.

Health Insurance If You Are Unemployed

The COBRA mentioned above is in force whenever you leave a job, whether it's to take another job (as discussed above), or to stop working entirely. In fact, if you are forced by your health to stop working, COBRA requires that you cannot lose your health insurance for 36 months after you stop working. Unfortunately, again, you can lose your health insurance if you can't pay for the premiums. People who have lost their jobs for health reasons may qualify for Medicare, which will pay some medical bills (but not prescriptions), but only after 2 years of being unable to work (!). So, some patients are caught in a difficult bind: too sick to work, unable to afford medical insurance, and with 24 months to wait until they can get Medicare. Some states have "over 21" programs that will pay for CF-related medical bills for people over 21 years old in this difficult 24-month waiting period. These programs are a big help, although they don't have unlimited resources, and have some arbitrary rules about what is and isn't covered. In Pennsylvania, for example, CF medical bills are covered (doctor's bills, most medications, etc.), but if you have CF diabetes, the state won't pay for your insulin or other diabetes-related expenses, even though the CF caused the diabetes. Your CF center staff is likely to be very knowledgeable about all these rules, and is there to help.

Social Security Disability Insurance

Everyone who is employed pays into the federal Social Security fund, designed to help people who become unable to work. If you become unable to work, you may be eligible to receive income from Social Security. The amount you receive depends on how long you've worked and the amount of money you've put into the fund. A downside of this program is that—while it gives some income—it does not give health insurance for the first 2 years someone is on the program. After 2 years, you may qualify for Medicare, which is a form of health insurance (see previous paragraph).

Some patients who have lost their jobs because of their health may qualify for public assistance (Welfare), even if they are getting monthly Social Security Disability checks. For some, however, their income may be too high to qualify for public assistance. Your CF center social worker should be able to help you through the maze of public and private organizations set up to help. Or, you can call your local Social Security office or Public Assistance office.

EDUCATION

Many adults with CF choose to continue their education beyond high school, and some attend trade schools; many graduate from college and even get advanced degrees.

One of the main ways in which CF affects an adult's education is in the decision of whether to leave home to attend college. Leaving home is an exciting and valuable experience for many young adults, with CF or without. It is a time to establish one's independence and even to help "invent" a new personality. It can mean leaving unwanted parts of the past behind and fitting in with a new set of friends. Unfortunately, for too many people with CF that has meant trying to leave CF behind: Not wanting to be different, so not wanting to tell anyone about CF can also mean not doing treatments, not taking medicines, not taking care with nutrition, and so on. In too many cases, it has been possible to ignore CF until it's been too late. There are far too many young adults who have let their health slide and have realized what their parents and physicians had been saying all along about taking care of themselves only after they have suffered irreversible lung damage. Far too many adults have come to us and said, "I wish I had listened, and taken care of myself, but I thought I knew everything, and I never believed I could get sick. Now I wish I had it to do over again . . ."

Leaving home most often means leaving behind the people who perform daily chest physical therapy (CPT) treatments, which, in turn, means that a replacement must be found (either a replacement person to help with the treatments or a replacement form of airway clearance, using a technique you can do on your own). Much of the CPT can be done oneself, especially if you use the Flutter (see Chapter 3, *The Respiratory System*) or percussor vest or mechanical percussors with straps or extension handles, but some young adults feel more secure with a treatment performed by someone else, and may feel that their parents do the best CPT. They are probably right. After all, it is very likely that no one cares as much about your health as you and your parents do. However, there are ways to get adequate help with CPT. Many college health services will offer assistance in this realm. Some schools that have PT students or respiratory therapy students may be able to arrange for these students to help give treatments. College students often have close friends who learn how to administer treatments. Others have placed more emphasis on an aerobic exercise program or on "huff" techniques that are easier to perform on oneself than the traditional CPT.

The Flutter and the vibrating vest (see Chapter 3, *The Respiratory System*) have freed many people from dependence on others for effective airways clearance treatments. Some CF physicians will accept 15 to 20 minutes each day of vigorous exercise as a substitute for CPT. Whatever one chooses, it is extremely important to find some way to keep up with treatments and to not give in to the temptation to skip them in the excitement of being away on one's own, perhaps for the first time. There are always reasons to skip a treatment (test tomorrow, party tonight, etc.), and while it's fine to skip an occasional treatment, this cannot become a habit. A problem with many treatments, including CPT and other airway clearance techniques, is that you may not feel much better after them; what's important is their cumulative effect over many days, weeks, and months. So you may well skip a treatment and not notice any dire consequences. If this happens, it's easy to let yourself slip into a habit of skipping treatments. Unfortunately, many people have noticed their lungs being worse from skipping treatments only after irreparable harm has been done to them. Then it's too late. So, it's important to try to keep up with all your treatments. It's also important to keep up with good nutrition, which many young adults have let slide when their parents (usually especially their moms) are not there to nag them or to cook for them.

While we're on the topic of nonhealthful temptations, it's important to mention two others, namely, smoking and drinking. It should be obvious (but isn't always) that smoking (cigarettes particularly, but also probably marijuana) is bad for anyone's lungs, and especially so if one has underlying lung disease, like CF. There is definite evidence that secondhand cigarette smoke (that is, someone else is doing the smoking, and you're breathing in the extra smoke that just happens to be in the air around) is harmful to patients with CF; it stands to reason that active smoking is that much worse. Smoking will absolutely disqualify you for a lung transplant if you should ever decide that you want one. Alcohol in moderation is probably not bad, but you should discuss it with your physician, because there are some medications, including some antibiotics, that interact badly with alcohol.

Many states have vocational rehabilitation offices or bureaus [offices of vocational rehabilitation (OVRs) or bureaus of vocational rehabilitation (BVRs)] that provide educational and occupational counseling and financial assistance for students after high school. These programs used to be extremely helpful, with some of them automatically paying college tuition for anyone with CF, but many are now suffering from slashed budgets and may not be able to provide as much assistance as in years gone by. They may still be able to give helpful guidance on career selection, though, and are worth checking out. Your CF center social worker should be able to tell you about these resources, or you can call your state Department of Labor and Industry Office of Vocational Rehabilitation.

EMPLOYMENT

Men and women with CF have had—and succeeded at—many different kinds of jobs, including physician, CF research scientist, lawyer, race car driver (at least one woman!), basketball coach, school teacher, computer repair technician, farmer, homemaker, and so forth. CF may well influence one's career choices. It is important to consider your current physical condition and what your physical condition will be in several years as you make occupational plans. In general, a relatively sedentary job is better over the long haul than one that is physically demanding. This does not mean that a sedentary life is preferable, but rather that one should exercise during nonwork time. It also doesn't mean that physical labor is bad, but rather it makes sense to plan for a time when you might not be as strong as you are when you are starting employment. Then, if you should become ill or weakened, it would not jeopardize your job and would only affect your leisure time exercise regimen. Jobs involving constant exposure to dust, chemical fumes, or smoke should be avoided. If you're thinking about teaching school, especially younger children, you should keep in mind the possible danger of near constant exposure to an ever-changing array of respiratory viruses.

CAREERS IN HEALTH CARE

Many people with CF are interested in careers related to health care. This makes a lot of sense and patients have much to contribute, as they have much knowledge of and experience with various aspects of the health care system. Jobs in health care often have good benefits, too. Furthermore, many health care careers have the possibility of transition to administrative roles, which are less physically demanding than active roles in direct patient care can be. This may be desirable if the patient/employee's health and stamina decline. However, there can also be a down side (can't there always?). As we just suggested, some health care careers are very physically demanding, perhaps too much so for someone with limited endurance. Infection control is another major consideration, for both the patient with CF and the potential employer. Frequent exposure to multiple respiratory viruses, as happens in pediatrics, is not helpful to patients with CF. The other side of the coin is that patients with CF who cough may pose a risk to patients they care for, particularly if those patients have any problems with their immune system. Thus, the decision to pursue a career in health care requires a great deal of thought.

If someone is not able to continue to do full-time work, some employers may be able to offer part-time work. Some patients have been able to do some of their work at home, particularly with the help of a computer modem and/or fax machine.

The Americans with Disabilities Act (ADA) of 1990 is a very important law for people with CF to know about. This is a federal law that protects people with disabilities from being discriminated against, including in the workplace. What "disability" means for this law is different from what it may mean in other settings. There have been many people who have applied for Social Security Disability (see below) and have been denied those benefits because they weren't sick or "disabled" enough. Yet, these people may still be covered by the ADA. For this law, the definition of a person with a disability is someone who

- "has an impairment that substantially limits one or more major life activities; or
- has a record of such an impairment; or
- is regarded as having such an impairment."

People with CF, even those who are not dreadfully ill, may qualify. Here's how: CF may be considered to give a "substantial limitation" to the "major life activities" of breathing, eating, or walking. This may be true even if with treatment, you breathe, eat, and walk well. The disability determination must be made without considering the effects of treatments. Even for someone who has absolutely no limitation from CF, the ADA may provide protection for you from the situation where an employer or union official thinks you're limited. Of course, if anyone (from CF or other cause) becomes too sick too work, then the employer can fire that person. But before an employer can fire you because you are unable to do your job, the ADA requires that "reasonable accommodation" be made to allow you to continue to work. This "reasonable accommodation" includes such things as job restructuring, changing work hours, and giving additional sick time (paid or unpaid). This might mean allowing you to start work later in the morning, to allow for morning CPT. Unless there is something crucial about your job that requires it to be done very early, and doing it later would mean a hardship for your employer, you may have the right to have your work hours changed. Another possible "reasonable accommodation" would be getting 2 weeks more sick leave for a hospital admission.

Applying for a Job

Patients often wonder what they should do about mentioning their CF in a job interview. Most lawyers and disability rights experts think it's not a good idea to volunteer the information during an interview. If you do mention your CF, and aren't offered the job, it will be hard to know (or prove) whether it was the employer's feelings about CF that caused you to lose the job. On the other hand, if you don't mention CF, and are offered the job, but then the job offer is withdrawn after the employer finds out you have CF, it's easier to prove that the offer was withdrawn because of CF, and that's illegal. If you are asked point blank during an interview if you have a disability, it gets tricky. Employers are allowed to ask if you will be able to do what's required for a specific job, but are not allowed to ask if you have a disability. If you tell an interviewer that it's illegal to ask if you have a disability (which is true), you could lose the job because of an "attitude" problem, whereas if you lie and say you don't have any problem, then you put yourself in a compromised position if and when it ever comes out that you have CF. In actual fact, in most cases, the question won't come up.

MARRIAGE AND FAMILY

About half the patients with CF over 25 years of age marry, and most of these marriages succeed, with a lower divorce rate than in the general population. Decisions about raising a family are definitely difficult if one partner has a life-shortening disease that limits fertility. Women with CF have a more difficult time conceiving than women without CF, and 98% of men with CF are sterile. Careful consideration must be given to the potential parents' long-term health, and difficult issues must be faced such as the possible death of one parent, which would leave the other a single parent and the child or children with only one parent. If it is the woman who has CF, the possible effects of pregnancy on her health must be considered. Pregnancy has often caused dramatic deterioration in the health of women with CF if their lungs were not in excellent shape at the outset. Similarly, in women with severe lung disease, the chances of having a miscarriage, stillbirth, premature birth, or birth of an abnormally small baby are increased. In addition, both parents must keep in mind that raising a child is hard, tiring work: occasionally up all night with crying or minor illnesses, giving the child attention for much of the day, and being exposed to the many different viruses that all children bring home from day care or school. These can be difficult stresses and strains on the parent with CF, especially if he or she is the one doing most of the child care. Finally, with either parent having CF, the baby might have CF. The child will have gotten one abnormal CF gene from the parent with CF, and whether he or she ends up with CF depends on whether the other parent passes on an abnormal CF gene as well. The chances of this happening are presented in Table 11.1. Because of the dangers to the mother and baby, a number of women with CF lung disease have been advised not to get pregnant or to terminate a pregnancy. This can be hard advice to hear, and has made some women sad and/or angry, particularly if they had their hearts set on having children. Both partners must be willing to discuss all the issues around the important decision of whether to have children or not. It certainly is okay to decide not to have children.

Infant Feeding: Breast Versus Bottle

Women with CF who do have babies may be interested in breast-feeding their infants. Breast milk from women with CF is perfectly normal and healthful for the infants. Breast-feeding may put a strain on the mother, however, and may put both a nutritional and energy drain on her. If a woman is having trouble maintaining her own nutrition, breast-feeding may add to her difficulty of keeping her weight up. Bottle-feeding infant formulas will also provide excellent nutrition for the baby, and will spare the CF mother that extra calorie drain. It will also make it possible for both parents to share the joy (and work) of feeding, including middle-of-the-night feedings.

Many couples in which the husband has CF have decided to adopt children, and some have decided to have children through artificial insemination. New, expensive, high-tech methods have made it possible for a few men with CF to father children, as discussed earlier in this chapter.

Sex

Most couples with one partner with CF are able to have fulfilling intimate relations, including an active healthy sex life. As you've already learned, men with CF have blocked or incompletely formed *vas deferens*, making it as though they had had a vasectomy. They can have sexual intercourse normally, only no sperm come out. Similarly, although women with CF have more difficulty getting pregnant than women without CF, they too usually have normal sex lives. For both men and women, coughing spells can be disruptive during intimate times, and this may on occasion be a problem. Some patients with CF with more advanced disease have a harder time breathing when they are lying flat on their backs. If this is a problem that interferes with sex, different positions can be used. Just as oxygen can help people breathe more easily when they exert themselves in other ways, it can also be helpful for people who otherwise become short of breath during intercourse. Other small adjustments can make a big difference to the partner with CF if he or she has advanced lung disease that has interfered with a couple's sex life: Consider timing your sexual activities for when you feel good. Many people with CF lung disease are not at their best in the early morning before a good aerosol and airway clearance session, so sex first thing in the morning may not be such a good idea for such a person. Similarly, some people feel short of breath and tired after a big meal, so think about giving yourselves a while to digest before planning exertion of any kind, including in bed. Finally, an aerosol and airway clearance may help make sex less taxing for the patient with CF and therefore more enjoyable for both partners.

PSYCHOLOGICAL ISSUES

The overall psychological health of patients with CF is excellent. Professionals have been impressed at the low rate of depression and the excellent ability to cope among patients with CF who have a life-shortening disease that—for some—makes employment difficult, decreases fertility, and presents so many physical and financial obstacles. Most patients do extremely well psychologically and emotionally. They are models of a very realistic, healthy, positive outlook.

Nevertheless, some patients with CF will be sad, and some will be depressed. These feelings can interfere with people's ability to work, to sleep, and to function in many different ways. These feelings should not be ignored, because in most cases, they can be helped with counseling or medication. If you experience depression or other difficult emotions that make it hard for you to carry on, you should let your doctor or social worker know, because you are certainly not alone, and there is an excellent chance that you can get effective help.

DEATH

This book contains a whole chapter on the difficult subject of death. We mention the subject briefly here because it is an area of particular concern to adults. More adults than children with CF die each year, and the death rate for adults is much higher than that for children (in 2001, 74% of patients with CF who died were 18 years or older). However, perhaps surprisingly, the chances of dying at any given age do not seem to keep increasing for every year you age: In one recent year, the mortality rate for 10-year-olds with CF was 0.012 (meaning that of every 1,000 10-year-olds with CF, about 12 died), while it was 0.054 for 20-year-olds, but only 0.047 for 30-year-olds, and 0.045 for 41-year-olds. Furthermore, if you look at PFT results to try to predict who will die, you find big differences between children and adults, in favor of the adults: For any given PFT number, a child with that number will be more likely to die than an adult with the same number. An example is the FEV_1: about 27% of children 6 to 17 years old who had an FEV_1 between 30% and 40% of normal died within 2 years, while only 18% of those aged 18 to 44 years died within 2 years. The same difference holds between children and adults for most PFT values. Experts speculate that a child who has a low PFT (bad bronchial blockage) may be sicker and have somehow more rapidly worsening lungs than an adult who has taken up to 30 more years to develop the same amount of blockage. So, adults with CF, even with fairly severe lung disease, have staying power. Nonetheless, some do die, and adults with CF have to face the issue.

Adults may have spouses, children, and jobs to consider and personal and financial affairs to get in order. Adults will also be forced to confront issues like life support when they are hospitalized, since federal and state laws now require any adult who is admitted to the hospital to be informed of his or her right to make "advanced directives." These are decisions about what medical treatments they will or will not accept, including "artificial ventilation, artificial feeding, and artificial hydration."

Adults may have to decide whether they want to consider lung transplantation. Many patients have found this decision to be the most difficult they've ever faced, and thinking about it to be among the most stressful tasks they've ever undertaken. The stakes are so very high, with possible positive outcomes so positive, and possible negatives so very negative (these are discussed at some length in Chapter 8, *Transplantation*). Add to this the seeming irreversibility of the decision and the time pressure patients have felt to make the decision, and you have a recipe for a difficult and emotional time. It must be stressed that either decision—for or against transplantation—can be the right one for different people.

COMMUNICATING WITH OTHER ADULTS WITH CYSTIC FIBROSIS

Many people with CF are interested in meeting others who might be going through similar trials and tribulations. Some communication with other CF adults happens through the CF center, just through the coincidence of being in the clinic waiting room at the same time or being hospitalized at the same time. CF center physicians, nurses, and social workers can give you names of other patients/families who have expressed a similar interest. (Of course, not everyone wants to get together with other patients.) Many local Cystic Fibrosis Foundation branches used to have get-togethers for families, but because of increased concern about sharing bacteria that may be dangerous along with sharing good times, there are many fewer of these social functions these days. Since it appears that physical contact, or extremely close proximity, is usually required for transmission of bacteria, CF centers now encourage their adults to avoid physical contact with other patients with CF and, for example, to forego the usual handshake when they meet other patients with CF. There are several newsletters and Internet websites that are aimed particularly at (and run by) adults with CF. Newsletters come and go, and are often driven by one dedicated person, so your CF center or the Cystic Fibrosis Foundation may be able to give you up-to-date information on these newsletters and websites. The opinions expressed in the newsletters and on the websites do not always coincide with what CF physicians might believe, so we urge you to discuss treatment issues with your physician. We include here several websites and newsletters that have been helpful to some adults with CF:

1. Newsletter of Cystic Fibrosis Worldwide: write to editor Sam Hillyard, c/o 1 The Cottages, Southill Road, CARDINGTON, Bedfordshire, MK44 3TF, England; e-mail her at: editor@cfww.org; the website for this organization is: www.cfww.org (Cystic Fibrosis Worldwide)
2. CF Roundtable (a publication of the United States Adult Cystic Fibrosis Association: USACFA Inc., P.O. Box 1618, Gresham, OR 97030-0519)

SUMMARY

Most patients with CF now live well into their adult lives. Adulthood with CF brings challenges of living independently, perhaps facing declining health and the possibility of dying, but also the satisfactions that can come with approaching life with a positive attitude and succeeding at many different tasks in one's personal, family, educational, recreational, and career paths.

15

Death and Cystic Fibrosis

THE BASICS

1. Many people with cystic fibrosis (CF) think about death, and most will die of their CF, and not of old age.
2. People with CF do not choke to death on their mucus.
3. Death is not painful for people with CF.
4. Death is seldom sudden or unexpected for people with CF.

It has been stressed throughout this book how well people live with cystic fibrosis (CF) and how much better and longer their lives are now than they were just a few decades ago. Advances in treatment and the exciting research progress promise even better things to come. In the meantime, people do still die from CF. In fact, until a cure is found, it is probable that most people with CF will die from their disease, and not of old age. In order to dispel some common misunderstandings and fears about dying, this chapter will discuss what happens when someone dies from CF.

Most people who die from CF die because their lungs have become so damaged that they can no longer perform the work of bringing in oxygen and eliminating carbon dioxide. At this point, the level of these gases in the bloodstream will be inappropriate. All body tissues need oxygen to stay alive, so when the oxygen level is too low, life is impossible. When the carbon dioxide level rises, it acts first like a sedative and then like a general anesthetic, putting the person to sleep. If the carbon dioxide levels become extremely high, the person may sleep so deeply that the breathing efforts become very weak. This can happen to such a degree that the carbon dioxide builds up even further and the oxygen drops down even further, causing the person to die.

When someone's lungs are seriously damaged, both oxygen and carbon dioxide levels may be inappropriate; however, often one of these dominates. In some people, the low oxygen level is the factor that is most apparent in their final hours or days. When this is the case, unless something is done to alter the situation, it is an extremely uncomfortable condition. "Air hunger" is a term that is used to describe how someone feels if the oxygen level is too low. This condition is very distressing, both for the patient and for family and friends who find themselves unable to relieve the suffering. Fortunately, even when the lungs are so damaged that nothing can be done to prevent the person's death, most often something can be done to relieve that terrible feeling.

The other problem that can occur is that the carbon dioxide level can become dangerously elevated. In this case, the high carbon dioxide level serves as a sedative, and the patient is relaxed, often asleep for much of the time. These people are not suffering. As the condition progresses, the person may fall very deeply asleep, as though under a general anesthetic. In this situation, the person may be difficult or impossible to awaken, may not respond to people in the room, and may die in his or her sleep. This is more difficult for people who are watching and waiting with the patients than for the patients themselves, since they are not uncomfortable.

WHAT CAN BE DONE?

If someone's oxygen level is low enough to be causing terrible air hunger and distress, one relatively simple thing is to give more oxygen to breathe. Although this is an obvious thing to do, it is not always done because of physicians' concerns about its effects on how the brain controls breathing. You'll recall from Chapter 3, *The Respiratory System*, that when someone's lungs are badly damaged, and the carbon dioxide level has been high for some time, a low oxygen level may become the brain's main signal to keep breathing. Conscientious physicians will be concerned that if extra oxygen is given, it may raise the blood oxygen level enough that the brain will respond by inhibiting the signal to breathe hard. Breathing will then get progressively shallower, and the carbon dioxide level will build higher, putting the patient to sleep, perhaps so deeply that he or she will die.

There are several fallacies in these concerns. The first is that even when someone's carbon dioxide level has been high for some time, receiving extra oxygen *rarely* lowers the breathing level. Sometimes it even improves it (probably just by giving needed oxygen to the breathing muscles). The second essential point is that at this time, the primary concern should be for the patient's *comfort*, and sedating the person slightly by allowing the carbon dioxide to build up may, in fact, be helpful. The extra oxygen may change the situation from one in which low oxygen dominates, making the patient suffer, to one in which high carbon dioxide dominates, making the patient sedated and comfortable.

Another treatment for people who are suffering from low oxygen levels is the careful administration of a medication that can relieve the anxiety and discomfort. Morphine is the best drug for this purpose and is extremely effective. Its main danger is that too much of it can oversedate people to the point where they fall so deeply asleep that they don't wake up. Given carefully, the drug is not likely to cause this problem and is very likely to relieve otherwise unbearable suffering. Its effects are often like those just discussed of administering oxygen: Morphine and/or oxygen can sedate someone whose oxygen levels are intolerably low, making that person much more comfortable. Each medication alone or in combination with the other may also oversedate. Almost always, if a person is likely to be dying, the primary concern should be for the person's comfort.

MYTHS ABOUT DYING WITH CYSTIC FIBROSIS

There are a number of widespread misunderstandings about dying with CF that are important to mention and correct.

Choking

"My Child (or I) May Choke on Thick Mucus and Die."

It is certainly true that thick mucus is a problem for people with CF and that some children and adults with CF have very hard coughing spells when it can look (and feel) as though they won't be able to catch their breath. However, *people with CF do not die by choking on their mucus*. In fact, a sudden unexpected death in CF is extremely rare. People with CF do not go to bed well and die during the night.

Predictions

"Doctors Know When a Person with Cystic Fibrosis Is Going to Die."

It is possible to know that someone is getting sicker and that his or her pulmonary function has been declining for several months. Some statistics enable physicians to say that someone with these numbers for pulmonary function tests (PFTs) has a 50% chance of dying within the next 2 years. There are no PFT results (or other test results) that can give a higher than 50% likelihood of dying within the next 2 years. In extreme conditions, experienced CF physicians may be able to say that someone is so sick that he or she is not likely to live many more hours or days. *It is never possible to predict the exact timing of death.* Physicians who have worked with patients with CF for any length of time have seen patients who they thought could not possibly make it *through the night*, pull through and recover sufficiently to live for months or even years longer. For this reason, many CF physicians believe that when someone is extremely ill and is unlikely to recover, it is still worth giving as much treatment as possible to enable the lungs to recover [usually intravenous (IV) antibiotics, aerosols, and postural drainage]—*if these treatments do not interfere with the patient's comfort.* Certainly, very invasive and uncomfortable procedures and treatments, such as using a tube in the trachea and a mechanical ventilator, are not justifiable if the chances of recovery are extremely small. On the other hand, relatively simple treatments such as IV medications, which might give a person the slight chance of recovery and which would not interfere with comfort, should be given.

Pain

"Dying from Cystic Fibrosis Is Very Painful."

If someone is dying with a very low oxygen level, that sensation of suffocation can be terrible. However, that sensation can most often be lessened considerably by giving oxygen and sometimes a sedative, perhaps morphine. There is usually no physical pain.

"It's Better to Die at Home than in the Hospital."

Don't all of us—if we have to die—want to die among loved ones, in a familiar setting, without strangers being present and without suffering intrusive treatments? This can be arranged in most hospitals, though. When the patient, family, and physician have discussed all these matters and agreed on the approach, the procedures and medications necessary to keep the patient comfortable can be handled much more readily in the hospital. For extreme circumstances, the support of the hospital staff can be very comforting to patients and their families. In some communities, Hospice may be able to provide many of the necessary services, medications, and support in the home.

"It's Important to Keep Fighting."

Very often, when someone with CF is dying, that person has lived for many years (usually decades) with the disease, has done much to stay well (exercise, airway-clearance treatments, medications, etc.), and has been recognized as fighting against the odds. Family, friends, and the patients themselves think of them as "fighters," in the very positive sense of that word. Too often, however, in a family's grief over losing a very special person, they may convey to that person the idea that they must keep fighting, and not give in. It is usually not intended this way, but the message may come across that if the patient dies, he or she has let down the family. Sometimes, after a long fight, patients may need permission to let go, and rest. They need to know that they don't have the burden of supporting their surviving family.

TRANSPLANTATION AND DYING

While the advent of lung transplantation for patients with CF has brought hope to many, and has extended the life of some, it has greatly complicated the dying process for many others. If someone is dying, and is awaiting a transplant, there can be conflicting goals: For the dying patient, it has been traditionally believed that the humane approach was to stress *comfort*, even if that meant fewer days of life. For the hopeful transplant candidate, the goal sometimes changes to extending life day-by-day as long as possible until donor organs become available. In some centers, this life extension has included measures as drastic as tracheostomy and mechanical ventilation (often in a center hundreds of miles from home). Patients and families can be in a very difficult bind: Do they forego the chance of extended life—with renewed health—that transplant represents, in favor of a peaceful, calm, and relatively comfortable death, or do they forego that peace, calm, and comfort for the possibility of years more of good life? The 2- to 3-year waiting list for donor lungs has made this decision all the more difficult.

PATIENTS' CONCERNS ABOUT DYING

Adolescents and adults with CF (and occasionally younger children with CF) may worry about death. It is important for them to have someone to be able to talk with about these concerns. Very often, they may be worried because a friend or acquaintance has died, and it may be reassuring for them to hear of ways in which they are different from the person who died and that they are not in danger of dying soon. On the other hand, it may be that their concerns are very realistic and that they are in fact close to the end of their lives. In either case, it is extremely important for them to be able to confide in someone, express their fears, and have their questions answered.

It is tempting for people who care a lot about patients to reassure them and to try to cheer them up and turn their thoughts away from death and dying. It's fine to look on the bright side of things as much as possible, but you don't do a child (or adult) a service by refusing to talk about worries on his or her mind. It may be that just listening and being supportive can relieve someone tremendously. Many people have thoughts and worries about their own death, and it is helpful for those thoughts to be discussed openly. *It is not helpful, however, to* **force** *a discussion of death on someone who is not ready for it.* Parents, close friends, physicians, and other personnel at the CF center may be the people chosen to share in this kind of discussion.

The questions that children have about death may range from whether they will be in pain (on this point they can be reassured) to whether they will see their dead relatives. A family's religious beliefs will have a strong influence on what they will want to tell children about those questions.

REACTIONS TO THE DEATH OF SOMEONE WITH CYSTIC FIBROSIS

When a loved one dies, family and friends have many different kinds of feelings. Sadness and grief for the lost loved one, and for the suffering that he or she might have gone through, are often accompanied by feeling sorry for oneself for having to go on without the person who has died. There is also commonly a feeling of relief, especially if the death comes after a prolonged difficult period. This relief may cause guilt, but it is a perfectly normal and healthy feeling. Parents who have lost a child with CF may have some renewed sense of guilt for having "caused" the CF, or for not having done more for their child. Again, these feelings are normal, but must be balanced by the realization that *no one causes a genetic disease* and that, in most cases, families have done an outstanding job in caring for their children. It may be time to remember that until recently, all children with CF died before school age, and if their child lived a good life beyond that, it represents an improvement, due in great part to the parents' treatment.

Parents with other children with CF may be especially sad to think that what one child has just gone through will be repeated for the surviving sibling(s). This may be true. It is also true that treatment continues to improve, and surviving children may be able to be spared some of what their sibling has just gone through.

Surviving brothers and sisters have complex reactions, which may be confusing to them. They will be sad, of course. They may have a frightening feeling that they were somehow to blame for their brother's or sister's death because of "bad thoughts" they had had. It is important for them to know that all children at some times wish that their siblings were dead, or out of the way, so that they can have their parents' attention and love. They might be feeling especially guilty because they had wished these things and had felt that their parents favored the sick child. They need to know that these thoughts are normal, and that they are not bad for thinking them, and that they did not cause their sibling's death. It can be helpful to point out ways in which the surviving child was special to the sibling who has died.

If the surviving sibling has CF, he or she may be especially frightened about his or her own fate. In this case it is helpful to point out any differences that could indicate a better prognosis for the surviving child, and to assure him or her that you and the physicians will do everything they can to keep him or her well for as long as possible. It is important to give the child the chance to express worries, however, and give reassurances that you'll be with him or her.

POSTMORTEM EXAMINATIONS (AUTOPSIES)

A physician may request permission for performing an autopsy. This is very difficult to think about. The postmortem examination is very important when it was not clear why the patient died. In these cases, important information may be discovered, which may make it somewhat easier for surviving family members and friends. It is also possible that something will be discovered that could benefit other children or adults with CF.

ORGAN DONATION

When someone has died, it can provide a small bit of comfort to know that he or she may still be able to help someone who is alive but suffering. Organ donations for transplantation may offer this solace. Patients with cystic fibrosis have been able to donate their eyes to enable others to see and their hearts to enable others with terminal heart disease to live.

RESEARCH

As everyone who is reading this book now knows, the basic defect for CF is still not completely understood, and there is no cure for CF, but many scientists around the world are working toward these ends. In some cases, the research can only be carried out with tissues from someone with CF. This means that it may be possible for organs from someone with CF to be donated to a research laboratory in order to help answer the questions about CF to help future generations of people with CF. The fact that many, many patients and their families have asked that their organs or tissue be donated for CF research has been part of the reason we've learned so much about CF, and have come so much closer to improved treatments, to the point where we can think about a *cure*.

16

Research and Future Treatments

THE BASICS

1. Cystic fibrosis (CF) research has increased our understanding of CF and has led to the development of new treatments.
2. Basic researchers (scientists in the laboratory) are now examining the different CF gene mutations, how CF interferes with salt and water transfer, how CF cells might be made to act like they didn't have CF through drug therapy, and how to cure CF cells with gene therapy.
3. Clinical researchers (researchers working with patients) are evaluating new ways of fighting infection, decreasing airway inflammation, thinning CF mucus, bypassing or correcting the defective CF protein, and transferring healthy CF genes into patients' cells.
4. Both researchers and patients have important responsibilities for CF research.
5. New treatments soon will be available for fighting infection, reducing inflammation, thinning mucus, and digesting food and absorbing its nutritional components, continuing to improve the outcome for patients.
6. New, powerful approaches to treating CF are in development that may be able to prevent CF symptoms by correcting the function of the defective CF protein or using alternative chloride channels in cells to get the job done.
7. One day, gene therapy may cure CF.

Despite the tremendous improvement in the quality and length of life of patients with cystic fibrosis (CF) and the major advances in our understanding of the basic defects in CF cells, it is impossible to estimate when CF will be cured. The only way that CF therapies will continue to improve is through research, just as the current achievements in treatment were derived from previous research. Investigations into the numerous complex facets of CF have become some of the most exciting areas in all of science. In fact, many outstanding scientists have been attracted from other fields to direct their attention toward solving the problems of CF. This chapter reviews the main areas of current CF research and progress, the direction for future research, and the potential future treatments that are being explored.

Medical research is divided into two general categories—*basic* and *clinical*. Basic research, sometimes called "bench" research because it usually takes place in a laboratory, concerns itself with tissues, cells, and even molecules. Clinical research deals directly with people, examining the effects of diseases or treatments on individual patients or groups of patients. Scores of clinical research projects related to CF are continually being conducted. They may deal with any one of the problems seen with CF or its treatment. Some of the projects involve very few patients; others involve national or even international cooperative efforts involving many researchers and hundreds of patients.

Both basic research and clinical research are essential for a complete understanding and satisfactory treatment of any disease. In the current era of CF research, there is great cooperation and overlap between basic and clinical research; for example, basic scientists work on ways to alter cells or deliver genes to cells in the laboratory, and, if successful, these techniques are carefully evaluated by clinical researchers to see if the new therapeutic approach is effective and safe in people with CF. You can read more about the Cystic Fibrosis Foundation–supported network of research centers set up to facilitate this translation of basic research discoveries into new treatments, the *Therapeutic Development Network* (TDN), in Chapter 17, *The Cystic Fibrosis Foundation*.

In the following sections, we discuss the basic and clinical research approaches that are being carried out in different CF-related categories. You can think of these categories as the steps of the disease, beginning with the defective gene and ending with associated symptoms. Treatments in one category may affect another. For example, a drug that helps clear CF mucus may also lead to improved control of airway infection and inflammation. And a drug that corrects the basic defect [i.e., the gene or the cystic fibrosis transmembrane conductance regulator (CFTR) protein] may prevent the other symptoms from even developing. Much of the background for this chapter can be found in Chapter 1, *The Basic Defect,* Chapter 3, *The Respiratory System,* and Chapter 11, *Genetics.*

THE CYSTIC FIBROSIS GENE

Basic Research

Because CF is an inherited disease, finding the gene that causes it in 1989 was an extremely important step toward unraveling the mysteries of the disease and coming closer to solving them. As you'll recall from Chapter 11, *Genetics,* the CF gene directs the production of the CF protein, CFTR. You might say that the gene carries the blueprint for the CFTR protein. The normal blueprint is actually a series of DNA letters. When the letters are joined together, they form words and sentences. If letters are scrambled, then the sentence no longer makes sense. In the cell, if the DNA letters are changed, the resulting protein will no longer "make sense," or work properly.

Scientists have identified more than 1,000 different changes (mutations) in the CF gene's DNA that can be abnormal and produce CF. (Of these 1,000, most are quite rare, and 25 mutations account for more than 90% of mutations seen in patients.) Work continues to identify how the different mutations in the CF gene determine the different defects in the cells.

But (as you'll recall from "Different Mutations: Different Diseases?" in Chapter 11, *Genetics*), the types of CF gene mutations probably do not tell the whole story behind the characteristics of a patient's disease. Researchers are identifying other genes that may modify the course and the severity of CF. "Modifier" genes are an area of intense study; scientists are exploring the effect of these genes on the degree and range of a patient's symptoms. Modifier genes may help explain why two patients with exactly the same CF gene mutations may develop different symptoms or levels of disease progression. Identification of key modifier genes may lead to the development of exciting new ways to treat CF.

Past research has demonstrated that it is possible to correct a CF cell by adding a healthy CF gene to it. This was done first in the laboratory and has since been shown to be successful at correcting cells in patients—but only for a short period of time. Basic researchers are working to make gene therapy a reality for people with CF by developing various methods of transferring the healthy gene into airway cells. They are also working to overcome the barriers to the success of this complicated process, maximizing safety for the patient, and extending the therapeutic effect of the healthy gene once it has successfully gotten into the CF cell.

Scientists have come up with several creative methods of getting healthy genes into CF cells. First, the scientists have to find something that can carry a healthy gene into the affected cells. This "something" that carries a gene into target cells is called a "vector." Most gene transfer research has been performed using viruses as vectors. These viral vectors are attracted to cells lining the airways (epithelial cells). By attaching the healthy CF gene to modified versions of these viruses and aerosolizing this virus–gene combination into the lung, scientists hope that the healthy gene can be delivered directly and safely to airway cells. The viruses need to be modified so that they don't cause infection, which is what viruses are used to doing; don't multiply out of control; and don't cause inflammation.

Gene therapy for CF has turned out to be more complex than expected, but researchers are working to surmount every obstacle that arises. For example, some viral vectors, although modified, were found to trigger an immune response in patients' airways, causing inflammation, and limiting adequate transfer of the healthy gene. Therefore, scientists are working on ways to modify the virus to make it less likely to be recognized by the body as a "foreign invader," to tone down the body's immune response, or to use a nonviral vector to carry the gene into CF cells.

Some work has been done using specialized fat particles called *liposomes* instead of viruses as the vectors to which a healthy gene could be attached and which could carry that gene into affected cells. Another exciting approach is with the use of specially *compacted DNA*. Some researchers have devised ways of packing the gene material tightly together with the resulting material so small that it may not need a vector at all to get into the target cells, but may be able to squeeze through pores in the cells' nucleus (see below).

Another direction of CF gene therapy research involves the route of gene delivery. Currently, investigational CF gene therapy is delivered directly to the cells lining the inside of the lung, by aerosolization. Several researchers are looking for ways to enable healthy genes to be delivered into the bloodstream and have the gene taken up only by the cells in the body that need it. Theoretically, advantages to this route of administration include the ability to treat parts of the lung that are physically blocked from an aerosol's reach (for example, by mucus or damaged tissue) as well as the possibility of treating the CF cells in other organs affected by CF, including the pancreas and liver.

Clinical Research and Future Treatments

There are currently several clinical trials going on around North America and Europe using various vectors to deliver healthy CF genes to the airways of patients with CF. Although these studies have the eventual goal of paving the way to CF gene therapy, it would be inaccurate to say that the trials going on now are actually gene "therapy" trials, because these trials are not really *therapy* (treatment); no one who goes into the current trials expects to be made more healthy. Rather, these are experiments primarily to see if it is possible to get the healthy gene into cells in living patients with CF and to make the cells act as though they no longer have CF and not cause harmful reactions. Therefore, we refer to these experiments as gene "transfer" trials, and try to avoid calling them gene "therapy," so that we do not give the mistaken impression of being a lot closer to a cure than we really are.

In many of these studies, the nose is the first site targeted, followed by the lung. The nose is used initially because the cells lining the nose are the same as those lining the inside of the lungs and are readily accessible.

At the time of this writing, two promising methods of CF gene transfer were working their way through clinical trials in patients via the Cystic Fibrosis Foundation's TDN of specialized centers.

The first of these uses an *adeno-associated virus* (AAV) vector to deliver the CF gene to the airways by aerosol. In early studies, it seems to be safe and is showing preliminary signs of improvements in patients' health. Hopes are high for this CF gene transfer system, but there are still many more rigorous steps to satisfy before it can be submitted to the Food and Drug Administration (FDA) for approval as a new therapy.

A more recent CF gene therapy entry in clinical trials—*compacted DNA*— does not require a vector to carry its gene particles into the CF cell nucleus. The tiny size of the compacted gene fits through the pores of the nuclear membrane on its own. Having no vector should be an advantage, because sometimes the body mounts an inflammatory response against gene transfer vectors, which may prevent successful gene transfer.

CYSTIC FIBROSIS TRANSMEMBRANE CONDUCTANCE REGULATOR FUNCTION

Basic Research

Exciting research is being conducted in laboratories worldwide to figure out exactly how the malfunctioning CFTR protein does not permit chloride secretion through CF epithelial cells and why sodium seems to be overabsorbed through airway cells (which also affects the flow of water). Scientists are learning why these defects lead to the problems that occur in the organs and glands affected by CF and, finally, what might be done to reverse these cell transport abnormalities. Some scientists are investigating whether the transport of other ions (tiny particles that carry an electric charge) besides chloride and sodium are affected by the abnormal CFTR protein.

You may recall from Chapter 1, *The Basic Defect,* that the CFTR protein is produced within the cell, then must fold into a particular shape so that it can be transported to the cell membrane, where it does its job of allowing chloride to exit the cell. You may recall further that some of the CF gene mutations create a situation where the CFTR protein does not get to the cell membrane, but if it is artificially placed there by researchers, it is able to work, to a certain degree. Various chemicals and conditions (e.g., cool temperature) have been identified that help get the altered CF protein from where it is made to where it belongs. Research is being conducted to identify and assess chemicals that patients might be able to take as medications that could get the CFTR protein to the cell membrane in millions of airway cells, when otherwise those proteins would be stuck in the interior of the cell where they do no good.

One powerful new approach that basic researchers are taking to find new ways to "fix" CFTR is called *proteomics*. Proteomics is the science of the complete analysis of proteins to uncover their locations, control, and functions. It is believed that many protein–protein interactions are involved in determining the processing, regulation, and function of the CFTR protein. By identifying and studying all of the other proteins in CF cells, the researchers hope to find which ones play a role in CFTR's functioning or malfunctioning in CF. Once this is known, researchers will find ways to target the relevant proteins with new therapies, with the goal of making the CFTR protein behave normally, regulating a healthy balance of salt and water at CF cell membranes.

Another new strategy to fix CFTR is called *structural genomics*. This is a science that helps to determine the precise three-dimensional structure (shape) of proteins within cells. Researchers are determining the three-dimensional structure of CFTR in CF cells and non-CF cells. The structure of the normal CFTR protein can then be compared to the abnormal CF protein's structure, giving chemists a tool to help in the design of drugs to correct the malfunctioning CFTR.

Clinical Research and Future Treatments

Scientists in universities and industry have developed special "screens" to identify drugs that could get CFTR to behave normally or to find other means to improve the ion transfer in CF cells, potentially preventing CF symptoms from developing. They have identified several promising compounds that are undergoing further evaluation to determine if they are suitable to move forward in clinical testing.

In the meantime, several therapies to correct the function of the CFTR protein—or even bypass it through alternate means of getting chloride through the cell membrane—are progressing through clinical trials. Several interesting therapies aimed at stimulating the CFTR protein to act properly are in clinical trials, including *gentamicin,* and a combined therapy of *phenylbutyrate* and *genistein.* In some cases, these therapies may be specific to certain CF gene mutations. For example, phenylbutyrate/genistein is being tested in patients with *ΔF508* CFTR, the most common CF gene mutation. It appears that phenylbutyrate can improve CFTR's trafficking (i.e., move it to the cell surface). Once there, genistein seems to have the ability to activate the protein further, to fulfill its role as a chloride channel.

The drug gentamicin appears promising for patients with *premature stop mutations,* which include several CF gene mutations containing the letter "X," such as *G542X* and *W1282X.* In these gene mutations, synthesis (production) of the CFTR protein is halted before it is complete. Gentamicin, an antibiotic in the aminoglycoside family (see Appendix B, *Medications*) may be able to suppress the premature "stop!" signal. This may partially restore the production of functional CFTR protein in patients with these specific gene mutations. This innovative approach continues to be evaluated in patients in multicenter clinical trials, and additional compounds that may be more potent are in early development.

Ultimately, a combination of therapies, such as a sodium-absorption blocker and a chloride-secretion enhancer may be used to correct the ion-transport defect in CF cells.

AIRWAY FLUID/MUCUS COMPOSITION

Basic Research

Although you cannot see the abnormal CF gene and protein with the naked eye, you can certainly see the results of the disordered salt and water balance in the CF airway. Abnormally thick and sticky airway mucus characterizes CF and encourages chronic infections. Many scientists are closely examining the composition of the fluids in CF airway, including the proteins found in the mucus, for better understanding of the disease process in CF and to find new ways to treat it.

Defective CFTR results in too little chloride secretion *into* the airways from the cells and too much sodium absorption *from* the airway into the cell. The net result is dehydration (drying) of airway secretions, making airway mucus harder to clear, and setting the stage for airway infection and inflammation. Therefore, correcting these abnormalities should improve the ability of CF airways to be cleared.

Clinical Research and Future Treatments

Researchers are exploring the role that the mucus-secreting *submucosal* glands play in the abnormal composition of airway fluid and mucus in CF. One exciting new mucus-inhibiting drug being evaluated in people with CF is Lomucin (Genaera Corporation, Plymouth Meeting, PA). This oral drug appears to block excess mucus production (and may also be useful for asthma and other chronic respiratory and sinus disorders). Preventing the production of excess mucus may open the airways and ease breathing, among other benefits for CF. Lomucin targets a protein, hCLCA1, which was identified through genomics research to be a regulator of abnormal mucus production.

INS37217 (Inspire Pharmaceuticals, Durham, NC) is believed to bypass CFTR function by activating an alternative ion channel that moves chloride and water in and out of the cells lining the lungs. This enhances the lung's ability to clear mucus. Early clinical trials have shown that INS37217 is well tolerated and appears to increase sputum expectoration and improve lung function.

CHRONIC CYSTIC FIBROSIS LUNG INFECTIONS

Basic Research

Basic scientists using new *genomics* technologies are increasing our understanding of why the CF airways are prone to chronic infections, especially with *Pseudomonas aeruginosa. Genomics* is the science of understanding how genes influence biological activity—so in CF, it is studying how the CF gene—and other genes—and their alterations make cells and organs act normally and abnormally. In this case, the genes that are of special interest are the genes of the *Pseudomonas* bacteria.

All of *P. aeruginosa*'s genes were recently mapped on a tiny computer chip. Using this microchip tool, researchers are determining the functions of each of the nearly 6,000 genes that make up this organism. Those genes that are found to be essential for survival of *P. aeruginosa* may be possible to use as targets for new antibiotics to kill the *Pseudomonas* organisms.

A special set of *P. aeruginosa* genes that are receiving a lot of attention among CF researchers are referred to as *quorum sensing* genes. Quorum sensing is the process whereby certain bacteria can send chemical signals by which other bacteria can tell how many of them there are in the vicinity. When they sense a certain density of bacteria (a certain number in a particular neighborhood), the bacteria can respond by creating a protective coating, called a *biofilm,* which shields the bacteria from antibiotics and the body's host defenses. Researchers are looking for ways to target the protein products of these genes in a way that would allow antibiotics to work more effectively. For example, a new antibiotic might be able to fool the bacteria into thinking there wasn't a "quorum"—there weren't enough similar bacteria around—to start making the protective biofilm. In this case, without the protective biofilm, even old antibiotics might be able to penetrate into the bacteria and kill them.

Clinical Research and Future Treatments

Although new antibacterial therapies that are produced from basic research are probably still years away, other new antiinfective approaches against *P. aeruginosa* and other bacteria and respiratory viruses are being evaluated in clinical trials today. These approaches include novel anti-infectives, drugs that are already FDA-approved for other conditions, vaccines, and new formulations of older drugs.

Many CF clinical researchers are working to evaluate drugs that are already on the market for other diseases and conditions to see if they have value in treating CF. For example, the widely prescribed oral antibiotic *azithromycin* was successfully added to the CF arsenal, because a recent study showed it could improve lung function and body weight and to decrease hospitalizations in patients with CF. Another readily available antibiotic, *aztreonam,* is being developed for possible use in an inhaled form. This drug kills *P. aeruginosa,* and it may also kill *Burkholderia cepacia* (see Chapter 3, *The Respiratory System,* for discussion of these bacteria).

INFLAMMATION

Basic Research

In the airways, inflammation naturally results from the body's defense against bacteria and other invaders. The body produces an *immune response,* usually a beneficial and necessary reaction, to fight infection or other perceived threats. This immune response includes *inflammation,* with white blood cells being sent to the site of invading bacteria. These white blood cells release chemicals that can help kill bacteria. However, in CF, the immune response, including the release of chemicals from white blood cells, is more intense and prolonged than in people without CF, and injures lung tissue as well as killing bacteria.

The overactive immune response of CF is an area of very active investigation. Presently, researchers are trying to understand why the immune response in the CF lung does not slow down and stop, as it should. In addition, scientists are examining which chemical signals from the lung are important in starting the CF immune response. Blocking these signals would decrease the destructive inflammatory process.

Clinical Research and Future Treatments

Inflammation is a part of many other diseases besides CF. In the same way described in the lung infection section, antiinflammatory therapies that are already on the market are also being tested for their use in CF. The Cystic Fibrosis Foundation calls this a "low-hanging fruit" strategy, because these potential new treatments can be "harvested" for CF use fairly quickly, because they have already successfully completed many of the time-consuming steps of clinical trials. In particular, researchers are looking at antiinflammatory drugs being used for diseases such as asthma, rheumatoid arthritis, and Crohn's disease.

OTHER CLINICAL RESEARCH

Studies to enhance the understanding and treatment of many other important aspects of CF, including nutrition, CF-related diabetes, CF-related bone health, reproduction, lung transplantation, methods of airway clearance, measures to assess patients' health status, exercise, and psychosocial aspects, also are ongoing. Following are just a few examples.

Gastrointestinal System and Nutrition

Most people with CF must take numerous capsules containing pancreatic enzymes with every meal and snack to help them digest their food. A new type of pancreatic enzymes is now in clinical trials with patients, and may offer advantages over the currently available enzymes. TheraCLEC-Total (Altus Biologics, Cambridge, MA) may be more effective yet require fewer pills and may be available in a liquid formulation.

Exercise Tolerance

Exercise tolerance has its own category (and its own chapter: Chapter 10, *Exercise*) because it seems to affect—and be affected by—many other factors. Research into exercise has shown that exercise testing can be helpful in assessing a patient's progress before and after treatments of various kinds (hospitalizations, exercise training programs, etc.). Exercise testing also can identify patients whose oxygen level may drop while they are active.

Research in exercise tolerance has led to the understanding that most patients with CF can exercise safely and receive the same benefits that their classmates and friends receive from a regular exercise program. Important research with regard to salt loss during exercise in the heat has led to the recognition that people with CF can replace that salt perfectly well on their own without salt tablets or other forced salt replacement. It also was found that a patient's fitness level as measured in an exercise test correlated more closely than any other measure with the patient's likelihood of surviving for the next 8 years. Researchers continue to work to determine the type of exercise that is most helpful for patients with CF and whether exercise can improve lung function or delay its deterioration.

Psychology and Education

Research in several centers is examining the psychological adjustment of patients with CF and their families. Several studies have shown that individuals with CF and their families are remarkably well adjusted, and other studies are directed at understanding these strengths so that people with other chronic illnesses might benefit. Additional research is focusing on the best ways to educate children with CF about their illness.

RESEARCH ETHICS

Investigators' Responsibilities

Many medical researchers feel a responsibility to do what they can to answer questions that will ultimately lead to better health and less suffering for people. They also have the responsibility of conducting their research so that its drawbacks are clearly outweighed by the potential benefits. For clinical research, the drawbacks are expense, patients' inconvenience, discomfort, and possibility of toxic side effects. All federally funded research is evaluated for the balance of risks and benefits by Institutional Review Boards (sometimes called Human Rights Committees) of the hospital or university where the research is taking place.

Patients who are asked to participate in research must be given complete and understandable explanations of the research, including its possible risks and benefits. In most cases, patients or legal guardians must sign a consent form, saying that they do understand and that they are participating voluntarily.

To enhance patient safety in the clinical trials it supports, the Cystic Fibrosis Foundation formed the *Data Safety Monitoring Board.* This is an unbiased, independent group of CF physicians, an ethicist, pharmacists, and biostatisticians that serves in a "watchdog" capacity to protect patients and ensure the highest standards in clinical research. Among their duties, these clinical trial overseers review all research studies performed under the TDN for reports of side effects and can call for a clinical trial to be placed on hold or stopped if they have concerns.

Patients' Responsibilities

Patients and their families have responsibility, first of all, to themselves. People have an absolute right to refuse to participate in research, for whatever reason they might have. It is worth mentioning, though, that for a disease like CF, where there is no animal that has the exact disease, and where there are relatively few patients with the disease (approximately 30,000 in the entire United States), it is essential that some people with the disease volunteer to help with research. If no one volunteers, the encouraging progress that is being made will come to a halt.

Individuals who do participate in studies, and their families, often feel that they reap large benefits from being an essential part of the research team that will eventually control CF. Yet, it is unfair for the burden of all the research studies to fall on a small group of people who participate time after time, while others never help. Patients associated with a large CF care center are likely to have many research projects from which to choose, so they may easily participate in some, while skipping others. In 2001, about 1,813 patients (8.5% of all patients followed in U.S. care centers) at participated in clinical research. Because of the recent discovery of promising new CF therapies ready for clinical evaluation, more and more CF care centers are now offering individuals with CF the opportunity to participate in an ever-expanding variety of clinical trials.

TISSUE NEEDED FOR CONTINUING RESEARCH

In the laboratories, investigators are working with tissues from the body to answer many of CF's critical questions. Progress has been phenomenal, yet it could be even faster if there were enough tissue to work with. Even now that there are genetically engineered animals with abnormal genes, and very good experimental CF cell lines, they are not the same as humans with CF. That means, for much of the research, tissue must still come from people with CF. Nasal polyps that are removed because they were blocking up the nose can be used, and lungs and livers that are removed from patients with CF who are getting transplants provide a rich source of tissue for research. Still more is needed. Organs can be used from patients who die, but few patients or families are aware of this possibility, and often CF physicians hesitate to bring up this potentially painful topic to a grieving family around the time of the death of a patient.

SUMMARY

The participation and collaboration of an ever-increasing number of superb scientists and patients with CF has meant that basic and clinical research has answered many questions about CF and its treatment. The research to date is paying off with improved treatment that will continue to enhance the length and quality of patients' lives. The continued enthusiasm of researchers and patients will ensure that we will eventually understand CF completely, have optimum treatments and—one day—a cure. In many ways, the critical factor continues to be the willingness of the CF patient community to participate in ongoing clinical trials.

17

The Cystic Fibrosis Foundation

THE BASICS

1. The Cystic Fibrosis Foundation is a national organization that raises money to support cystic fibrosis (CF) research and specialized patient care throughout the United States.
2. CF Foundation–funded research has been very helpful in increasing our understanding of CF, leading to better therapies.
3. The CF Foundation promotes the development of new CF therapies through the Therapeutics Development Program.
4. The CF Foundation sponsors fellowships and other awards for physicians and scientists early in their careers.
5. The CF Foundation accredits and funds a national network of CF care centers that give patients access to a team of CF experts from various specialties.
6. The CF Foundation provides patient education through printed materials, videos, the CF Foundation Web site (www.CFF.org), and a toll-free telephone information line.
7. The CF Foundation advocates for patients' rights in government legislation.
8. The CF Foundation has a mail-order pharmacy subsidiary to facilitate access to CF medications and equipment. This subsidiary also works with medical insurance companies to promote adequate insurance coverage for individuals with CF.

The mission of the Cystic Fibrosis Foundation is to fund the research to find a cure for cystic fibrosis (CF), as well as to improve the quality and length of life for people with CF by developing new means to treat and control this disease. Established in 1955 by a small group of parents and caregivers of CF-affected children, the CF Foundation has grown into a voluntary health organization that sponsors 119 specialty CF care centers, ten distinguished CF research centers, 14 specialized CF clinical trial centers, a comprehensive CF drug discovery and development pipeline (the Therapeutics Development Program), and many other innovative programs to ensure that its lifesaving mission is fulfilled.

The CF Foundation is recognized as a pioneer among health charities and has been emulated by many other organizations. In fact, CF Foundation support for biomedical research has led to many scientific breakthroughs, including discovery of the gene that causes CF, landmark gene therapy research that has since been applied to other diseases, and new life-extending drugs. By taking control of the future of CF and through aggressively pushing CF research forward, the CF Foundation has redefined the role of the health charity.

FUND-RAISING

The CF Foundation receives no federal or state funds for its programs. Therefore, it fulfills the task of supporting medical research and specialized patient care with its own fund-raising programs. Fund-raising is managed at the CF Foundation's national office and implemented through a network of more than 80 chapters and branch offices across the country. These local fund-raising chapters, working with thousands of volunteers and staff, stage special events throughout the year—from black-tie dinners to bowl-a-thons and, most prominently, the annual GREAT STRIDES walk-a-thon. The CF Foundation consistently is ranked high by consumer and trade publications among nonprofit health organizations for efficiently using the money it raises to work on behalf of people with CF.

The CF Foundation's national office has a state-by-state listing of fund-raising chapters, available upon request and posted on the Web site: *www.cff.org*. The volunteers throughout the country who get involved in fund-raising for the CF Foundation—many are not even personally affected by CF—are truly the lifeblood of the organization. None of the advances in CF research and care would have been possible without the hard work of these dedicated individuals. As the momentum continues to build toward a cure, the invaluable role of CF Foundation volunteers is more critical than ever.

MEDICAL/SCIENTIFIC PROGRAM

The CF Foundation uses a variety of funding mechanisms to support CF research, including grants to fund multidisciplinary research centers, individual grants for basic and clinical research studies, graduate and postgraduate research training programs, matching grants to biotech companies to pursue CF drug development, and support of small- and large-scale clinical trials to evaluate new CF treatments. The pursuit of new CF therapies makes the medical/scientific program the primary focus of the CF Foundation. In 2002, the CF Foundation invested $104 million into its wide-ranging medical programs.

PEER REVIEW

To ensure that the CF Foundation invests in the best and most promising research, it uses a model review system for evaluating each proposed project. A committee of scientific experts carefully reviews research applications; the proposals are judged on the quality of the science and the potential importance to understanding CF and bringing the CF community closer to a cure. In most cases, full funding and/or renewal of each project is contingent on achievement of research milestones along the way. The investigators are required to submit progress reports on a regular basis detailing work accomplished, problems encountered, and achievement of objectives.

CYSTIC FIBROSIS DRUG DISCOVERY AND DEVELOPMENT

For nearly five decades, the CF Foundation's medical research program has built a strong platform of knowledge about the disease. But, because CF affects a relatively small number of people, most large drug companies with the state-of-the-art technology to translate this knowledge into the creation of lifesaving drugs have been hesitant to get involved. The potential "market" for the drug would yield only a small return on their investment.

In 1997, the CF Foundation turned this challenge into an opportunity by launching the ambitious Therapeutics Development Program (TDP). CF Foundation leadership and a dedicated community of CF experts and drug development specialists created a unique business model—a virtual drug company—to make certain that new therapies to improve the outlook for people with CF are developed as quickly as possible.

The basics of the TDP are to offer matching grants to biotechnology firms with areas of expertise relevant to the creation of CF drugs, and then to offer them the use of an established network of CF care centers, where clinical trials of these new drugs can be carried out expertly and efficiently in patients with CF. Already, several completely novel CF drug candidates have been discovered through these efforts, and these drugs are moving steadily through the early stages of development.

Typically, it takes 10 to 15 years and more than $800 million for a new drug to be developed. The TDP is expected to move drugs faster and at far less expense than these industry averages. In fact, the TDP is on target to develop new CF drugs in 7 to 9 years, at less than $70 million per drug. Cutting-edge technology, including *genomics* (the science of understanding how genes influence biologic activity—so in CF, it is studying how the CF gene—and other genes—and their alterations make cells and organs act normally and abnormally) and access to libraries of millions of chemical compounds for rapid screening and potential development into CF drug candidates, is allowing the TDP researchers to chart unprecedented scientific territory.

CLINICAL RESEARCH

The CF Foundation's Clinical Research Program, established in 1983, supports treatment-oriented research. The CF Foundation has initiated many large-scale clinical trials involving thousands of people with CF. These studies have provided important information that has helped to refine CF care. The most critical component of CF clinical research is the individuals with CF who volunteer to participate in this research.

The clinical research program's intent is twofold. The first part of the program involves clinical trials of promising new treatments, which are developed and managed by the CF Foundation and its medical advisors, and sometimes involve pharmaceutical companies. These studies require the participation of many CF Foundation care centers and hundreds of individuals with CF to evaluate new CF therapies. These trials generally represent the final stages of evaluation before new treatments are submitted to the Food and Drug Administration (FDA) and, if approved, subsequently made available to patients.

Second, it supports individual research studies, submitted through the CF Foundation's grants program, that are conducted through the network of CF Foundation care centers. Through this mechanism, the CF Foundation has helped to carry out important studies on the effects of exercise and nutrition on lung function, for example.

As mentioned in the *Drug Discovery and Development* section, the CF Foundation has established a specialized network of CF care centers with the infrastructure to expertly and efficiently carry out CF clinical trials. These research sites are called *Therapeutics Development Centers*. Today, there are more promising CF drugs in clinical trials than ever before. It is particularly exciting that several of the drug candidates now in clinical trials target the root cause of the disease—the CF gene and its defective protein product—rather than treating only the symptoms. (See Chapter 16, *Research and Future Treatments,* for more information.)

One of the reasons the number of promising drugs in CF clinical trials is surging is the CF Foundation's "low-hanging fruit" initiative. Many CF researchers are exploring drugs that are already FDA-approved for other diseases and may have potential for CF. This is a relatively quick way to bring new treatments to patients that will improve their length and quality of life. An example of this is the well-known antibiotic azithromycin dihydrate, which in 2002 was shown in a CF Foundation–supported clinical trial to improve patients' lung function, decrease by nearly half the number of days in the hospital, and increase body weight. (See Chapter 16, *Research and Future Treatments,* for more information.)

Patient safety is a top priority in CF Foundation–supported clinical research. Not only must studies be approved by the Institutional Review Boards at the facilities where they are performed, but also, the CF Foundation's independent Data Safety Monitoring Board carefully oversees each study.

In addition, clinical data compiled in the CF Foundation Patient Registry (a confidential database) on every patient seen in the care center network are invaluable resources for drug evaluation in patients with CF. The data provide information leading to patient selection for trials and trial design. Furthermore, it keeps track of important factors, including effects of new CF drugs in the CF population as a whole, after the drugs are approved by the FDA. The Patient Registry allows researchers to identify important trends in the patient population. For instance, the Registry now clearly shows that nearly 40% of all individuals with CF are aged 18 years or older.

Cystic Fibrosis Foundation Research Centers

In 1981, the CF Foundation established an innovative network of research centers focused on CF, a complex disease that requires many scientists from different fields of research working together. This Research Development Program is the first such initiative supported by a voluntary health organization and is endorsed by the federal government's National Institutes of Health (NIH).

These ten research centers supported by the CF Foundation feature top-notch scientists who are exploring many different aspects of the disease. Over the years, their landmark research has identified the CF gene and its protein product, determined abnormalities in CF cells, and uncovered the mechanisms of lung infection and lung damage in CF. Moreover, these centers also have been responsible for developing novel research methods and producing highly targeted scientific tools and resources that will help scientists throughout the country pursue their own studies that will lead to new therapies to treat CF.

The CF Foundation also supports specialized laboratories that are working to fine-tune knowledge about the bacteria, viruses, and fungi that cause lung infections in CF, so that their treatment can be improved. The CF Referral Center for Susceptibility and Synergy Studies, at Columbia University, in New York, analyzes samples of antibiotic-resistant bacteria from patients with CF throughout the country, and works to find strategies to kill these difficult bacteria in the laboratory, including experimentation with combinations of antibiotics. The CF Foundation National Laboratory and Repository on *Burkholderia cepacia*, at the University of Michigan in Ann Arbor, confirms identification of strains of this rare but potentially dangerous type of bacteria for patients at CF care centers. The storage and cataloguing of these samples also serve as vital resources for urgently needed *B. cepacia* research.

In addition, CF Foundation–funded functional genomics centers are using cutting-edge technology to seek new ways to treat CF lung infections (see *Chronic Cystic Fibrosis Lung Infections—Basic Research* in Chapter 16, *Research and Future Treatments*).

Individual Research Grants and Fellowships

Besides supporting multidisciplinary research centers, the CF Foundation also recognizes the importance of stimulating and funding research by individual investigators. To that end, the CF Foundation pushes the field of CF to the forefront of cutting-edge science and clinical research by offering a number of avenues for research support. Grants for training new investigators and caregivers to apply their skills to CF is another priority of the CF Foundation. More information on these grants may be obtained from the CF Foundation Web site: *www.cff.org.*

COLLABORATION FUELS SUCCESS

The CF Foundation also devotes considerable effort to monitoring scientific advances in many different diseases and encouraging these "outside" scientists to become involved in CF-related research. This is accomplished through special scientific meetings, interaction with professional societies, and preparation of informational materials for the scientific community at large. The CF Foundation's annual North American Cystic Fibrosis Conference attracts thousands of scientists and caregivers from around the world to discuss the latest advances in CF research and care. This lively forum also encourages collaboration and provides a high level of information exchange to propel the field forward.

Periodically, smaller gatherings of researchers and/or clinicians take place to achieve very specific goals. Consensus conferences, for example, are convened by the CF Foundation a few times a year to update clinical practice guidelines about areas of patient care, such as nutrition and infection control. Medical knowledge is growing at an unprecedented rate; therefore, experts from several related fields present and review all of the latest research on a topic and then work to agree on recommendations to ensure that patients with CF are receiving the most up-to-date care. These guidelines become mandatory practice for all CF Foundation–accredited care centers.

The CF Foundation's efforts have contributed to a dramatic increase in the overall scientific interest in the field of CF among leading researchers. This has been evident in the growing number of research proposals submitted to, and supported by, the CF Foundation and the NIH, as well as the actual advances made toward understanding the disease.

CYSTIC FIBROSIS FOUNDATION CARE CENTERS

The CF Foundation care center program is a nationwide network of currently 119 medical institutions (see Appendix F) where individuals with CF can seek diagnosis, comprehensive specialized care, and long-term follow-up from professionals knowledgeable in the latest CF treatment advances. Most centers are associated with major medical schools and teaching hospitals and offer a range of outpatient and inpatient services. As part of this care network, centers must meet specific CF Foundation requirements in terms of staff, facilities, and services. Centers are regularly reviewed and visited by the CF Foundation Center Committee.

At these centers, patients with CF have access to a team of CF experts from all of the relevant medical and psychosocial disciplines; team members work together to deliver the comprehensive care that this complex disease requires. Staff at these care centers, including pulmonologists, gastroenterologists, nurses, dietitians, and respiratory therapists, have specialized training related to CF. In addition, the CF Foundation keeps these professionals up to date on research and advances in care through special meetings, publications, and a password-protected Intranet.

The CF Foundation care center network serves as a resource for specialized care and emotional support of individuals with CF and their families. For example, psychosocial therapy is available for patients and their families to hope them cope with the impact of CF in their lives. Social service workers provide guidance for health insurance issues and other challenges. In addition, these centers are an important resource for research on CF, and provide the ideal environment for conducting clinical research on new CF treatments. Furthermore, the CF Foundation care centers are an important part of the education and training of health care professionals who are interested in CF.

The care center network of the CF Foundation has been heralded as one of the finest models for taking care of patients with a chronic disease. The existence of these centers has greatly contributed to the improvement in the life expectancy and the quality of life for patients with CF.

PARTNERSHIP WITH THE NATIONAL INSTITUTES OF HEALTH

Beyond the CF Foundation, some research related to CF is also funded by the NIH, the leading supporter of biomedical research in the world. The CF Foundation has carefully designed its programs to complement those CF-related programs of the NIH. The CF Foundation also interacts regularly with the NIH staff to identify additional research opportunities related to CF and to encourage science in these areas. The CF Foundation's efforts have led to a series of NIH research meetings on CF and to a dramatic increase in the NIH support of CF studies. The CF Foundation will continue to work closely with the NIH to identify research opportunities and to support promising new studies.

OTHER CYSTIC FIBROSIS FOUNDATION EFFORTS TO IMPROVE QUALITY OF LIFE

The CF Foundation's Public Policy and Patient Affairs Programs address legislation and social concerns affecting individuals with CF. The CF Foundation actively participates in developing and monitoring legislation at the federal and state levels to promote and protect the needs of people with CF and their families. A primary emphasis has been to advocate for increased federal investment in biomedical research. Activities include testifying on Capitol Hill to support enhancing the budget of the NIH and orchestrating national letter-writing campaigns to Congress and the administration.

Other activities and issues pursued by the CF Foundation's Public Policy and Patient Affairs Programs include the following:

- Produced the comprehensive *Advocacy Manual: A Clinician's Guide to the Legal Rights of People with Cystic Fibrosis* for the social workers and other staff at the CF care centers. This guide covers important issues that patients face including health insurance, education, and employment.
- Worked with patients and CF care centers to write letters to state policy leaders and Departments of Health to advocate for the continued funding of Children with Special Health Care Needs, a government program whose health care benefits have been extended by law in some states to patients with CF over age 21. This program has been facing budget cuts in several states.
- Worked with volunteers and the U.S. Congress to designate a "National Cystic Fibrosis Awareness Week," spreading awareness about CF and the need for increased support of medical research both to Congress and to the general public.
- Filed a petition to the Environmental Protection Agency (EPA) to regulate the manufacture and use of *B. cepacia* complex—bacteria that are potentially dangerous for people with CF—in products for the environment (This petition was filed in response to a proposal in the agricultural industry for widespread spraying of *B. cepacia* on crops.) In response, the EPA published a proposed "Significant New Use Rule" that would give them an opportunity to evaluate new uses of *B. cepacia* and, if necessary, to prohibit or limit that activity.
- Developed a recommended program of measures to prevent the spread of infections among patients. This includes a set of evidence-based medical guidelines for CF care centers and rules regarding patient participation in CF Foundation events to protect against cross-infection.

Education is another cornerstone of the CF Foundation's programs—not only education of patients and their families, but also of the public and the caregivers at the CF care centers. The CF Foundation produces a variety of materials, available free of charge, including the national newsletter, *Commitment*; consumer fact sheets that cover information about CF, from health insurance guidance to nutrition; and videotapes about CF health care and research. The latest news about research developments and CF Foundation activities and general information about CF can be obtained through the Web site *www.cff.org* or by calling (800) FIGHT-CF or (301) 951-4422.

Cystic Fibrosis Services, Inc., the CF Foundation's national pharmacy subsidiary, makes all CF drugs available to people with CF by mail order. CF Services also advocates on behalf of the patients to facilitate coverage from insurance companies for their CF prescriptions. In addition, CF Services educates patients and their families about CF through a newsletter called *Homeline* and community outreach efforts. Patients and their families can register and renew prescriptions online at the CF Services Web site *www.cfservicespharmacy.com,* or by calling (800) 541-4959.

DIRECTIONS FOR THE FUTURE

Although it is impossible to predict when medical research will provide the answers needed to "control" CF, the CF Foundation approaches the future with an increasing sense of optimism, challenge, and vigor. The steadfast support for research efforts to understand CF and to develop therapies will further improve the lives of individuals with CF. This strategy will continue to stimulate innovative research and to involve outstanding scientists in the expanding realm of CF science.

To support its aggressive medical/scientific plans, the CF Foundation is implementing new approaches to raising funds at the local and national levels. There are many types of opportunities for volunteers to play an active role in this endeavor. To be even more effective, the CF Foundation also seeks to involve more members of the community in its efforts. Patients and families may be linked to the CF Foundation through the local fund-raising chapter as well as the CF care center. To learn more, please see the list of chapters and centers in Appendix F.

The future directions of the CF Foundation will continue to be shaped by its ultimate goal—to find a cure for CF. The outlook for individuals affected by this disease grows brighter every day. The ingredients necessary to reach this goal—the base of scientific knowledge, the research technologies, and the medical/scientific manpower—are now available. Having many of the world's brightest scientists dedicated to CF research, plus the tireless devotion of patients with CF and their families to raise funds to support this research and to participate in clinical trials, makes a formidable team that will defeat this disease.

Appendix A

Glossary of Terms

aerosol A mist for inhalation, usually containing medicine. Aerosol mists may be made by an air compressor that blows air through a nebulizer, which contains liquid medicine, or may come from a handheld spray can.

airways The tubes that carry air in and out of the lungs. These tubes begin with the nose and mouth and include the trachea (windpipe), bronchi, and bronchioles.

alveoli The air sacs of the lung where gas exchange takes place.

anastomosis A surgically created junction between two structures. An example of an anastomosis is the junction formed between the donor and recipient airways during a lung transplant.

anorexia Loss of appetite.

anticoagulant A drug that prevents blood clots.

atelectasis Incomplete expansion of a portion of the lung, usually caused by mucus plugging.

BAL An abbreviation for bronchoalveolar lavage.

b.i.d. An abbreviation meaning "twice a day."

baseline One's normal state of health. The baseline or usual level of functioning includes a number of considerations, such as the amount of cough, exercise tolerance, and breathing effort. One's baseline health is often referred to for comparison. For example, after a pulmonary exacerbation, the goal of treatment is to return someone to his or her baseline state of health.

bicarbonate An acid-neutralizing juice that is normally produced by the pancreas.

biopsy A small tissue sample of an organ. For example, after liver transplantation, the physician may wish to examine a piece of the transplanted liver; the piece obtained is known as a biopsy sample. "Biopsy" can also be used as a verb: Taking the small piece of the organ is called a biopsy.

blood gas The level of oxygen and carbon dioxide in the bloodstream, especially in the arteries. The term "blood gas" is also used to refer to the test and to the actual measurement of oxygen and carbon dioxide.

bronchi The tubes through which air travels between the trachea and the bronchioles.

bronchioles The smallest airways, connecting the bronchi to the alveoli. These airways differ from the bronchi in that they are smaller and have no cartilage to support them.

bronchoalveolar lavage Washing a fluid (usually sterile salt water) into a small airway through a bronchoscope and then sucking the fluid back into a container. The fluid mixes with cells and other materials in the airway and allows them to be examined in the laboratory.

bronchoscope An instrument that allows someone to look into the trachea and airways. There are two major types of bronchoscopes. The "rigid" bronchoscope is a steel tube that is placed through the mouth and into the trachea and airways. The "flexible" bronchoscope is a softer rubber and plastic bronchoscope that can be placed into the trachea and airways through the mouth, nose, or endotracheal tube.

bronchoscopy Looking into the airways using a bronchoscope.

bronchus Singular of bronchi.

cardiopulmonary bypass A heart–lung machine used during cardiac surgery temporarily to take the place of the heart and lungs.

cardiovascular system The heart and blood vessels.

central line A kind of intravenous catheter that extends into a very large vein, or even into the heart.

cilia The tiny hairs in the nose, trachea, and bronchi, which, through their coordinated movement, help keep the airways clean.

chromosome Threadlike structures carrying all of the body's 5,000 genes.

clubbing An abnormal shape to the tips of the fingers and toes that is associated with many different conditions, including cystic fibrosis.

cyst A fluid-filled sac.

dehiscence The breakage of an anastomosis.

diaphragm The main breathing muscle. The diaphragm is located at the bottom of the lungs and separates the chest from the abdomen.

digestion The process of breaking foods down into particles that are small enough to be absorbed through the intestinal wall into the bloodstream.

DNA "Deoxyribonucleic acid"—the basic blueprint of the body's structure and function.

donor A person donating tissue for transplantation; the person from whom a transplanted organ comes.

ectasia Abnormal distention or enlargement. Bronchiectasis is abnormal widening of the bronchi.

-emia A suffix meaning "in the blood." Thus, hypoxemia means lower than normal oxygen level in the blood.

enzymes Chemicals that help perform biologic processes in the body; "enzymes" usually refer to digestive enzymes, which are the chemicals formed in the pancreas that break down food into absorbable particles.

esophagus The tube that connects the mouth to the stomach.

fellow A physician in training for a subspecialty. A fellow has completed medical school, internship, and a specialty residency.

fibrosis Scarring.

flaring Nasal flaring.

gas exchange The process of bringing oxygen into the bloodstream and removing carbon dioxide.

gastroenterology The study of the structure, function, and diseases of the digestive system, including the esophagus, stomach (that's what the "gastro-" part refers to), and intestines (that's the "entero-" part). A gastroenterologist is a physician specializing in this area.

gastrostomy A surgical opening through the abdominal wall into the stomach. A tube is placed through this opening, which allows feedings to be given through the tube.

GE reflux Gastroesophageal reflux. A process in which fluid moves backward from the stomach into the esophagus.

gene A unit of DNA that directs to production of a protein. Genes are responsible for directing everything all the cells in the body do.

genomics The science of understanding how genes influence biologic activity.

graft Tissue from one person placed into a second person. An example is a lung graft, in which a lung from one person (donor) is placed into a second person (recipient).

heart failure A condition in which the heart is not able to pump its full load of blood, resulting in the backup of fluid. Heart failure is *not* heart *stoppage*.

hemoptysis Coughing up blood.

hep lock (see Glossary of Drugs in Appendix B). An intravenous needle whose end can be plugged while it is not being used for medication administration.

hyper A prefix meaning "more than normal." Thus, a hyperactive child is more active than normal.

hyperalimentation This term literally means "overfeeding," but actually refers to the method of giving extra nutrition through an intravenous.

hypo- A prefix meaning "less than normal." Thus, hypoxia means less oxygen than normal.

IM Intramuscular. A way of administering medicine by injection into the muscle.

immunosuppression Decreasing the immune response, usually using medications known as immunosuppressives.

intern A physician who has graduated from medical school and is training in a medical specialty such as pediatrics, internal medicine, family medicine, or surgery.

internal medicine The branch of medicine dealing with the general health of adults.

internist A medical specialist in internal medicine (not to be confused with an intern).

in vitro **fertilization** A procedure for uniting a sperm and egg outside the body, then implanting the fertilized egg in a woman's uterus.

-itis A suffix meaning "inflammation." Thus, bronchitis means inflammation of the bronchi.

IV Intravenous. This can mean the way a drug is given (IV) or the actual tubing used to give the drug ("the IV").

jejunostomy A surgical opening made through the abdominal wall into the jejunum. This opening is used to hold a tube for feedings, as is a gastrostomy.

jejunum The second part of the small intestine.

larynx The part of the upper airway that contains the vocal cords—the "voice box."

lobe The largest division of the lung. The right lung has three lobes and the left has two.

low-hanging fruit The research strategy that targets possible solutions likely to give fast results, for example, exploring drugs that are already approved by the Food and Drug Administration for other diseases and may have potential for cystic fibrosis.

lumen The inside of a tube. The lumen of the bronchial tubes is where the air flows.

lymphocyte A type of white blood cell. Lymphocytes are important in immune function and are involved in rejection of grafts.

MESA Microsurgical epididymal sperm aspiration. The procedure by which sperm can be removed from a man's testicle and used for *in vitro* fertilization.

mucociliary escalator A mechanism for keeping the lungs clear. Particles get trapped in the mucus, and the cilia move the mucus out of the lungs.

motility Movement. When used in reference to the intestines, this means the contractions of the muscles that help propel intestinal contents on their journey from esophagus to anus.

mucous Having properties like mucus. ("Mucus" is a noun; "mucous" is an adjective.)

mucus The slimy fluid secreted in many glands of the body and whose function appears to be to protect and lubricate.

mutation A change or alteration. Most often used to refer to a change in a gene that makes it abnormal.

nasal flaring Widening of the nostrils with each breath (often abbreviated, "flaring"). This is a sign that someone is working harder than normal to breathe.

nebulizer A device used with an air compressor that directs the compressed air past liquid medication, lifting the medication into a mist ("aerosol") for inhalation.

NG tube Nasogastric tube. A tube that passes through the nose into the stomach. This tube is used for feeding someone who can't eat, for continuous feeding during sleep, or for the administration of other substances such as medicines.

panresistant Resistant to all tested antibiotics.

peak The highest level that a drug reaches in the bloodstream.

PFT Pulmonary function test.

pneumothorax Collapsed lung caused by a hole in the lung. Air escapes from the lung through this hole, collects within the chest, and presses in on the lung.

proteomics Proteomics is the science of the complete analysis of proteins to uncover their locations, control, and functions.

pulmonary exacerbation An episode of worsening of the lung disease, usually caused by worsened bronchial infection.

pulmonology The branch of medicine dealing with breathing problems.

pulmonologist A physician specializing in the care of patients with breathing problems.

recipient A person receiving tissue for transplantation.

reflux The backward movement of fluid; this term is often used to refer to gastroesophageal reflux.

rejection The body's attempt to destroy transplanted tissue. Rejection is carried out by lymphocytes, which are immune cells capable of causing damage to foreign cells.

resident A physician who has completed medical school and is undertaking further training in a medical specialty.

resistant This term means "not killed by" when used to describe bacteria's relation to an antibiotic. For example, the statement, "*Pseudomonas* bacteria are resistant to penicillin," means that, in the laboratory, penicillin does not readily kill *Pseudomonas* organisms.

respiratory failure The condition in which blood oxygen levels are too low and blood carbon dioxide levels are too high.

retracting The pulling in of skin between the ribs with each breath, indicating hard breathing.

saline Salt water (see Appendix B).

sedation A state of reduced excitement, anxiety, and (often) a state of mildly reduced consciousness. Many drugs are used to produce sedation and are commonly used to decrease anxiety during medical procedures.

segment The second largest division of the lung. Each lobe is divided into several segments.

sensitive This term means "killed by" when used to describe bacteria's relation to an antibiotic. For example, the statement, "*Streptococcus* bacteria are sensitive to penicillin," means that, in the laboratory, penicillin kills *Streptococcus* organisms.

specialty (or medical specialty) One of the main branches of medical practice in which physicians can become trained and qualified. The specialties are pediatrics, internal (adult) medicine, obstetrics/gynecology, surgery, psychiatry, and family medicine. Physicians may focus their skills and training in more specialized areas, called subspecialties, such as pediatric pulmonology, cardiology, and neurosurgery. (A pediatric pulmonary specialist must first become a pediatrician; a neurosurgeon must first become a surgeon.)

sputum Mucus from the lungs that is coughed up and spit out.

stenosis Narrowing. In transplantation, stenosis can occur at an anastomosis, for example, where a donor bronchus is attached to the recipient bronchus.

stoma A hole, usually one created purposely by a surgical procedure. This word is often used as a suffix: tracheostomy is a hole made in the trachea; gastrostomy is a hole through the abdominal wall into the stomach.

TDN Therapeutics Development Network of the Cystic Fibrosis Foundation of the United States. A system of clinical research centers established to perform collaborative studies, especially on new drug treatments for cystic fibrosis.

TDC One of the centers in the TDN (Therapeutics Development Center).

toxicity Harmful effect(s). This term is often used to refer to the undesirable effects of a medication.

TPN Total parenteral nutrition. This term refers to nutrition given through an intravenous (same meaning as hyperalimentation).

trachea The tube that carries air from the mouth and throat into the chest, where it connects with the bronchi from each lung.

tracheostomy A hole placed in the trachea.

trough The lowest level that a drug reaches in the bloodstream (this level is found immediately preceding a dose of the drug).

urologist A physician specializing in problems of the urinary and genital tracts.

ventricle One of the two main portions of the heart. The right ventricle pumps blood through the lungs, and the left ventricle then pumps the blood to the rest of the body.

Appendix B

Medications

Your physician knows the most about your treatment needs and will prescribe the best medications for you. ***You should not take any medications without the advice of your physician.*** Contact your physician if you have questions about the medications described.

This appendix is organized according to the systems of the body; for example, the antibiotics used to combat lung infection are discussed under *Respiratory System Medications: Lungs*, and digestive enzymes are discussed under *Gastrointestinal and Digestive System*. There is a separate category for medications used specifically for people who have received an organ transplant. For each medicine discussed, there is information on how the drug is taken as well as possible side effects or dangers.

The most common method of taking the drugs described in this Appendix is by mouth. Some medicines can be given by injecting them into a vein (IV, for *intra*venous) or into a muscle (IM, for *intra*muscular). Others can be taken as aerosols, and breathed into the lungs or sniffed into the nostril, while still others may be applied directly to the skin.

A word about side effects: Every medicine has potentially serious side effects. There is no drug that has only good effects and absolutely no dangers. However, all the drugs discussed here have passed numerous tests, which, to most doctors and scientists, will mean that the drug's benefits outweigh their risks. Most people are able to take most of the medicines in this book without experiencing any serious problems. The "undesirable effects" noted for each drug are not meant to frighten you but to help you be as well informed as possible about your medications.

Drug names (generic names and the trade names given by the drug companies) are listed in the *Glossary of Drugs* at the end of Appendix B.

RESPIRATORY SYSTEM MEDICATIONS

Lungs

Antibiotics

Antibiotics are drugs used to fight infections caused by bacteria. They do not kill other kinds of germs, such as viruses and fungi. There are many different families of antibiotics, several methods of taking antibiotics, and certain unwelcome effects with which you should be familiar. These areas are all discussed below.

Perhaps two introductory words should be said about antibiotics and undesirable effects: The first is that antibiotics kill or control bacteria; that is their job, and they are usually very good at it. However, antibiotics can't tell good bacteria from bad. Everyone does have some good bacteria in the body, especially in the mouth and intestines. Among other things, these good bacteria keep people from becoming overrun with fungi and yeasts. Sometimes while someone takes antibiotics, the good bacteria are killed along with the bad. When this happens, a yeast infection can take hold, with a cheesy-looking material in the mouth or vagina. The condition is referred to as *thrush* when it occurs in the mouth. Generally, these yeast infections are easily dealt with, but your doctor needs to know about them in order to prescribe the right medicine (usually nystatin). The same problem of killing the good bacteria can also cause trouble in the intestines, and some patients develop diarrhea from antibiotics.

The last point to mention is that with the availability of so many new medicines, it is possible that new side effects can appear that have not been seen or recorded. If you develop any disturbing symptoms or problems shortly after you've started taking a new antibiotic, it may be from the new drug and you should let your doctor know about it.

Penicillins

This family was first used in the early 1940s and was one of the earliest groups of drugs to be used to fight infection in people. The number of drugs included in this family has grown tremendously over the past 30 years. New members of the penicillin family keep appearing, so it is impossible to list them all. Although the members of the penicillin family have distinct, individual personalities, there are a number of shared characteristics. The most important of these is that if you are allergic to any one penicillin, there is a strong chance that you will be allergic to all of them.

1. *Penicillin.* The first in its family (as you might have guessed from the name), this drug kills many germs, especially *Streptococcus* (*Strep*) and *Pneumococcus* (the "pneumonia germ"). These bacteria are not the major problem bacteria for patients with cystic fibrosis (CF). The most common causes of bronchial infections in patients with CF are *Haemophilus*, *Staphylococcus* (*Staph*), or *Pseudomonas* organisms, and penicillin is usually not effective in treating these infections.

   How taken: Penicillin can be given by mouth, by IV, or IM.

   Undesirable effects: Allergic reactions to penicillin can be mild, but can also be very serious. Any of the drugs in this family can cause a reaction in someone who is allergic to penicillin. Penicillin injections are painful.

Other than these two problems, penicillin is remarkably gentle to the human body while being brutally hard on the unwelcome bacteria.

2. *Ampicillin.* Ampicillin kills most *Haemophilus* (also called *H. flu*) in addition to the bacteria that penicillin kills. It does not usually kill *Staph* or *Pseudomonas* organisms.

    How taken: Ampicillin is most commonly taken by mouth. It can also be given by IV or IM injection.

    Undesirable effects: Loose stools are fairly common in people taking oral ampicillin. A skin rash may appear in some people, too, even if they are not actually allergic to the penicillins.

3. *Amoxicillin.* This is a slightly different version of ampicillin; it kills the same bacteria, but is given only by mouth and is less likely to cause diarrhea.

4. *Augmentin.* This combines amoxicillin with another chemical, clavulanic acid, and makes it effective against *Staph* in addition to the usual bacteria that are killed by amoxicillin.

5. *Methicillin, oxacillin,* and *nafcillin.* These three drugs have been modified so that they kill *Staph* very well. They do not usually kill *Haemophilus* or *Pseudomonas* organisms.

    How taken: These drugs are used mostly by IV, but can also be given IM. Oxacillin and nafcillin have some effect if taken orally (but not as much as cloxacillin or dicloxacillin, discussed next).

    Undesirable effects: These drugs are irritating to the tissues where they are injected. They can cause discomfort as they go into a vein.

6. *Cloxacillin* and *dicloxacillin.* These are also good anti-*Staph* drugs, used only by mouth. Otherwise they are similar to the other anti-*Staph* penicillins.

7. *Carbenicillin, ticarcillin, piperacillin, mezlocillin,* and *azlocillin.* These are anti-*Pseudomonas* drugs. They generally do not kill *Staph*, but they do kill *Haemophilus*.

    How taken: Almost always given IV. They can be given IM, but most people feel this is not a practical way to administer the drugs over the relatively long period of time (1 to 3 weeks or longer) for which they are usually used. Carbenicillin can also be given by mouth for treating bladder infections, but none of the drug gets to the lungs if it's taken by mouth. Therefore, orally, it is not effective in treating CF *Pseudomonas* bronchial infections. Occasionally, these drugs are given by inhalation.

    Undesirable effects: In addition to the possibility of allergic reactions in people who are allergic to penicillin, and the irritation these drugs can cause when they are injected, there are some other problems that occasionally arise. These medicines can make liver tests appear abnormal; fortunately, however, the problem is only with the laboratory result and not with the liver itself. The liver continues to function normally, and if the medicine continues to be given, the test results will return to normal. These antibiotics can also interfere with the function of platelets (blood cells that are responsible for proper clotting of blood).

8. *Timentin.* This combines clavulanic acid with ticarcillin , the way Augmentin combines it with amoxicillin, to make the ticarcillin effective against *Staph* in addition to *Pseudomonas* and *Haemophilus* organisms.
9. *Zosyn.* This is similar to Timentin, in that it takes an anti-*Pseudomonas* penicillin—piperacillin, in this case—and combines it with a chemical (tazobactam in this case, instead of clavulanic acid) that enables the drug to kill *Staph* in addition to *Pseudomonas* organisms.

Sulfa Drugs

These were the first antibiotics ever used to fight infections in people, and they still have many uses.

1. *Sulfisoxazole.* This drug can help in some infections with *Haemophilus*, but it is of little use in fighting *Pseudomonas* organisms.
   How taken: By mouth.
   Undesirable effects: Problems with this drug are not common. Some people have allergic skin reactions.
2. *Trimethoprim–sulfamethoxazole. (TMP-SMX)* This is a combination of two drugs. Trimethoprim is not a sulfa drug, but the combination is quite effective in treating several kinds of bacteria, usually including *Haemophilus*. It is not usually effective for infections caused by *Staph* or *Pseudomonas*.
3. *Erythromycin/sulfisoxazole.* This is another combination product including a sulfa drug (sulfisoxazole) and a nonsulfa (erythromycin) that is quite effective in treating several kinds of bacteria, usually including *Haemophilus, Strep,* and *Staph*. It is not usually effective for infections caused by *Pseudomonas*.

Aminoglycosides

This family includes gentamicin, tobramycin, neomycin, kanamycin, amikacin, and netilmicin. Many kinds of *Pseudomonas* infections can be treated effectively with these drugs, especially with gentamicin, tobramycin, amikacin, and netilmicin. These drugs seem to be particularly helpful in killing *Pseudomonas* if they are given with an anti-*Pseudomonas* penicillin.

How taken: Almost always given by aerosol or IV or IM injection since these antibiotics are not absorbed well into the bloodstream if they are taken by mouth. Shots into the muscle with these drugs are not as painful as those with the penicillins.

Undesirable effects: The two main problems with these drugs are their effects on the kidney and the ears. These problems are usually (but not always) avoidable if the blood levels of the drug are checked and dosages adjusted to keep the blood levels in what is considered the safe range. (Levels do not need to be checked if gentamicin or tobramycin is used by inhalation, since almost none of the drug gets absorbed into the bloodstream from the bronchi.) The kidney problems are usually just abnormal laboratory results and are not uncomfortable for the patient. The ear problem is worsened hearing. The harmful kidney effects usually disappear if the drug is stopped (or the dosage reduced). If the drugs are continued after the hearing or kidney damage has begun, there can sometimes be serious and permanent damage.

Chloramphenicol

This is one of the most powerful and effective antibiotics available for use in patients with CF. Because of its side effects (see below), it is no longer available in the United States, except under very special circumstances. It kills *Haemophilus*, some *Staph*, and another family of bacteria called anaerobes (bacteria that live without oxygen). It generally does not kill *Pseudomonas*. Despite this fact, it often is helpful in patients with CF whose main infection seems to be *Pseudomonas*. It is not known if this is because those patients have other bacteria that are not found on culture (like the anaerobes, which are difficult to culture in the lab). Because of its serious side effects, it should never be taken without your doctor's direct instruction.

How taken: By mouth or IV.

Undesirable effects: This drug has developed a bad reputation because of some real dangers and because of a lot of misuse. Some pharmacists who are not aware of its benefits in patients with CF may even try to convince you not to take it! There are two main problems with chloramphenicol, both having to do with the body's production of blood: In rare instances (less than one case in 40,000 courses of treatment), the production of blood cells may be shut off completely and irreversibly. If this happens, it is nearly always fatal. Another much more common blood-production problem is that, in many people, taking large doses for more than 2 weeks can result in the slowing down of the production of blood cells and lead to anemia. This problem is very different from the complete shut off of blood production, for this slow production always returns to normal after the drug is stopped. Most doctors check blood counts in their patients on "chloro" to detect if blood cell production is slowing down. There are a few other less common, nuisance-type problems, including a tingling feeling in the fingers and some rashes. Rarely, it can cause blurry vision and very rarely, blindness. Most of the serious problems with chloramphenicol have arisen when it is used inappropriately. Furthermore, there is strong evidence that this drug can be extremely effective in treating patients with CF lung infection when other antibiotics have not helped. Most CF doctors believe that the strong chances of its helping to stop or limit lung damage outweigh the small chance of a serious problem with it. However, it has become difficult to obtain because it is rarely used in non-CF patients.

Cephalosporins

This family of antibiotics is growing even faster than the penicillins. Most members of this family are helpful in combating infections with *Strep*, *Staph*, and *Haemophilus*. Some of the newest members of this family have some activity against *Pseudomonas*. To preserve space, only a few of the more commonly used cephalosporins are listed here (but a more complete listing is in the glossary).

How taken: Cephalexin and cefaclor are both taken by mouth only. Cephalothin, cephaloridine, ceftazidime, and cefotaxime are given only by injection (IM or IV).

Undesirable effects: About one third of people who are allergic to penicillins will also be allergic to cephalosporins. Other problems are fortunately not common, but include diarrhea or other stomach/intestinal upset.

Macrolides

These drugs include erythromycin, clarithromycin, and azithromycin. They are commonly substituted for penicillin in people who are allergic to penicillin. They kill *Strep*, many *Staph* and *Haemophilus* organisms, and several other bacteria that aren't big problems in CF. They may or may not kill *Pseudomonas*, but may decrease the inflammation caused by *Pseudomonas*. It is possible that one or more of the macrolides will kill *Pseudomonas* in the airways even though they don't kill it in the bacteriology laboratory.

How taken: Macrolides are most often taken by mouth, but IV forms are also available.

Undesirable effects: Abdominal cramping is sometimes an effect of these drugs, and some years ago, there was a scare about liver damage with some macrolide preparations. It now seems that liver damage is not very likely with this medicine.

Tetracyclines

The tetracyclines were among the first drugs available that had any effect against *Pseudomonas* organisms. They are no longer as helpful as they once were because many bacteria have become resistant to their effects. There are still some *Pseudomonas*, *Staph*, *Haemophilus*, and *Strep* bacteria that are sensitive to tetracyclines.

How taken: The tetracyclines are usually taken by mouth, but can be given by IV or IM injection.

Undesirable effects: The main undesirable effect of tetracycline, one that's known to those CF patients in their 30s and older, is that if it's given to people between the ages of approximately 4 months and 8 years, it can permanently stain their teeth a grayish/brownish/yellow color. Twenty years ago, physicians knew about the tooth problem, but often didn't have any other antibiotics to give, so they had to use a tetracycline. Fortunately, today there usually is another antibiotic available, and tetracycline should almost never be used in young children. Other side effects include allergic reactions, intestinal upset, and a rash that is made worse by being exposed to the sun.

Quinolones

This family of antibiotics has some activity against *Pseudomonas* organisms in the lung, even when the drugs (especially ciprofloxacin) are taken by mouth.

How taken: Several of these medications can be taken by mouth.

Undesirable effects: Remarkably few side effects have been recognized with these antibiotics. To date, intestinal upset has been seen occasionally. Another problem seems to be that bacteria become resistant to the quinolones very soon after the patient starts to take them (within a week or two). Young animals given these drugs have developed some problems with the cartilage in their joints, so most physicians are reluctant to prescribe the drugs for young children. These drugs may also cause a skin rash with sun exposure.

Imipenem and Meropenem

These drugs have activity against *Pseudomonas*, *Staph*, and *Haemophilus* organisms and seem relatively safe and effective.

How taken: These drugs are given by IV.

Undesirable effects: *Imipenem* can make the vein tender, and may cause nausea, particularly while it is running in; meropenem seems less likely to do either.

Aztreonam

This drug is one with some anti-*Pseudomonas* activity; it seems to be safe and effective.

How taken: Aztreonam is taken by IV injection.

Undesirable effects: The side effects of this drug have been few and not very serious. They have included diarrhea, nausea, allergic reactions, and tenderness at the site of injection.

Antiviral Medications

Although antibiotics do not kill viruses, a few drugs do.

Amantadine and Rimantadine

These drugs are used to treat or prevent influenza, especially in someone who has not received the flu vaccine (especially those who can't receive the flu vaccine because of severe egg allergy).

How taken: These are both taken by mouth, starting (for treatment) immediately after influenza has been diagnosed, or (for prevention) throughout the flu season.

Undesirable effects: These medicines are generally well tolerated.

Drugs for Respiratory Syncytial Virus

Respiratory syncytial virus (RSV) is a common respiratory virus that can cause severe disease, especially in infants with underlying lung problems. Three main drugs have been used: two for prevention, one for treatment; and none has been overwhelmingly successful.

Palivizumab (Synagis). Palivizumab (Synagis) has been used to prevent RSV in sick tiny infants. It has been used in CF, but its benefit has not been proven.

How taken: This drug is given by IM injection once a month for the whole influenza season

Undesirable effects: Although the drug is usually well tolerated, there can be local reactions at the site of injection, "cold" symptoms, rash, diarrhea, or vomiting.

Respigam. Respigam (RSV immune globulin) is also given to prevent RSV.

How taken: This drug is given by IV infusion once a month for the whole influenza season.

Undesirable effects: There can be allergic reactions, wheezing, dizziness, rash.

Ribavirin. Ribavirin has been used to treat RSV pneumonia.

How taken: This drug is given by aerosol. The treatments last 12 to 18 hours each day.

Undesirable effects: Wheezing and shortness of breath can occur, and it is difficult to administer the aerosols for as long as they need to be given each day. The tubing used to deliver the medicine often clogs.

Antifungal Medicine

There is usually not much call for antifungal medicines in patients with CF, but in the case of ABPA (allergic bronchopulmonary aspergillosis), killing some of the *Aspergillus* organisms can help decrease the allergic reaction to these fungi. One medicine that has become available for this task is *itraconazole* (*Sporanox*).

How taken: itraconazole is usually taken by mouth. In rare cases, it can be given IV.

Undesirable effects: This drug is usually well tolerated, but can have a long list of side effects, including fatigue, fever, itchiness, abdominal pain, and liver damage.

Bronchodilators ("Asthma Medicines")

Some people with CF also have asthma, or a condition like asthma, where the bronchi can become partly blocked for a time when the bronchial lining becomes inflamed and swollen and the muscles surrounding the bronchi squeeze down. Bronchodilators are medicines that open (dilate) the bronchi by relaxing the muscles around them. The medicines are effective in treating bronchospasm once it starts and help to prevent it from occurring. Some of these drugs can be taken by inhalation, some by injection (either IM, IV, or under the skin), some by mouth, and some by several different methods. Bronchodilators seem to help some people with CF, while not being effective in others.

Beta-Agonists

This is the name applied to a class of very helpful bronchodilators, including albuterol (that's what it's called in the United States; it's called salbutamol in the rest of the world) and others. Levalbuterol (Xopenex) is newer preparation of albuterol, very heavily marketed, that is not needed for most patients, but may decrease side effects in those few patients who do have trouble tolerating albuterol.

How taken: These drugs are best taken by inhalation (either from a hand-held canister-type nebulizer—usually called *a metered-dose inhaler*, or just MDI—or from the air-compressor type of aerosol machine). They can also be taken by injection or by mouth (pills or liquids), although the beneficial effects tend to be less and the side effects more than if they are used by inhalation.

Undesirable effects: The three main undesirable effects of this class of drugs are (a) shakiness, which often goes away with continued use of the drugs; (b) overactiveness (getting "hyper"), a fairly uncommon side effect; and (c) stimulation of the heart, causing it to speed up, which can be somewhat annoying. It may also cause an irregular heartbeat, which can be dangerous. Dangerous effects are uncommon if the drugs are taken by mouth or by inhalation. In the 1960s, a number of deaths were reported in patients with asthma who used their handheld nebulizers of beta-agonists too much. It's not clear what caused these deaths, but there are two likely reasons: It may have been the chemical used to make the aerosol, and not the bronchodilator itself, or, it may have been that patients got such good relief from the inhalations that they didn't see their doctor for a very serious asthma attack, but instead kept puffing on their aerosols, even when the effect lasted a shorter and shorter time. When they finally did try to go for help, they were too sick. Today, the vehicle for delivering the aerosol is safer. However, there is still a danger if a patient with asthma or CF tries home-prescribed antibiotics, bronchodilators, and so forth. While they may seem to work at first, they can lead to serious consequences. Talk to your doctors about medicine changes, in order to avoid dangerous combinations or dosages and to avoid overlooking a serious problem for which you should be seen.

Theophyllines

This family of bronchodilators is a large one that is used much less frequently now they were before good inhalational bronchodilators were available. There may be some confusion dealing with dosages and preparations, since almost every drug company has its own version of theophylline, with a similar name but different dosage. In addition, people process theophyllines at different speeds. In one person, 100 mg may reach a good level in the bloodstream and stay there for a long time, while in another, it may give only a low level and be gone quickly. For this reason, doctors often like to check a blood level of theophylline, to see if someone needs more or less than the average to reach a level in the bloodstream that is effective and safe.

Some theophyllines are short acting and are eliminated from the body quickly. Others are released slowly and stay in the body longer. The short-acting theophyllines usually need to be given four times a day (about every 6 hours), while the slow-release or sustained-release kind can be given three times a day (every 8 hours) or even (especially for older children, adolescents, and adults) twice a day, and still keep a good blood level for many hours.

How given: Theophylline can be given in the vein ("aminophylline"), or by mouth as a liquid, tablet, or capsule. There are preparations that can be given rectally, like an enema. Usually the rectal kind is not as safe, since it's harder to predict just how much will be absorbed into the bloodstream.

Undesirable effects: There are two main side effects: Some people get stomach upset with this family of medicines, and may lose their appetite, or even vomit. Nausea or vomiting can be important signs that the person is getting too much theophylline. People with CF may be more likely than other people to have this stomach upset with theophyllines. Some children also become agitated or overactive when they get too much of this drug. These side effects are quite common. However, if the drug is started (or restarted) at a very low dosage and then raised very slowly, most people will be able to tolerate relatively high levels of the drug. A very large overdose can cause seizures (convulsions), a danger that, fortunately, is rare.

Antiinflammatory Medications

Steroids

Steroids, also called "corticosteroids," are cortisone-like drugs whose name strikes fear in the hearts of many people because of the serious side effects caused by improper use. Actually, steroids can be extremely useful and very safe if used properly. In fact, everyone's body makes these drugs themselves and they are extremely important in maintaining health. They are very potent agents for decreasing inflammation and swelling within the bronchi (and else-where). In asthma, they also seem to increase the sensitivity of the body to the effects of the beta-agonist drugs. The inhaled, nonabsorbed steroids have become the "front-line" treatment around the world for people with asthma. It's not yet clear if they will also be helpful for people with CF, but early reports are encouraging.

How taken: Steroids can be taken by mouth (pills or liquid), by IV injection, or by inhalation. The inhaled steroids, budesonide, fluticasone, beclomethasone, triamcinolone, and others, affect the bronchi by *preventing* inflammation and bronchoconstriction, much more than by reversing inflammation and bron-choconstriction once they've started. Almost none of the inhaled steroid is absorbed into the bloodstream, so it has very little toxic effect on the rest of the body. There are many different schedules for taking steroids. They can be given several times a day, once a day, or once every other day. They can be given for a brief period—a 3- to 5-day "burst"—or for months. The schedule depends on the drug being used, what it is being used for, and the characteristics and needs of the person taking it.

Undesirable effects: There are many possible effects including greatly increased appetite and swelling ("chipmunk cheeks"), acne, slowed growth in height, increased possibility of developing diabetes, eye cataracts, bone brit-tleness, and difficulty in fighting infection. In general, the lower the dose and the shorter the length of time steroids are given the less likely one is to develop side effects. When these drugs are used by mouth or injection for longer than a week, the body begins to detect them and seem to say, "Well, we don't need to make any more of our own." If the drug is then stopped abruptly, the body is left without the protection of its own steroids. For this reason, if steroids are required for more than a week or two, you can't suddenly just stop the drug; instead, you need to reduce (taper) the amount you take over several days or even weeks (depending on how long you've been on them, and how used your body has become to receiving them from an outside source) so that your body gradually gets used to the idea of having to make steroids on its own again. If the drugs are used for less than a week (or even two), they can be stopped abruptly with an extremely small likelihood of side effects. Another way to get around most of the side effects is to take the drugs every other day. This gives the body a day to recover between doses. In some cases, when steroids are really needed, a patient may not be able to tolerate being off them for that in-between day. The inhaled steroids have very few side effects. One is the devel-opment of yeast infection in the mouth. This can be avoided by gargling, or even just brushing your teeth, after each dose. Some studies have shown a slowing of height growth in children taking inhaled steroids over a long time, but even in those studies, the children's eventual height is *not* affected. The *rare* child on inhaled steroids shows the same side effects that long-term oral or injected steroids cause.

Cromolyn and Nedocromil

These drugs don't actually relax the muscles around the bronchi, but may be very effective in preventing certain bronchoconstricting chemicals from being released in the body. They seem to help about 60% of patients with asthma or asthma-like conditions. There is no way of telling which patients will be helped by them, except by trying.

How taken: These drugs are almost always taken by inhalation, either from a liquid aerosolized in a regular air compressor/nebulizer, or—most commonly—from a handheld metered-dose inhaler.

Undesirable effects: A few patients may have some bronchial irritation from these medicines if they are inhaled in the powdered form. Otherwise, they are unlikely to cause any trouble.

Leukotriene Inhibitors

Leukotrienes are chemicals that are important in the cascade of reactions that cause inflammation. A whole class of drugs has been developed that interfere with the actions of various leukotrienes, including montelukast and montelukast.

How taken. These drugs are taken by mouth.

Undesirable effects. Headache is relatively common in patients taking these drugs.

Mucolytics

Lysis means destruction or decomposition of a substance, so *muco*lytics are drugs that destroy or break down mucus. Since much of the lung trouble in CF has to do with extra thick mucus, a completely safe and completely effective mucolytic for the lung would be wonderful. There isn't such a drug now. However, one comes closer than anything previously available. When one drug, DNase (Pulmozyme) is put in a glass test tube with CF lung mucus, it breaks down the mucus, making it much more watery, and easier to move. It seems to help some patients, and even has improved lung function in several hundred patients over a period lasting 6 months. Other patients have not had measurable improvements in pulmonary function, but have felt better. Very few patients are harmed by it. Not everyone with CF is helped by it, and it is impossible to predict who will benefit. This difficulty in predicting response goes both ways. That is, you might expect it to help only those patients who are clearly bothered by a lot of thick mucus. And, it does help many patients like that. But, it also helps improve pulmonary function in some patients whose lungs are in quite good shape, without lots of extrathick mucus. It is extremely expensive ($12,000 per year).

How taken: This drug is always given by inhalation.

Undesirable effects: A very few patients with very severe lung disease and a large amount of thick mucus may have trouble handling that mucus if it is suddenly all liquefied at once. This is uncommon.

Mucomyst (Acetylcysteine)

This is another mucolytic, one that's been in use for decades. Like DNase, it is highly effective in breaking down CF mucus, in the test tube. Unlike DNase, it seems to have adverse effects on a number of patients. In many people, this drug causes bronchial irritation with production of more mucus. In others, it causes bronchospasm. Some physicians prescribe an aerosolized bronchodilator along with Mucomyst to try to prevent bronchospasm. Mucomyst smells like rotten eggs and is expensive.

Oxygen

Most people with CF don't need any more oxygen than the amount that is in the regular air around us. Air is 21% oxygen, and at sea level, this generally provides plenty of oxygen for most people's bodies. If the lungs are severely affected by disease, or when someone is at high altitude—including in a commercial airliner, whose cabins are pressurized to be like an altitude of 5,000 to 8,000 ft—or when someone with moderate lung disease is exercising, it may be difficult for enough oxygen to enter the bloodstream. In these cases, people can breathe extra oxygen—air with 25%, 30%, 40%, or more oxygen. When someone's blood oxygen level is very low, it is remarkable how much better a little extra oxygen can make him or her feel.

How taken: This drug is always taken by inhalation (but you knew that). Oxygen can be kept in metal cylinders of different sizes. Small "B-cylinders" are about 3½ inches across and 16 inches high, and weigh about 6 lb when full. If someone is using 5 liters (L) per minute (see below), these cylinders last 44 minutes. Other cylinders are shown in Table B.1.

Cylinder	Time (at 5 L/Min)	Size (Inches)	Weight, lb (Full)
B	44 min	3 ½ × 16	6
D	70 min	4 ¼ × 20	10
E	2 h	4 ¼ × 30	14
M	11 h	7 ⅛ × 46	82
G	17 h	9 × 51	127
K	23 h	9 × 55	150

Oxygen can also be stored in liquid form. Liquid oxygen tanks hold much more oxygen in the same space than oxygen gas. Different-sized tanks of liquid oxygen are also available (Table B.2).

Cylinder	Time (at 5 L/Min)	Size (Inches)	Weight, lb (Full)
Stroller	3 ½ h	3 ½ oval	9.5
L-30	86 h	12 × 35	120

One other way of giving extra oxygen in the home is with an oxygen extractor or concentrator, which takes in regular room air and gets rid of the parts of air that are not oxygen (mostly nitrogen), resulting in almost pure oxygen. This method is expensive, and the machines are bulky and somewhat noisy, but for someone who needs oxygen much of the time, it may be cheaper and more convenient than using many small tanks.

Just how much extra oxygen you breathe depends on how the oxygen gets from the tank to your lungs. The main methods are mask and nasal cannula. The mask takes the pure oxygen from the tank and mixes it with varying amounts of room air to deliver 25%, 30%, 35%, 50%, or even 100% oxygen. Nasal cannulas, which consist of a flexible plastic tube with two short plastic prongs at the end that stick a short way into the nostrils, can deliver different amounts depending on how high you set the flow of oxygen from the tanks: for every liter per minute of oxygen flow, you add about 3% to 4% oxygen above room air. That means that if the flow is set at 4 L per minute, you get $4 \times 3 = 12\%$ or so above room air (room air has 21% oxygen), or $12 + 21 = 33\%$ oxygen. There are some newer methods that some adults are finding more convenient and less noticeable to other people than the old methods. These include nasal cannulas that come through eyeglasses (and therefore have just a little bit of tubing sticking out the end of the eyeglass nosepiece), and oxygen through a tiny tracheostomy (a small hole placed surgically in the neck; this way, the tubing can go under the clothes, and the tracheostomy itself can be hidden under a turtleneck or scarf). Other methods include oxygen tents, which surround the whole upper body; oxygen hoods, which surround the whole head; and single nasal tubes (with one thin tube going into the nostril). Most of these last methods are useful mainly for babies, and therefore are not used very much in CF, since babies with CF usually don't need extra oxygen.

Amount needed: Your doctor may want to do a "blood gas" or check a "pulseox" to see how much oxygen you have in your blood before he or she decides whether you need extra oxygen. The blood gas test involves taking blood from an artery (usually the radial artery, at the wrist), and is therefore somewhat more painful than most blood tests, which are usually taken from a vein (closer to the skin surface than arteries). However, if some lidocaine or other local anesthetic—like EMLA cream—is used, this is not a painful test, and it can be very important. The pulseox is a less painful (and slightly less informative) test you've probably had done when you've done pulmonary function tests (PFTs). This shines light through the finger and the computer calculates your blood oxygen level. To understand how much extra oxygen is needed, you have to understand how the brain directs breathing. This is discussed in Chapter 3, *The Respiratory System*.

Undesirable effects: The main danger of oxygen is giving so much that it turns off the signal to breathe. Oxygen is also very dry, even when it's been humidified (as it should always be before it's breathed), and can make the mouth and nose uncomfortably dry. Too much oxygen can be toxic to lung tissue (this is not a problem with less than 40% oxygen). The problem you might have heard of concerning eye damage from oxygen is true only in premature babies.

Addiction: Some people worry that once they start on oxygen they'll become addicted in the way that someone gets addicted to morphine or heroin. This does not happen. People whose lungs are bad enough that they need extra oxygen feel much better when they take that oxygen, and they won't want to stop taking it while their lungs are still in that condition. But if the lung disease improves, and extra oxygen is not needed any more, people don't continue to desire the extra oxygen because the body is now supplying it. If the lungs cannot improve, the person will continue to want to use the oxygen, but this is not an addiction.

Other worries about oxygen. Some people worry that needing oxygen is a bad sign—"the beginning of the end," or some such. It certainly does indicate that someone's lungs are in worse shape, but many people need oxygen for a few days or weeks, and then are able to get back to doing well without extra oxygen.

Cough Medicines

There are two main kinds of medicines that usually are referred to as "cough medicines." One of these is the *expectorants*. Expectorants are intended to make it easier to bring up mucus from the lungs. This is a good idea, but unfortunately, these drugs don't work. The other kind of cough medicine is the *cough suppressant*, that is, a drug that controls the cough center in the brain, and says, "don't cough, no matter what is in the lungs that needs to come up." This is usually a terrible idea, especially for someone with CF. Some drug preparations are available that combine these two types of cough medicine, which have opposite goals! In most cases, including most patients with CF, cough is an important defense mechanism that keeps the lungs clear of substances that shouldn't be there. Cough is a sign that something is wrong, but efforts should be directed at what is wrong. If someone is coughing because of bronchospasm, a bronchodilator will relieve the bronchospasm, and thus stop the cough; in a sense, it is a good kind of cough medicine. Similarly, if someone with CF is coughing because infection in the bronchi has gotten out of control, antibiotics are probably needed; they may control the infection and thus stop the cough. Other kinds of cough medicines are rarely useful.

Upper Airway

Polyp Medicines

Many people with CF have nasal polyps, which are growths of extra tissue (not cancer) in the nose. Usually these cause no problems except mild stuffiness, but they can get large enough to be seen at the end of the nose or block one side of the nose so you can't breathe through it. A few medicines have been used to shrink polyps, and some people believe that they work. These medicines include antihistamines, decongestants (like Neo-Synephrine), and steroid sprays (like Rhinocort, Nasalide, and Nasonex). A person with nasal allergy symptoms may also be helped by some of these same nasal sprays.

Sinus Medicines

On radiologic (x-ray) examination, most patients with CF appear to have abnormal sinuses. Usually this bothers the radiologist more than it bothers the patient. Sometimes the patient may have symptoms from inflammation in the sinuses, in which case the nasal steroids mentioned above under "Polyp Medicines" can help. Occasionally, there can be actual sinus infection (sinusitis), which may be a nuisance to the patient. In these cases, doctors may prescribe antibiotics and/or a decongestant.

Allergy Medicines

Allergies can cause problems with the upper respiratory system (stuffy, sneezy nose) or lungs (congestion, wheezing) or both. Patients with CF are somewhat more likely to have allergies than are people without CF. It is often very difficult to tell if an upper or lower airway problem is caused by infection or by allergy. Complicating the matter is that either one can probably make the other worse, so that constriction of the bronchi from a pollen allergy will make it harder to clear mucus from the bronchi and make it easier for infection to get out of control.

Antihistamines

Histamine is a chemical that is released from white blood cells in response to different things including irritation and allergy. Its release can cause many of the problems we associate with allergies: runny nose, itchy nose, constricted bronchi, hives. Antihistamines do not stop the release of histamine from the blood cells, but they do help to block its action in the nose, skin, and so forth.

How taken: These are most commonly taken by mouth but can be given by injection.

Undesirable effects: The most common and often the most troublesome side effect from these drugs is drowsiness. They can also cause a dry mouth. At least one antihistamine, cyproheptadine (Periactin) can cause an increased appetite. This can be good in some people with CF.

Decongestants

These drugs are supposed to make the nose less stuffy. Although they are used by millions of people, there is not very much scientific evidence that they work.

Some decongestant nasal sprays can temporarily open blocked nostrils. If they are used for more than a few days, they can cause "rebound" inflammation and blockage of the nose that is just as bad as the inflammation the cold caused.

Allergy Shots

This is a very controversial topic. Most pulmonary specialists believe that allergy shots may be helpful for nasal allergies but not for bronchial allergies (asthma), while many allergists believe that they sometimes can be helpful for asthma too. There is nothing about CF that makes someone more or less likely to respond well to allergy shots than anyone else.

THE HEART

The heart is not directly affected by CF, and most people with CF have very good hearts. Therefore, there usually is no need for heart medications. However, if someone's lungs become badly diseased (from CF or any other cause), the heart may not be able to pump all the necessary fluid through the diseased lungs. When this happens, two types of medicines are sometimes used: diuretics and digitalis.

Diuretics

These drugs help the kidneys get rid of extra fluid that may have built up in the body because of the heart's inability to pump all of the fluid. Most doctors agree that when someone has heart failure because of severe lung disease, it is very important to cut down on the amount of fluid that the heart is asked to pump. This is accomplished through restricting the amount of salt and fluid consumed and through careful use of diuretic medicines.

Furosemide

How taken: Furosemide (Lasix) can be taken by mouth (tablet, liquid) or by injection (either IM or IV).

Undesirable effects: Furosemide causes the body to lose potassium in addition to other salts and this can upset the body's salt balance if used in high doses every day for too long. This effect can be lessened by an every-other-day schedule in people who tolerate this schedule. The drug can also do too much of a good thing—in eliminating too much excess fluid, it may actually dehydrate the patient. Furosemide has been associated with some cases of hearing problems, which are usually reversible. Occasionally, someone who is allergic to sulfa drugs may be allergic to furosemide.

Spironolactone (Aldactone)

This drug is less powerful than furosemide, but keeps the body from losing potassium.

How taken: Oral tablets.

Undesirable effects: Any diuretic may cause excess loss of water (dehydration) and salt balance problems. Spironolactone may also give some gastrointestinal (GI) upset. A rash is sometimes seen. It may cause breast enlargement and/or impotence in men. These effects are nearly always temporary and disappear when the drug is stopped.

Thiazides

How taken: These diuretics are usually taken by mouth (tablet; although a liquid preparation is also available). Rarely, they may be given by IV, but not by IM injection.

Undesirable effects: These are quite safe and usually there are no problems. Textbooks do list many possible reactions, including GI upset, dizziness, fatigue, headache, anemia, weakness, muscle spasms, and gout.

Digitalis

This drug has been known for centuries and is very effective in making the heart contractions stronger. It is not clear whether it is helpful in people whose heart problems are mainly caused by lung problems.

How taken: Digitalis preparations can be taken by mouth (tablets or liquids) or by IV injection.

Undesirable effects: Too much digitalis can be very dangerous and can cause heart beat irregularities, confusion, visual problems, vomiting, diarrhea, headache, and weakness.

GASTROINTESTINAL AND DIGESTIVE SYSTEM MEDICATIONS

The main problem in the GI and digestive system is the thick mucus that blocks the ducts of the pancreas and prevents the digestive chemicals (enzymes) from reaching the intestines where they mix with the food that has been eaten. If these digestive enzymes are not available, the food cannot be digested, that is, broken down into particles small enough to be soaked up into the bloodstream through the wall of the intestine. As a result, a lot of the food (especially the fat) will not be available to the body and will pass out into the stools. Most (but not all) patients with CF have this problem. Another GI problem is that the intestines' own mucus is very thick, which can sometimes lead to blockage of the intestines.

Digestive Enzymes

These enzymes come from the pancreas of animals. They have changed what used to be a serious, even fatal, problem into a nuisance problem. With enzyme type and dosage properly adjusted, most patients with CF are able to absorb most of what they eat (even the fat). Thus, they are able to get the nutritional value from the food that would be lost without the enzymes. Enzymes are discussed fully in Chapter 6, *Nutrition*.

Antacid Drugs

Excess stomach acid can cause several different types of problems in anyone, and at least one additional problem if someone has CF. Too much acid interferes with the activity of digestive enzyme medicines. The way this happens is that the stomach acid may spill over into the small intestine, preventing the coating around each enzyme bead to dissolve where and when it's supposed to, in the duodenum.

Too much acid can also help cause ulcers. Occasionally, the stomach acid can reflux (go backward) up into the esophagus causing heartburn (the burning discomfort felt when the esophagus becomes irritated from acid). Drugs that prevent the stomach from making too much acid, or drugs that neutralize the acid once it is made, may be helpful for any of these problems. There are two main kinds of drugs that prevent the stomach from making too much acid, histamine-2 (H_2) *blockers* and *proton pump inhibitors*.

Histamine-2 Blockers

In addition to playing an important (and nasty) role in allergic reactions, histamine also plays a role (sometimes nasty) in the production of stomach acid. One class of medications, the H_2 *blockers*, can help prevent this part of what histamine does.

Cimetidine

Cimetidine (Tagamet) is one of the most prescribed drugs in the world, largely because it is very effective in decreasing the production of stomach acid.

How taken: Cimetidine is almost always taken by mouth, in a tablet or liquid form, usually before meals and before bed.

Undesirable effects: This is a very safe drug. Mild diarrhea, headache, or swelling of breasts have been seen in people taking cimetidine, but none of these problems is common.

Ranitidine

Ranitidine (Zantac) is a close relative of cimetidine and has largely taken over from cimetidine on the international hit list for popular drugs. It can be taken at a lower dosage, less frequently, with comparable effects to cimetidine.

Famotidine

Famotidine (Pepcid) is yet another H_2 blocker antacid.

How taken: Famotidine is also taken by mouth.

Undesirable effects: This is also a safe drug, with side effects similar to the others in its class.

Proton Pump Inhibitors

An important step in acid production depends on a pump in the cell membrane of acid-secreting cells. Drugs that slow down or stop this pump are called *proton pump inhibitors* (PPIs) and are among the most potent acid blockers known. Proton pump inhibitors include *omeprazole* (Prilosec), *lansoprazole* (Prevacid), and *esomeprazole* (Nexium).

How taken: These drugs are taken by mouth.

Undesirable effects: These are safe drugs. Mild diarrhea and headache occur in some people taking them.

Various Antacids

These medicines, taken by mouth as chewable tablets or the more effective liquid form, do not influence how much acid is produced by the stomach, but they can neutralize the acid once it's formed. They include Maalox, Mylanta, and Tums.

Antireflux Drugs

Several drugs may be helpful for patients with gastroesophageal reflux. Antacid treatment is usually used, and even if it doesn't decrease the amount of fluid that refluxes from the stomach into the esophagus, the fluid that does reach the esophagus will be less acidic, and therefore probably less damaging. A few drugs may actually decrease the amount of fluid that refluxes.

Metoclopramide (Reglan)

This drug may help reduce gastroesophageal reflux by two of its effects: It strengthens the grip of the muscle at the bottom of the esophagus, and it increases the speed with which the esophagus and stomach empty, leaving less there to back up into the esophagus.

How taken: Metoclopramide is taken by mouth

Undesirable effects: This drug can cause diarrhea. Its most worrisome side effect is that it can cause abnormal movement of the face and tongue. If the medicine is not stopped when this symptom appears, it can become permanent.

Erythromycin

Erythromycin, one of the macrolide antibiotics, increases the motility of the stomach, helping it to empty more quickly. An empty stomach has less fluid available to reflux.

How taken: Erythromycin is taken by mouth.

Undesirable effects: Too much erythromycin can cause abdominal cramping.

Anticonstipation Medicines

Constipation is seldom a problem in patients with CF, but it does occur occasionally. Failure to pass any stool can be an important sign of a dangerous intestinal obstruction called meconium ileus in a newborn infant and DIOS (distal intestinal obstruction syndrome) in someone older.

Enzymes

Before more drastic measures are undertaken, it usually helps to make sure the digestive enzyme dosage is appropriate, since very bulky, poorly digested stools may make blockage more likely.

Dietary Fiber

Someone who has difficulty passing bowel movements may benefit from increasing the amount of fiber in the diet. Foods high in fiber include fruits and some vegetables; bran is an especially good source of fiber. Breakfast cereals with bran should have at least 4 grams (g) of dietary fiber per serving to be effective (this information is included on the side panel of the cereal box; if the information isn't there, it's likely that there is very little fiber in the cereal).

Mineral Oil

On some occasions, a physician may prescribe oral mineral oil to help pass stools.

Bowel Stimulants

If someone is not completely blocked up, some medications that stimulate intestinal contractions may help the bowels to empty. Senna (Senekot) is one such laxative.

Enemas

With more blockage, enemas may be needed to help wash out the lower intestines. Generally, several types of enemas can be used in different situations. Always check with your doctor to be sure it's safe to use an enema, and to find out which kind.

Gastrografin Enemas

Severe intestinal obstruction is a serious matter that used to be treatable only with surgery. Fortunately, many cases can be treated in the hospital with special enemas. Gastrografin (and several similar products) is a substance that can be used for an enema and has several useful properties. It shows up on radiographs, so the radiologist can see the outline of the bowel to make sure there is not another problem causing intestinal blockage and to ensure the enema is going far up into the intestines so that it will work. It's very slippery, allowing it to slip by the blockage. It also acts like a sponge, pulling in lots of fluid from the rest of the body to help make the stools stuck in the bowel become more watery and easier to move out.

How performed: These enemas always must be done where there is x-ray equipment and a radiologist. This usually means they are done in the hospital. Most children who need them are sick enough to need to be in the hospital anyway.

Undesirable effects: These enemas are somewhat uncomfortable, as is true of any enema, but they can provide prompt relief from the abdominal pain from intestinal blockage. The main danger of this procedure is that so much fluid is pulled into the bowel from the rest of the body that the patient can become dehydrated. For this reason, most doctors will not perform this procedure on an infant unless the baby has an IV line in place, with fluids running in.

Miscellaneous

1. Miralax (polyethylene glycol): A powder that can be mixed with any liquid and then drunk. It works very well to "flush out" the intestines.
2. Lactulose (Cefulac, Chronulac): Medicines taken by mouth that pull fluid into the intestines to help make the bowel contents more watery and easier to move.

3. Golytely: A salty liquid that can be drunk in large quantities to "flush out" the intestines.
4. Colace: A stool softener.

Antibloating Medications

Some patients with CF have trouble with abdominal bloating. This may be caused by the thick mucus in the intestines, which can surround little air bubbles and does not let the little bubbles get together to make a single bubble that is big enough for a burp. Some drugs containing simethicone (Mylicon, Silain) may help dissolve some of that mucus and allow a gentle upward or downward explosion of that air, relieving the pressure and discomfort. These drugs are taken by mouth (tablets or drops) and are very safe.

Liver Medications

Ursodiol (Actigal), also referred to as ursodeoxycholic acid, is a bile acid that seems to help liquefy the secretions that otherwise block the smallest ducts within the liver and gallbladder. It is taken by mouth and is very safe. Usually, patients with CF liver disease may need to take more vitamins than usual.

Vitamins

These are not really drugs and should be a regular part of the diet. Four vitamins (A, D, E, K) are "fat-soluble," meaning that they dissolve in fat and are only absorbed in the body when fats are absorbed. Thus, patients who have trouble absorbing fats may have low levels of these vitamins. For this reason, most nutrition experts agree that patients with CF should probably receive supplements of these vitamins, at least some of the time. Vitamin D can probably be supplied from regular multivitamin preparations, but vitamin K, vitamin A, and vitamin E need to be taken separately. Your physician may periodically check your blood levels of the various vitamins. Some people feel quite well, and yet are deficient in several vitamins. For the vitamin E, most preparations you can buy will not work for someone who has trouble absorbing fats, and a form that is partly dissolvable in water needs to be used.

Growth and Appetite Stimulants and Supplements

Hormones

Most of the drugs used to stimulate appetite and growth are anabolic steroids and androgens (male hormones). They are used with increasing frequency, but have not been conclusively shown to be safe or effective in patients with CF. These medications include *growth hormone*, *testosterone*, and *megestrol* (*Megace*), actually a female hormone.

How taken: These hormones can be given by injection (mostly) or (some) taken by mouth.

Undesirable effects: Although the experience with growth hormone and megestrol seems much more benign than the other hormones (mostly the male hormones), it is too early to say with certainty that they are safe and effective. The complications of the male hormones are too numerous to list completely, are worrisome, and can actually result in stopping growth sooner than it would have stopped naturally (as these hormones increase bone growth, they also close the growth plate of the bones—the part of the bones where growth takes place—more quickly than normal). Other undesirable effects include fluid retention, hirsutism (increased hairiness), baldness, various genital disturbances (too big, too little, too excitable, not excitable enough), acne, sleeplessness, liver disease, nausea, ulcer-like symptoms, and finally, disqualification from the Olympics.

Diet Supplements

Many different kinds of diet supplements are available, from vanilla milk shakes and ice cream sundaes to expensive "elemental" (predigested) formulas. These are discussed in Chapter 6, *Nutrition*. These supplements usually have high calorie contents. They seem to be helpful in some people, whereas in others, the number of calories taken in with the supplements is balanced by the number of calories not eaten in the regular meals. High-calorie recipes (of regular food) can be found in Appendix D of this book. Some CF programs have been successful in helping patients gain weight and height by running nighttime feedings of these dietary supplements through a stomach tube while the patients sleep. Such a program, of course, should never be undertaken without your doctor's knowledge and cooperation.

How taken: Some of these can be sprinkled on top of regular meals; some can be eaten between meals. Others are designed to be given through a tube (mostly because they taste so bad, but also because they can be given very slowly while the patient sleeps).

Undesirable effects: The supplements may interfere with normal mealtime appetite. The tube feedings require a tube, which can be somewhat uncomfortable and/or inconvenient. Several tubes can be used, including a nasogastric tube, which goes through the nose ("naso-") into the stomach ("gastric"), and is usually put in each evening and removed in the morning. Another kind of tube is a permanent tube placed by a surgical operation that makes a hole or stoma in the wall of the abdomen directly into the stomach (a gastrostomy tube) or into the second part of the small intestine, the jejunum (a feeding jejunostomy tube). Possible problems from these nighttime feedings include overfilling the stomach.

TRANSPLANT-RELATED DRUGS

Antirejection Drugs

Steroids

(See "Antiinflammatory Medications," page 318, for more on steroids.) Steroids decrease inflammation, and they are important tools in preventing and fighting acute rejection (see Chapter 8, *Transplantation*).

Antilymphocyte Drugs

Lymphocytes are the white blood cells most responsible for rejection, so specific antilymphocyte drugs have been sought: If you decrease the rejection caused by the lymphocytes without interfering with other white blood cells trying to fight infection, that would be ideal.

Cyclosporine

This is the first very successful antilymphocyte drug used to help treat and prevent rejection.

How taken: This drug can be taken IV or by mouth.

Undesirable effects: This drug can cause high blood pressure, kidney damage, seizures, shakiness, hairiness, and excessive growth of the gums. Too much may lead to infection.

Tacrolimus (FK-506)

This drug is similar to cyclosporine, but may be a bit more effective.

How taken: This drug can be taken IV or by mouth.

Undesirable effects: This drug can cause high blood pressure, kidney damage, seizures, shakiness, hairiness, and headache. Too much may lead to infection.

Sirolimus

This drug is similar to tacrolimus, but is available only in oral form.

Antithymocyte Globulin

Antithymocyte globulin (ATG) is an antibody made by horses and directed against human lymphocytes.

How taken: This drug is given by IV.

Undesirable effects: The drug can cause fever and "flu"-like symptoms, including headache.

OKT3

This is a "bioengineered" antilymphocyte drug.

How taken: This drug is given IV.

Undesirable effects: The drug can cause fever and "flu-like" symptoms, including headache.

"Antimetabolites"

These drugs interfere with the body's ability to make white blood cells, so there are fewer cells around to reject an organ. (Of course, that also means there are fewer white blood cells to fight infection.)

Azothioprine (Imuran).

How taken: This drug can be given IV or by mouth.

Undesirable effects: The main side effect is too much of its desired effect, that is, the white blood cell count getting too low and therefore the body not being able to fight off infection. The platelet count may also go too low, and—since platelets are needed for proper clotting of blood—there can be abnormal bleeding.

Mycophenolate mofetil (CellCept)

This drug interferes with DNA production. It is taken orally, and has the same undesirable effects as Azothioprine.

GLOSSARY OF DRUGS

This glossary is a partial list of drugs that can be found under both their generic and trade names. Drugs that are discussed in this appendix contain references to the appropriate section. For example, Pen-Vee K is a form of the antibiotic penicillin, which is discussed under *Lungs: Antibiotics: Penicillins*.

Accolate (zafirlukast). A leukotriene-inhibitor antiinflammatory drug.

acetylcysteine A mucolytic (see page 321).

Actifed (triprolidine hydrochloride + pseudoephedrine hydrochloride). A decongestant/antihistamine combination (see page 324).

Actigal (ursodeoxycholic acid). A bile salt used to treat CF liver disease (see page 331).

acyclovir An antiviral drug.

ABDEK A multivitamin that includes vitamins A, D, E, and K.

ADEK A multivitamin that includes vitamins A, D, E, and K.

Adrenalin (epinephrine). A bronchodilator (see page 316).

Advair An inhaled combination of fluticasone (a steroid) and salmeterol, a long-acting bronchodilator).

Aerobid An inhaled steroid (see page 318).

Afrin (oxymetazoline hydrochloride). A decongestant (see page 324).

albuterol A beta-agonist bronchodilator (see page 317).

Aldactone (spironolactone). A diuretic (see page 326).

Allerest A decongestant/antihistamine (see page 324).

Alupent A beta-agonist bronchodilator (see page 317).

amantadine A medication that can help control infection with the influenza virus.

Amcill (ampicillin). An antibiotic (see page 309).

amikacin sulfate An aminoglycoside antibiotic (see page 312).

Amikin Amikacin sulfate, an aminoglycoside (see page 312).

aminophylline A theophylline bronchodilator (see page 318).

amoxicillin An antibiotic (see page 311).

Amoxil Amoxicillin (see page 311).

Amphojel (aluminum hydroxide gel). An antacid.

amphotericin A drug used to fight infection caused by fungi.

ampicillin An antibiotic. (see page 311).

Ancef (cefazolin sodium). A cephalosporin antibiotic (see page 314).

Aquamephyton A vitamin K preparation (see page 331).

Aquasol A A vitamin A preparation (see page 331).

Aquasol E A vitamin E preparation (see page 331).

Asbron A theophylline bronchodilator (see page 318).

Atgam An antithymocyte globulin for fighting organ rejection (see page 333).

Atrovent (ipratropium bromide). A kind of bronchodilator.

Atuss A cough medicine that includes a cough suppressant, an antihistamine, and a decongestant (see page 324).

Augmentin (amoxicillin/clavulanate potassium). An antibiotic (see page 311).

Avazyme (chymotrypsin). A digestive enzyme, useful only for digesting protein, and not fat (see page 326).

Azactam (see Aztreonam below).

azlocillin An anti-*Pseudomonas* antibiotic (see page 311).

Azmacort (triamcinolone acetonide). An inhaled corticosteroid.

azothioprine An antimetabolite, for fighting organ rejection (see page 334).

Aztreonam An anti-*Pseudomonas* antibiotic (see page 315).

bacampicillin HCl An ampicillin (see page 310).

Bactrim (trimethoprim–sulfamethoxazole). A combination antibiotic (see page 312).

Bactrim DS Double-strength Bactrim (see Bactrim).

Basaljel (aluminum carbonate gel). An antacid (see page 327).

beclomethasone dipropionate An inhaled corticosteroid.

Beclovent (beclomethasone dipropionate). A corticosteroid (see page 318).

Beconase   (beclomethasone dipropionate). A nasal steroid spray often used for polyps or nasal allergies (see page 323).

Beepen-VK   (penicillin). An antibiotic (see page 310).

Benadryl   (diphenhydramine hydrochloride). An antihistamine (see page 324).

Betapen-VK   (penicillin V potassium). An antibiotic (see page 310).

Biaxin   (clarithromycin). A macrolide antibiotic (see page 314).

Bicillin   (penicillin G benzathine). An injectable (intramuscular) penicillin (see page 310).

Bilezyme   A digestive enzyme combination containing protein-digesting enzymes but no fat-digesting enzymes. Also contains bile salts (see page 326).

bisacodyl   A laxative (see page 330).

bran   A very rich source of dietary fiber. Taken in pure form, it tastes like rabbit food, but is very effective in helping to prevent constipation (see page 329).

Brethine   (terbutaline sulfate). A beta-agonist bronchodilator (see page 317).

Bricanyl   (terbutaline sulfate). A beta-agonist bronchodilator (see page 317).

budesonide   An inhaled steroid.

carbenicillin   An anti-*Pseudomonas* antibiotic (see page 311).

Ceclor   (cefaclor). A cephalosporin antibiotic (see page 314).

cefaclor   A cephalosporin antibiotic (see page 314).

cefadroxil   A cephalosporin antibiotic (see page 314).

Cefadyl   (cephapirin sodium). A cephalosporin antibiotic (see page 314).

cefamandole   A cephalosporin antibiotic (see page 314).

cefazolin   A cephalosporin antibiotic (see page 314).

Cefobid   A cephalosporin antibiotic with some effect against *Pseudomonas* (see page 314).

cefoperozone   A cephalosporin antibiotic with some effect against *Pseudomonas* (see page 314).

cefotaxime   A cephalosporin antibiotic (see page 314).

cefoxitin   An analog derivative of a cephalosporin antibiotic (see page 314).

cefprozil   A cephalosporin antibiotic (see page 314).

ceftazidime   An anti-*Pseudomonas* cephalosporin (see page 314).

Ceftin   Cefuroxime.

Cefulac   (lactulose). An anticonstipation medication (see page 330).

cefuroxime   A cephalosporin antibiotic (see page 314).

Cefzil   Cefprozil.

Celbenin   (sodium methicillin). An anti-*Staphylococcus* antibiotic (see page 310).

Cenalax   An anticonstipation drug (see page 330).

cephalexin   A cephalosporin antibiotic (see page 314).

cephaloglycin   A cephalosporin antibiotic (see page 314).

cephaloridine   A cephalosporin antibiotic (see page 314).

cephalosporins   A family of antibiotics (see page 314).

cephalothin   A cephalosporin antibiotic (see page 314).

cephapirin   A cephalosporin antibiotic (see page 314).

cephradine   A cephalosporin antibiotic (see page 314).

Cerose   A combination of various cough medicines (see page 323).

Cerylin   A combination theophylline bronchodilator (see page 318) and guaifenesin expectorant (see page 323).

chloramphenicol   An antibiotic (see page 313).

Chloromycetin   (chloramphenicol). An antibiotic.

Chlor-Trimeton   (pseudoephedrine sulfate + chlorpheniramine maleate). An antihistamine (see page 324).

Choledyl   (oxtriphylline). A bronchodilator closely related to theophylline (see page 324).

cimetidine   An antacid preparation (see page 327).

Cipro   (ciprofloxacin). A quinolone antibiotic (see page 315).

ciprofloxacin   A quinolone antibiotic (see page 315).

Claforan   A cephalosporin antibiotic (see page 314).

clarithromycin   A macrolide antibiotic (see page 314).

Cleocin   (clindamycin). One of the aminoglycoside antibiotics (see page 310).

clindamycin   An antibiotic.

clotrimazole   An antiyeast medication, used for vaginal yeast infections.

cloxacillin   An anti-*Staphylococcus* penicillin (see page 311).

Cloxapen   (cloxacillin). A penicillin.

cod liver oil   A traditional source of vitamins A and D whose main advantage is its bad taste (see page 329).

codeine   A cough suppressant (see page 323).

coffee   A caffeine-containing popular drink. Caffeine is also found in Coca-Cola, Pepsi and in some cases serves as a bronchodilator (see page 316).

Colace   (docusate sodium). A stool softener (see page 331).

colistin   A very potent antibiotic, a relative of the aminoglycosides. Given intravenously it can have severe side effects including headaches and kidney damage.

Coly-Mycin S   (colistin sulfate). An antibiotic.

Contac   An antihistamine and decongestant (see page 324).

Co-Pyronil   (pyrrobutamine compound). An antihistamine and decongestant combination (see page 324).

Coricidin   An antihistamine and decongestant (see page 324).

Cotazym   (pancrelipase). A pancreatic digestive enzyme (see page 327).

Cotazym-B   A digestive enzyme with bile salts (see page 327).

Cotazym-S   An enteric-coated pancreatic enzyme (see page 327).

co-trimoxazole   A combination antibiotic (trimethoprim–sulfamethoxazole).

Co-Tylenol   A combination of decongestant, antihistamine, and cough suppressant with acetaminophen (see page 323).

Creon   (pancreatin). An enteric-coated pancreatic enzyme (see page 327).

Criticare   A nutritional supplement and formula that is very low in fat and includes protein that is predigested.

cromolyn   An inhaled medicine used to prevent bronchospasm (see page 320).

cyclacillin   "Twin brother" of ampicillin; an effective antibacterial agent (see page 311).

Cyclapen   cyclacillin.

Decadron   (dexamethasone). A steroid (see page 318).

Declomycin   (demeclocycline). A tetracycline antibiotic (see page 314).

Delatestryl   (testosterone enanthate). A male hormone sometimes used to stimulate growth and appetite (see page 331).

Deltasone   (prednisone). A steroid sometimes used to decrease bronchial inflammation (see page 318).

Demazin   (chlorpheniramine maleate + phenylephrine hydrochloride). A combination antihistamine–decongestant (see pages 323, 324).

demeclocycline   A tetracycline antibiotic (see page 314).

Demerol   [meperidine (pethidine) hydrochloride]. A narcotic painkiller and sedative.

Depo-Testosterone   A male hormone (testosterone) in injectable form sometimes used as a growth and appetite stimulant (see page 331).

De-Tuss   A combination cough medicine and antihistamine (see pages 323, 324).

dexamethasone   A steroid that is sometimes taken by aerosol inhalation (see page 318).

dextromethorphan (DM)   A cough suppressant (see page 323).

Dianabol   (methandrostenolone). An anabolic and male sex hormone sometimes used as a growth and appetite stimulant (see page 331).

dicloxacillin sodium   An anti-*Staphylococcus* penicillin (see page 311).

digitalis   A drug that strengthens heart contractions (see page 326).

digitoxin   A digitalis drug (see page 326).

digoxin   A digitalis drug (see page 326).

Dilaudid   (hydromorphone hydrochloride). A narcotic that is occasionally used for pain and for cough suppression.

Dimetane   (brompheniramine maleate). A combination cough medicine, antihistamine, and decongestant (see pages 323, 324).

Dimetapp   Similar to Dimetane.

diphenhydramine hydrochloride   An antihistamine (see page 324).

disodium cromoglycate   Cromolyn; used in treatment of bronchial asthma (see page 320).

diuretics   Medications that increase the kidneys' production of urine and thus help rid the body of excess fluid (see page 325).

DNase   A mucolytic (see page 320).

Donatussin   (chlorpheniramine maleate + phenylephrine hydrochloride + guaifenesin). A combination cough medicine, antihistamine, and decongestant (see pages 323, 324).

Dorcol   (guaifenesin + phenylpropanolamine hydrochloride + dextromethorphan hydrobromide). A cough medicine that includes a decongestant and a cough suppressant (see pages 323, 324).

doxycycline A tetracycline antibiotic (see page 314).

Dristan A decongestant (see page 324).

Dynapen (dicloxacillin). An anti-*Staphylococcus* antibiotic (see page 311).

dyphylline A form of theophylline bronchodilator (see page 318).

E-Mycin A macrolide antibiotic (see page 314).

EES (erythromycin ethylsuccinate). A macrolide antibiotic (see page 314).

Elixicon (theophylline). A theophylline bronchodilator (see page 318).

Elixophyllin A form of theophylline bronchodilator (see page 318).

EMLA cream A local anesthetic that can be put on the skin to numb a site for intravenous needle placement (322).

Ensure A calorie supplement (see page 332).

Entolase An enteric-coated digestive enzyme (see page 327).

Entolase-HP An enteric-coated digestive enzyme (see page 327).

enzymes Catalysts of chemical reactions; (see page 329).

ephedrine Sometimes used as a bronchodilator (see page 316).

epinephrine Adrenalin. Often used as an emergency bronchodilator, similar in some of its action to the "beta-agonists" (see page 317), but with more effect on the heart (speeds it up).

Erythrocin A macrolide antibiotic (see page 314).

erythromycin The original member of the macrolide family of antibiotics (see pages 312, 329).

ethacrynic acid A diuretic (see page 325).

fiber An important component of the diet (see page 329).

Fleet enemas Occasionally used for treating constipation (see page 329).

Flovent (fluticasone). An inhaled steroid.

Fluticasone An inhaled steroid.

Formeterol A long-acting bronchodilator.

Fortaz (ceftazidime). A cephalosporin antibiotic (see page 314).

furosemide A diuretic (see page 325).

Ganciclovir An antiviral agent.

Gantrisin (sulfisoxazole). A sulfa antibiotic (see page 312).

Garamycin (gentamicin). An aminoglycoside antibiotic (see page 312).

Gastrografin (meglumine diatrizoate). A substance that is occasionally used in the hospital for an enema (see page 330).

Gaviscon (aluminum hydroxide + magnesium carbonate). An antacid (see page 327).

Gelusil (aluminum hydroxide + magnesium hydroxide + simethicone). An antacid (see page 327).

gentamicin An aminoglycoside antibiotic (see page 312).

Geocillin An oral form of the antibiotic carbenicillin. The oral form of the medicine is not effective for lung disease (see page 311).

Geopen An injectable form of carbenicillin (see page 311).

Golytely A salty liquid that can be drunk in large quantities to "flush out" the intestines (see page 331).

guaifenesin   An expectorant (see page 323, *"Cough Medicines"*).

Halotestin   (fluoxymesterone). A male sex hormone sometimes used for growth and appetite stimulation (see page 331).

heparin   An anticoagulant; that is, a drug that prevents clotting of the blood. This is very useful when used in very small amounts in a needle in a vein. It can keep the blood from clotting up the needle so that the needle can be used for a long time for administration of intravenous antibiotics.

heparin lock   A needle that is inserted in the vein and periodically rinsed out with heparin solution. This enables the needle to be used for administration of intravenous antibiotics on an intermittent basis. Once rinsed out, the needle can be plugged up and just taped to the arm without any extra tubing connected to it, leaving the arm free.

Hep-Lock   The dilute heparin solution used in a heparin lock.

hetacillin   An antibiotic related to ampicillin (see page 311).

Hexadrol   (dexamethasone). A steroid sometimes used to decrease bronchial inflammation (see page 318).

Hycodan   (hydrocodone bitartrate). A combination cough medicine that contains a cough suppressant (see page 323).

Hycotuss   (hydrocodone bitartrate + guaifenesin). A multiingredient cough medicine that includes a cough suppressant (see page 323).

hydrocodone bitartrate   A narcotic sometimes used as a cough suppressant (see page 323).

hydrocortisone   A steroid occasionally used in different forms to decrease bronchial inflammation (see page 318).

Ilozyme   (pancrelipase). A pancreatic enzyme (see page 327).

imipenem   An anti-*Pseudomonas* antibiotic (see page 315).

Intal   (cromolyn sodium; see page 320).

Ipecac   A medicine used to induce vomiting (usually used after a child has accidentally ingested a poisonous substance).

isoetharine   A bronchodilator drug taken by inhalation (see page 316).

isoproterenol   An inhaled bronchodilator (see page 316).

Isuprel   (isoproterenol). A bronchodilator taken by inhalation (see page 316).

Itraconazole   An antifungal drug.

kanamycin   An aminoglycoside antibiotic (see page 312).

Kantrex   (kanamycin). An antibiotic (see page 327).

Keflex   (cephalexin). A cephalosporin antibiotic (see page 314).

Keflin   (cephalothin sodium). A cephalosporin antibiotic (see page 314).

Kefzol   (cefazolin sodium). A cephalosporin antibiotic (see page 314).

lactulose   An anticonstipation medication (see page 330).

Lanophyllin   A form of theophylline bronchodilator (see page 318).

Lanoxin   (digoxin). A type of digitalis (see page 326).

lansoprazole   A proton pump inhibitor acid suppressor (see page 328).

Larotid   (amoxicillin). An antibiotic (see page 309).

Lasix   (furosemide). A diuretic (see page 325).

Ledercillin (penicillin G procaine). A form of penicillin (see page 310).

Lincocin (lincomycin hydrochloride). An antibiotic.

lincomycin An antibiotic not commonly used in CF.

Lufyllin (dyphylline). A theophylline bronchodilator (see page 318).

Maalox An antacid (see page 328).

Marax (ephedrine sulfate + theophylline + hydroxyzine hydrochloride). A combination drug including a theophylline bronchodilator (see page 318) and another bronchodilator.

Maxair (pirbuterol). A beta-agonist bronchodilator (see page 317).

Medihaler-EPI An inhaled form of epinephrine or adrenalin (see page 317).

Medihaler-ISO (isoproterenol sulfate). An inhaled bronchodilator with iso-proterenol (see page 316).

Medrol Methylprednisolone, an oral steroid.

Megace Megestrol, a female hormone used for stimulating appetite.

Megestrol A female hormone used for stimulating appetite.

Merem Meropenem, an anti-*Pseudomonas* antibiotic.

Meropenem An anti-*Pseudomonas* antibiotic.

Metaprel (metaproterenol sulfate). A beta-agonist bronchodilator (see page 298).

metaproterenol sulfate A beta-agonist bronchodilator (see page 317).

methacycline A tetracycline antibiotic (see page 314).

methicillin sulfate An anti-*Staphylococcus* antibiotic (see page 311).

methyltestosterone A male sex hormone, sometimes used as a growth and appetite stimulant (see page 331).

metoclopramide A drug that increases the movement of foods through the gastrointestinal tract and that may decrease gastroesophageal reflux (see page 328).

Mezlin (mezlocillin). An anti-*Pseudomonas* antibiotic (see page 311).

milk of magnesia There are several different preparations: antacids (see page 311) and laxatives, which are used as an anticonstipation preparation (see page 329).

Minocin (minocycline hydrochloride). An antibiotic (see page 314).

minocycline A tetracycline antibiotic (see page 314).

misoprostol An antacid medication (see page 327).

montelukast A leukotriene inhibitor antiinflammatory drug (see page 320).

mucolytics Chemicals that break up mucus (see page 320).

Mucomyst (acetylcysteine). A mucolytic (see page 321).

Mycostatin (nystatin). A drug that kills yeast infections, which can appear when a patient is taking antibiotics. Mycostatin is occasionally prescribed when a child is taking antibiotics.

Mylanta (aluminum hydroxide + magnesium hydroxide + simethicone). An antacid (see page 328).

Mylicon (simethicone). An antibloating drug (see page 331).

Nafcil (nafcillin sodium). An antibiotic.

nafcillin   An anti-*Staphylococcus* antibiotic (see page 311).

Naldecon   A decongestant antihistamine combination (see page 324).

Nasacort   A nasal steroid (triamcinolone).

Nasonex   A nasal steroid (mometasone).

Nebcin   (tobramycin sulfate). An aminoglycoside antibiotic (see page 312).

nedocromil   An inhaled antiinflammatory medication closely related to cromolyn (see page 320).

neomycin   An aminoglycoside antibiotic (see page 312).

Neo-Synephrine   (phenylephrine hydrochloride). A decongestant (see page 324).

netilmicin   An aminoglycoside antibiotic (see page 312).

Novahistine   A combination of many ingredients, used for coughs and cold symptoms (see pages 323, 324).

nystatin   Used to fight yeast infections, which can appear when a patient is taking antibiotics.

omeprazole   An antacid drug (see page 328).

Omnipen   (ampicillin). An antibiotic (see page 311).

Orapred   An oral suspension preparation of the steroid prednisolone.

Organidin   (iodinated glycerol). An expectorant (see page 323).

oxacillin   An anti-*Staphylococcus* antibiotic (see page 311).

oxtriphylline   A theophylline bronchodilator (see page 318).

oxytetracycline   A tetracycline antibiotic (see page 314).

palivizumab   A drug to prevent respiratory syncytial virus (RSV) infection.

Pancrease   (pancrelipase). An enteric-coated digestive enzyme (see page 327).

pancreatin   A digestive enzyme (see page 327).

pancrelipase   A digestive enzyme (see page 327).

Panmycin   (tetracycline). An antibiotic (see page 314).

papase   A drug with some enzyme activity (see page 327).

Pediamycin   (erythromycin ethylsuccinate). A macrolide antibiotic.

Pediapred   An oral suspension of prednisolone, a steroid.

Pediazole   (erythromycin ethylsuccinate + sulfisoxazole acetyl). A combination antibiotic that contains erythromycin and a sulfa drug.

penicillin   An antibiotic (see page 310).

Pen-Vee K   A penicillin antibiotic (see page 310).

phenylephrine hydrochloride   A medication sometimes used in aerosols. It constricts blood vessels and may therefore cut down on swelling in the bronchi, by decreasing the blood flow to the bronchi.

piperacillin sodium   An anti-*Pseudomonas* antibiotic (see page 311).

Pipracil (piperacillin).   An antibiotic.

pirbuterol   A beta-agonist bronchodilator (see page 317).

Pneumovax   The so-called "pneumonia vaccine." This is useful for children who have a particular deficiency in their body defenses that enables them to become infected with a germ called *pneumococcus*, such as children with sickle-cell disease. Many physicians feel that it is of no particular value to patients with cystic fibrosis.

Polycillin　(ampicillin). An antibiotic (see page 311).

Polycose　A high-calorie diet supplement (see page 332).

Poly-Histine　A cough and cold preparation (see page 324).

Polymox　(amoxicillin). An antibiotic (see page 311).

polymyxin B　An antibiotic.

polymyxin-E　An antibiotic, also known as colistin, that is effective against *Pseudomonas*; however, it is often difficult to tolerate.

prednisolone　A steroid used to decrease inflammation (see page 318).

prednisone　A steroid used to decrease inflammation (see page 318).

Prilosec　(omeprazole). An antacid drug (see page 328).

Primaxin　(imipenem). An antibiotic with some activity against *Pseudomonas* (see page 315).

Principen　(ampicillin). An antibiotic (see page 311).

Prostaphlin　(oxacillin sodium). An anti-*Staphylococcus* penicillin antibiotic (see page 310).

Proventil　A beta-agonist bronchodilator (see page 317).

prunes　One of the best sources of dietary fiber, especially effective in combating constipation (see page 329).

Pulmicort　An inhaled form of budesonide, a steroid.

Quibron　A bronchodilator preparation that contains several different drugs, including theophylline (see page 318) and an expectorant (see page 323).

quinolones　A family of antibiotics (see page 315).

ranitidine　A medication that decreases the stomach's production of acid (see page 328).

Reglan　(metoclopramide; see page 328).

Rhinocort　A nasal form of the steroid budesonide.

rimantadine　An antiinfluenza drug.

ribavirin　An aerosol medicine that can help control some viral bronchial infections, especially bronchiolitis caused by RSV (respiratory syncytial virus).

Robitussin　(guaifenesin). A cough preparation consisting of an expectorant (see page 323).

rofecoxib　A nonsteroid antiinflammatory drug.

Rondec　(carbinoxamine maleate + pseudoephedrine hydrochloride). A cough and cold preparation (see pages 323, 324).

saline　Salt water.

salmeterol　A long-acting inhaled beta-agonist bronchodilator.

Senekot　(senna). An intestinal stimulant (see page 330).

Serevent　(salmeterol). A long acting inhaled bronchodilator.

Silain　(simethicone). An antibloating drug (see page 331).

Singulair　(montelukast). A leukotriene inhibitor antiinflammatory.

Slo-Phyllin Gyrocaps   A long-lasting theophylline bronchodilator (see page 318).

sodium chloride   Salt.

Somophyllin   A theophylline preparation (see page 318).

Spectrobid   A type of penicillin closely related to ampicillin (see page 311).

spironolactone   A diuretic (see page 326).

Sporanox   (itraconazole). An antifungal drug.

Staphcillin   (sodium methicillin). An anti-*Staphylococcus* antibiotic (see page 310).

steroids   Very potent drugs that are similar to the chemicals made in the body in the adrenal glands. They are very powerful and can be used safely for a short period of time for some purposes such as decreasing bronchial inflammation (see page 318). They are often used for other purposes, including growth and appetite stimulation (see page 331).

sulfamethoxazole   A sulfa antibiotic (see page 312).

Sulfatrim   A combination antibiotic trimethoprim–sulfamethoxazole (see page 312).

Sus-Phrine   (epinephrine). A bronchodilator medication with some beta-agonist activity. It is used only by injection, primarily for treating serious allergic reactions or an asthma attack (see page 317).

Sustacal   A nutritional supplement formula (see page 332).

Sustaire   A theophylline bronchodilator (see page 318).

Synagis   (palivizumab). A drug to prevent respiratory syncytial virus (RSV) infection (see page 316).

Tagamet   (cimetidine). An antacid drug (see page 327).

Tazidime   ceftazidime.

Tegopen   (cloxacillin sodium). An anti-*Staphylococcus* penicillin (see page 310).

terbutaline sulfate   A beta-agonist bronchodilator (see page 317).

Terramycin   (oxytetracycline). A tetracycline antibiotic (see page 314).

Testionate   A male steroid hormone used for growth and appetite stimulation (see page 331).

testosterone   The primary male hormone (see page 332).

tetracycline   An antibiotic family (see page 314).

Theo-Dur   A theophylline bronchodilator (see page 318).

Theolair   A theophylline bronchodilator (see page 318).

theophylline   A family of bronchodilators (see page 318).

ticarcillin   An anti-*Pseudomonas* penicillin (see page 311).

Tilade   (nedocromil; see page 320).

Timentin   An anti-*Pseudomonas* and anti-*Staphylococcus* antibiotic (see page 312).

tobramycin   An aminoglycoside antibiotic (see page 312).

Tornalate   (methanesulfonate). A beta-agonist bronchodilator (see page 317).

triamcinolone   An inhaled steroid (see page 319).

Triaminic (phenylpropanolamine hydrochloride + pheniramine maleate + pyrilamine maleate). A cold preparation (see page 324).

trimethoprim An antibiotic usually found in combination with a sulfa drug (see page 312).

Tussionex A cough mixture including an antihistamine; a narcotic cough suppressant (see page 323).

Ultrase A pancreatic enzyme supplement (see page 327).

Vancenase (beclomethasone dipropionate). A nasal steroid spray (see page 323).

Vantin A cephalosporin antibiotic (see page 314).

Veetid B-Cillin (penicillin). An antibiotic (see page 310).

Velosef A cephalosporin antibiotic (see page 314).

Ventolin (albuterol sulfate). A beta-agonist bronchodilator (see page 317).

Vibramycin A tetracycline antibiotic (see page 314).

Viokase (pancreatin). A digestive enzyme (see page 327).

Vioxx (rofecoxib). A nonsteroid antiinflammatory drug.

Vipep A nutritional supplement formula (see page 332).

Virazole (ribavirin).

Vital A nutritional supplement formula (see page 332).

Vivonex A nutritional supplement formula (see page 332).

Winstrol (stanozolol). A sex steroid hormone (see page 331).

Wycillin (penicillin). An antibiotic (see page 310).

zafirlukast A leukotriene-inhibitor antiinflammatory drug.

Zantac (ranitidine). Helps to decrease the stomach's production of acid (see page 328).

Zymase A digestive enzyme (see page 327).

Zyrtec (cetirizine). An antihistamine.

Zyvox (lenezolid). An antibiotic.

Appendix C

Airway Clearance Techniques

POSTURAL DRAINAGE TECHNIQUES

Infants

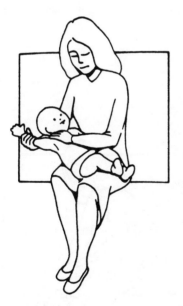

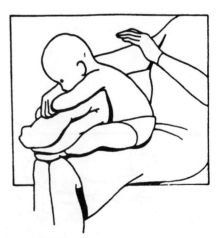

Figure C.1. Draining anterior apical segments.

Figure C.2. Draining posterior apical segments.

The material presented here has been reproduced with the kind permission of Dr. Beryl Rosenstein from his excellent booklet, The Johns Hopkins Hospital Cystic Fibrosis Patient Handbook (Beryl Rosenstein and Terry S. Langbaum, editors).

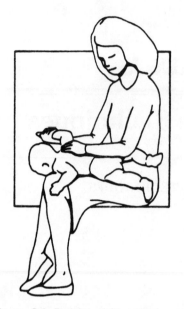

Figure C.3. Draining right posterior segment.

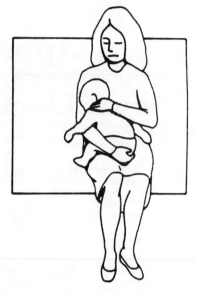

Figure C.4. Draining left posterior segment.

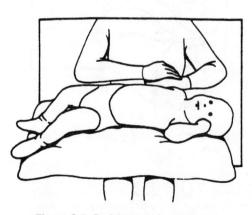

Figure C.5. Draining anterior segments.

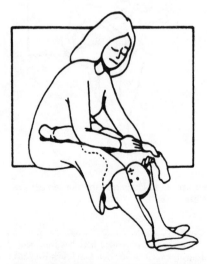

Figure C.6. Draining right middle lobe.

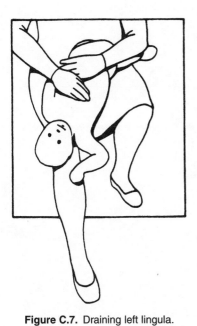

Figure C.7. Draining left lingula.

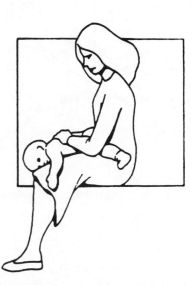

Figure C.8. Draining right and left superior segments.

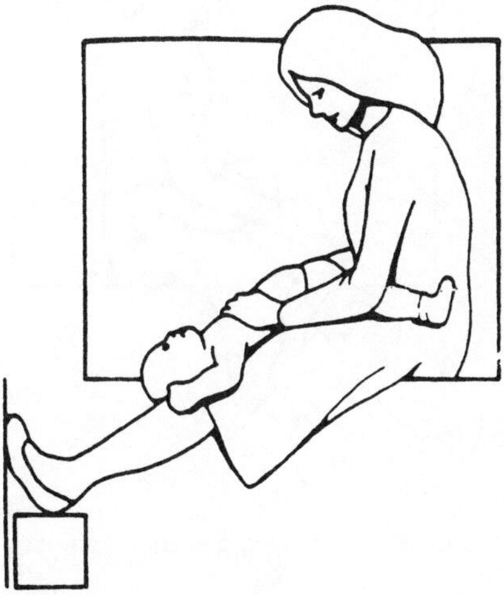

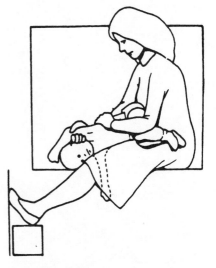

Figure C.9. Draining anterior basal segments.

Figure C.10 Draining left lateral basal segment.

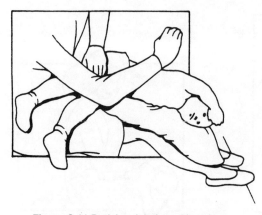

Figure C.11 Draining right lateral basal segment.

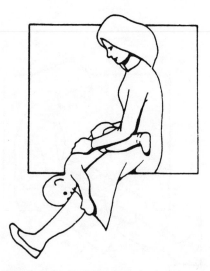

Figure C.12. Draining posterior basal segments.

Toddlers

The following points will be helpful in performing postural drainage (PD).

- Clap 1 minute—vibrate five exhalations—vibrate while huffing two to three times, cough, repeat once.
- Each session should last a maximum of 30 to 40 minutes.
- Always do treatment sessions before meals.
- Two to three sessions per day are usually recommended.

Other Considerations

Children may become frightened initially when given PD. As this treatment is very important, you should be encouraged not to apologize or sympathize for having to give this form of treatment. Children should understand, to the best of their ability, why the treatment is being done and accept it as part of the daily routine. Children should be encouraged to talk and sing, as this helps them to breathe. Children should not be offered rewards for future treatments. The drainage should be done with as little fuss as possible.

Your child does not need to dislike the time spent in physical therapy. You can make this time a pleasant, quiet opportunity to spend in conversation, or you can provide entertainment by playing records or tapes, or by doing drainage in front of the television.

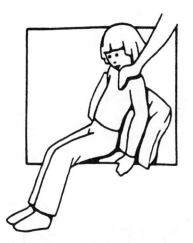 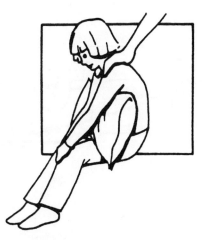

Figure C.13. Upper lobes, apical segments. *Sitting:* Lean back against pillow (30-degree angle) and clap below collar bone in front with cupped hands.

Figure C.14. Upper lobes, posterior segments. *Sitting:* Lean forward onto pillow (30-degree angle) and clap behind collar bone on the back. The fingers usually go a little over shoulders.

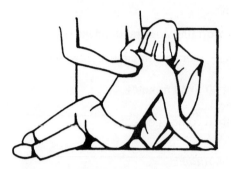

Figure C.15. Left upper lobe. *Bed elevated 45 degrees:* Head up, lying on right side. Place pillow in front, from shoulders to hips, and roll slightly forward onto it. Clap over left shoulder blade.

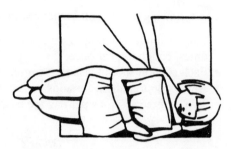

Figure C.16. Right upper lobe. *Lying on left side:* Place pillow in front, from shoulders to hips, or roll slightly forward onto it. Clap over right shoulder blade.

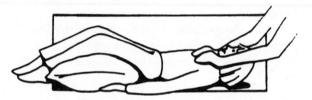

Figure C.17. Upper lobes, anterior segments. *Lying flat on back:* Place pillow under knees and clap just below where you clapped on apical segment.

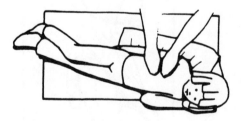

Figure C.18. Right middle lobe. *Lying on left side:* Place pillow behind from shoulders to hips (30-degree tilt) and roll slightly back onto it (one-quarter turn). Clap over right nipple.

Figure C.19. Left lingula. *Lying on right side:* Place pillow behind, from shoulders to hips, and roll slightly back onto it. Clap left nipple (30-degree tilt).

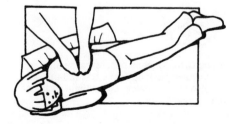

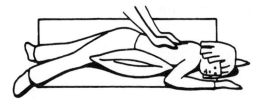

Figure C.20. Lower lobes, superior segments. *Bed flat:* Lying on stomach with pillow under stomach, clap at area of shoulder blades (apex of lower lobes).

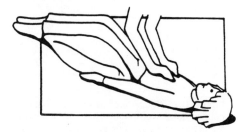

Figure C.21. Lower lobes, anterior segments. *Lying on back:* Place pillow under knees and clap on lower ribs (45-degree tilt).

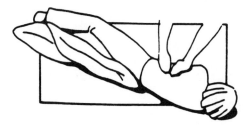

Figure C.22. Lower lobes, left lateral. *Lying on right side:* Knees bent, clap at lower ribs, keeping spine straight (45-degree tilt).

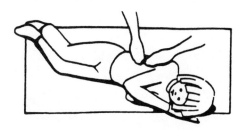

Figure C.23. Lower lobes, right lateral. *Lying on left side:* Knees bent, clap at lower ribs, keeping spine straight (45-degree tilt).

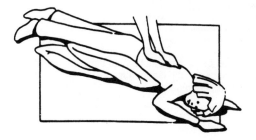

Figure C.24. Lower lobes, posterior segments. *Lying on stomach:* Place pillow under hips and stomach to make spine straight (45-degree tilt). Clap at lower ribs (stay off spine).

SELF SEGMENTAL BRONCHIAL DRAINAGE

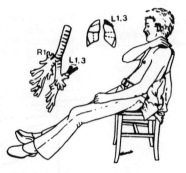

Figure C.25. Sit on a chair and lean backward on a pillow at a 30-degree angle. Clap with a cupped hand over the area between the clavicle (collarbone) and the top of the scapula (shoulder blade). The area for clapping shown in the diagram is for the *apical*-posterior segment of the left upper lobe, *L1,3.* The *apical* segment of the right upper lobe, R1, is drained in the same position, with clapping on the right side. Upper lobes: apical segments: *1;* apical-posterior segment; left: *L1,3;* apical segment; right, *R3.*

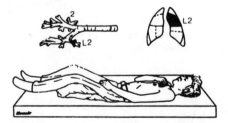

Figure C.26. Lie flat on your back (supine) on a bed or drainage table. Clap between the clavicle (collarbone) and nipple. The area for clapping shown in the diagram is for the *anterior* segment of the left upper lobe, *L2.* Upper lobes: anterior segments: *2.*

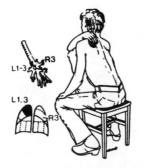

Figure C.27. Sit on a chair leaning forward over a folded pillow at a 30-degree angle. Clap over the upper back. The area for clapping shown in the diagram is for the apical-*posterior* segment of the left upper lobe, *L1-3.* The posterior segment of the right upper lobe, *R3,* is drained in the same position with clapping on the right side of the upper back. Upper lobes: posterior segments: *3,* posterior segment; right: *R3;* apical-posterior segment, left: *L1-3.*

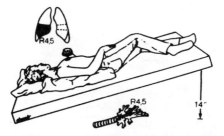

Figure C.28. The foot of the table or bed is elevated 14 inches (about 15 degrees). Lie head down on the left side and rotate one fourth of a turn backward. A pillow may be placed behind and back (from shoulder to hip). The knees should be flexed. Clap over the area of the right nipple. Women should use a cupped hand with the heel of the hand under the armpit and the fingers extending forward beneath the breast. The area for clapping of the right *middle lobe, R4,5,* is shown in the diagram. Right middle lobe: *R4,5;* lateral segment: *R4;* medial segment: *R5.*

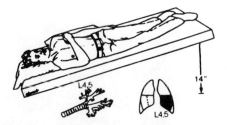

Figure C.29. The *lingular* segment of the left upper lobe, *L4,5,* is drained by lying in a head-down position on the right side and rotating 1/4 turn backward. Clap over the area of the left nipple. Women should use a cupped hand with the heel of the hand under the armpit and the fingers extending forward beneath the breast. A pillow may be placed behind the back for support. Lingular segment, left upper lobe: *L4,5;* superior segment: *L4;* inferior segment; *L5.*

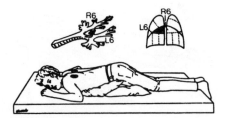

Figure C.30. Lie on your abdomen on a bed or table that is in a flat position with two pillows under your hips. Clap over the middle part of the back at the tip of the scapula (shoulder blade) on either side of the spine. The area for clapping of the *superior* segment of the left lower lobe, *L6,* is shown in the diagram. The *superior* segment of the right lower lobe, *R6,* is done in the same position, with clapping on the right side. Lower lobes: superior segments, *6.*

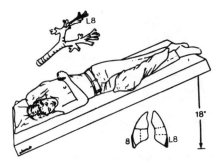

Figure C.31. The foot of the table or bed is elevated 18 inches (about 30 degrees). Lie on your side at a 90-degree angle in the head-down position with a pillow under your knees. Clap with a cupped hand over the lower ribs just beneath the axilla (armpit). The area for clapping shown is for drainage of the left *anterior basal* segment, *L8*. To drain the right *anterior basal* segment, *R8,* lie on your left side in the same position and clap over the right side of the chest. Lower lobes: anterior basal segments, *8.*

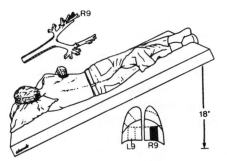

Figure C.32. The foot of the table is elevated 18 inches (approximately 30 degrees). Lie on your abdomen, head down, and rotate one-quarter turn upward from a prone position. Flex your upper leg over a pillow for support. Clap over the lower ribs. The area for clapping shown in the diagram is for the draining of the *right lateral basal* segment, *R9*. To drain the *left lateral basal* segment, *L9,* lie on your right side in the same position and clap over the lower ribs on the left side of the chest. Lower lobes: lateral basal segments, *9.*

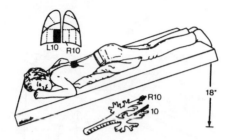

Figure C.33. The foot of the bed or table is elevated 18 inches (about 30 degrees). Lie on your abdomen, head down, with a pillow under your hips. Try to clap over the lower ribs close to the spine. The area for clapping shown in the diagram is for drainage of the *posterior basal* segment of the left lower lobe, *L10* . For drainage of the *posterior basal* segment of the right lower lobe, lie in the same position and try to clap over the lower ribs on the right side of the chest. This is a difficult area for some individuals to reach and you may want to obtain assistance in clapping in this position. Lower lobes: posterior basal segments, *10*.

FLUTTER TECHNIQUE

The flutter technique has been very successful for children, adolescents, and adults, and is done independently. A simple piece of equipment is needed, namely, the Flutter device. It can be purchased from Scandipharm (22 Inverness Center Parkway, Birmingham, AL 35242) or through many different pharmacies, including the national Cystic Fibrosis Foundation's pharmacy services.

The device (as you may recall from Chapter 3) is

> a handheld device, small enough to carry around in your pocket, that looks a little like a kazoo. It has a stainless-steel ball in it that vibrates up and down (flutters, you might say) as you blow into the tube. The vibrations are transmitted backward down through the patient's mouth into the trachea and bronchi, where they shake the mucus free from the bronchial walls.

Instructions for its use are as follows:

Sit with your back straight and head slightly tilted back so that your throat and windpipe are wide open. Some patients prefer to place their elbows on a table to help keep them from slouching.

Hold the Flutter so that the stem is parallel to the floor (this places the cone at a slight angle, enabling the ball to flutter and roll). You'll then try slightly different positions and see which gives you the most vibrating in your chest.

The inhalation step (breath in) is very important. Take in as big a breath as possible. Then HOLD that breath for at least 2 to 3 seconds.

Then, at the end of the breath-hold, place the Flutter in your mouth and begin to exhale at a constant speed. You should NOT breathe out as fast as you can, but try different speeds of blowing out, and see which speed makes the most fluttering feeling in your chest and helps you clear mucus best. While you're blowing out, keep your cheeks flat (don't let the vibrations be wasted on your cheeks; instead you want them to go to your lungs). While you're learning, you might hold your cheeks lightly with your other hand to keep them from vibrating.

Exhale as much air as possible. Really squeeze it out to help clean those small airways. This is a maximum effort (remember, not maximum hard blast, but maximum long breath out).

Leave the Flutter in your mouth and take in another big breath (through your nose) and repeat the whole Flutter breath several times.

Now, remove the Flutter, take in a big breath, hold it for 2 to 3 seconds, and "huff" out a breath, holding your mouth and throat open, and cough.

THE VEST

The vest also has been successful for many children, adolescents, and adults. It allows older children and adults to be independent in their airway clearance. The device is not easily portable and is very expensive. The instructions are as follows:

- Be sure that your vest fits properly.
- It's fine to do bronchodilator, saline, or steroid aerosols during vest treatments.
- It's probably wise to delay antibiotic aerosol treatments until after the vest treatment (to avoid coughing the antibiotic right out, before it's had a chance to work in the lower airways).
- Drink lots of fluid before treatments.
- Stop to cough and clear airways every 5 to 10 minutes.
- Use a comfortable pressure and frequency.

The main supplier of the vest is Advanced Respiratory (1020 West County Road F, St. Paul, MN 55126; tel.: (800) 426-4224; Web site: www.thevest.com).

OTHER TECHNIQUES

The following techniques are used more in Europe than in North America. What follows is just a brief description of each, along with the name, address, and telephone and fax numbers for an expert from the International Physiotherapy Group for Cystic Fibrosis (IPG/CF). This group has dedicated itself to educating people interested in airway clearance for patients with CF.

Positive Expiratory Pressure Mask

For the PEP mask (positive expiratory pressure) technique, the patient breathes through a special mask that has an exhale valve that requires some air pressure to open. It is thought that this expiratory pressure is transmitted back down the airways and helps to prop them open during the exhalation, allowing mucus to be pushed out along with the air (remember that usually during exhalation, the airways tend to narrow a little bit, so this keeps them open wider than they would normally be). Contact:

Meret Falk and Mette Kelstrup
Physiotherapists
Department of Physiotherapy
Rigshospitalet
DK-2100 Copenhagen
Denmark
Tel: 45-35-453545
Fax: 45-35-456717

Active Cycle of Breathing

This technique has three phases, breathing control (quiet breathing), thoracic expansion (deep breaths in), and forced expiration or huffs (quick, strong—but never violent—breaths out, with the mouth and throat open). Contact:

Jennifer Pryor and Barbara Webber
Physiotherapy Department
Royal Brompton Hospital
Sydney Street
London SW3 6NP
United Kingdom
Tel: 44-171-351-8056
Fax: 44-171-351-8950

Autogenic Drainage

Autogenic drainage involves a series of breaths controlled so that some are done with very little air in the lungs, some with a medium amount, and some with the lungs filled almost to capacity. This technique requires instruction by someone very skilled in its use before it can be effective in mobilizing mucus. Contact:

J. Chevallier, P.T.
Zeepreventorium
5 Koninkluke Baan
B8420 De Haan
Belgium
Tel: 32-59-233911
Fax: 32-59-234057

Exercise

Many people believe that vigorous exercise may be helpful to loosen mucus and to keep bronchi clear. Certainly, hard exercise, laughing, or crying often result in a coughing spell that brings up mucus, even in people who do not raise mucus during the traditional PD treatments. Since there is not yet any scientific evidence that exercise can successfully replace the time-honored PD treatments, it is best to encourage patients to be very active and to do their treatments. (Exercise is discussed at greater length in Chapter 10, *Exercise*.)

Appendix D

Some High Calorie Recipes

PASTA POT

By Stefani Czekaj

2 lb ground meat
2 medium onions, chopped
1 clove garlic, minced
1 (14 oz) jar spaghetti sauce
1 (16 oz) can stewed tomatoes
3 oz canned or fresh mushrooms
8 oz shell or spring macaroni
3 cups sour cream
8 oz provolone cheese, shredded
8 oz mozzarella cheese, shredded

Cook beef in skillet; drain excess fat. Add onions, garlic, spaghetti sauce, stewed tomatoes, and mushrooms. Simmer 20 minutes. Meanwhile, cook macaroni according to package directions; drain and rinse in cold water.

Pour shells into deep casserole, cover with tomato meat sauce. Spread sour cream over sauce and add provolone cheese. Top with mozzarella cheese. Cover casserole and bake at 350°F for 35 to 40 minutes. Uncover and bake until cheese melts and browns.

Yield: 10 servings
1 serving: 613 calories

Note: For higher calories use cheeses made with whole milk.

FETTUCCINI ALFREDO

By Kevin Helmick

1 (8 oz) package fettuccini, uncooked
½ cup melted butter
¾ cup grated Parmesan cheese
4 tbsp half and half
salt and pepper

Cook pasta according to package directions; drain well. In warm serving dish combine butter, cheese, half and half, salt and pepper. Add pasta to mixture. Gently toss to coat all fettuccini. Top with Parmesan cheese.

Yield: 4 servings
1 cup: 450 calories

SPINACH PASTA

By Peggy Tommarello

½ cup vegetable oil
1 tbsp butter
1 tsp salt
1 tsp basil
2 cloves garlic, halved
1 package frozen spinach, cooked
½ lb small shells, cooked and drained
1 (6 oz) can grated Parmesan cheese

Sauté first five ingredients; add cooked spinach. Mix well. Sauté for 7 to 10 minutes. Add cooked pasta and then the Parmesan cheese. Stir until pasta is coated; heat thoroughly. Serve hot.

Yield: 6 servings
1 serving: 363 calories

VEGETABLE PIZZA

2 packages crescent rolls
2 (8 oz) packages cream cheese, softened
1 cup mayonnaise
2 tsp onion powder
2 tsp dry dill, crumbled
2 cups chopped broccoli
2 cups chopped cauliflower
1 green pepper, chopped
2 tomatoes, diced and drained
2 medium carrots, shredded

Unroll and pat crescent rolls onto a cookie sheet to make crust. Bake at 350°F until light, golden brown. Cool. Combine the cream cheese, mayonnaise, onion powder, and dill. Spread over cooled crust. Top with the broccoli, cauliflower, green pepper, and tomatoes. Place shredded carrots on top. Cut in small triangles to serve.

Yield: 12 servings
½₂ recipe: 272 calories

SHRIMP SPREAD

8 oz cream cheese, softened
1 small onion, diced
¼ cup mayonnaise
1 (6 oz) can mini-shrimp
½ tbsp lemon juice
¼ tsp garlic powder
½ tbsp Worcestershire sauce
¾ cup cocktail sauce

Mix all ingredients except cocktail sauce. Refrigerate for at least 1 hour. When ready to serve, mound cheese mixture in middle of plate. Pour cocktail sauce over the mound of cheese. Serve with a favorite cracker. (Crabmeat can be substituted for the shrimp.)

Yield: 24 servings
¹⁄₂₄ recipe: 60 calories

ARTICHOKE PIZZAZZ

By Karen Ketyer

1 (14 oz) can artichoke hearts, drained and chopped
1 cup grated Parmesan cheese
1 cup shredded mozzarella cheese
1 cup mayonnaise
2 tbsp chopped green onion
1 dash garlic powder

Combine all ingredients and put in a 1½ quart casserole dish or quiche pan. Bake at 350°F, for 25 to 30 minutes. Serve hot with a sturdy cracker.

Yield: 1 quart
¹⁄₂₀ recipe: 88 calories

PEANUT BUTTER ROUND-UPS

By Amanda Ogden

1 cup shortening
1 cup granulated sugar
1 cup brown sugar, firmly packed
2 eggs
1 cup peanut butter
2 cups all-purpose flour
½ teaspoon salt
2 tsp baking soda
1 cup quick rolled oats

Mix the ingredients one at a time in order of recipe; mix well. Place a teaspoonful of mixture on cookie sheet. Press with fork. Bake at 350°F for 10 to 12 minutes.

Yield: 6 dozen balls
1 ball: 85 calories

LEMON BARS

By Louise Bauer

1 cup (2 sticks) butter
2 cups all-purpose flour
3 tbsp granulated sugar
2 (8 oz) packages cream cheese
2 cups powdered sugar
2 small packages lemon pudding and pie filling (not instant)
1 medium container Cool Whip
chopped nuts

Combine butter, flour, and sugar like a pie dough. Pat into bottom of jelly-roll pan or cookie sheet. Bake at 325°F for 15 minutes. Cool.

Blend cream cheese and powdered sugar with electric mixer. Spread on cooled crust.

Cook pudding according to package directions. Spread on top of cream cheese layer. Let gel. Cover with Cool Whip and sprinkle with chopped nuts, if desired. Cut into bars to serve.

Yield: 24 bars
1 bar: 260 calories

MILKY WAY CAKE

By David Orenstein

1 lb of Milky Way bars
1 cup buttermilk (or plain yogurt)
3 sticks margarine
½ tsp baking soda
4 eggs
2 tsp vanilla
2<fr1/2> cups flour
<fr1/2> cup chopped nuts
2 cups granulated sugar
2 cups powdered sugar

Melt about 11 oz of the candy bars and one stick margarine in double boiler until smooth; set aside. Cream granulated sugar and one stick margarine; add eggs one at a time, beat until smooth; add flour, buttermilk (or yogurt), and baking soda. Add Milky Way mix, 2 tsp vanilla, and nuts. Bake in greased and floured bundt pan or angel food pan for 1 hour 20 minutes at 325°F.

Frosting: Melt remaining candy bars (about 5 oz) and the other stick of margarine in double boiler until smooth, add little vanilla and powdered sugar until desired thickness, add a little milk if necessary. This cake should be stored in the fridge, but it probably won't need to be stored long!

Yield: 12 servings
1 serving: 705 calories

ORENSTEIN FAMILY BROWNIES

By Florence, Jacob, Herbert, and David Orenstein and Miriam Sumner

4 1-oz cubes unsweetened baking chocolate
1 cup butter
3 eggs
2 cups sugar
1 cup flour
1 cup chopped walnuts
½ tsp vanilla (optional)
(raisin lovers can add ½ to 1 cup raisins)

Preheat oven to 350°F. Grease large flat cookie pan (about 10 × 15 inches) with closed ends.

Melt chocolate and butter over hot water, add sugar, then eggs, flour, and walnuts (and vanilla and raisins, if you're using them).. Spread in pan. Bake 20 to 30 minutes.

Yield: 24 pieces
1 brownie: 175 calories, but no one can eat one.

GERMAN APPLE PIE

By Michelle Gruskos

1 cup flour
1 cup sugar
¾ cup melted butter
1 egg
½ cup finely chopped walnuts
½ cup raisins
enough sliced apples to fill 9-inch pie pan
cinnamon mixture (1 tbsp sugar + 1 tsp cinnamon)

Preheat oven to 350°F. Fill pie pan with sliced apples. Sprinkle cinnamon sugar mixture over. Mix all other ingredients in bowl and spread over apples. Bake at to 350°F for 45 minutes

Yield: 6 big pieces
1 piece: 387 calories

STICKY DATE PUDDING

By Jenny Cooper, Sydney, Australia

6 oz dates, stoned & chopped
1 tsp baking soda
10 oz boiling water
4 tbsp butter
6 oz caster (very fine) sugar
2 eggs
6 oz flour
½ tsp vanilla

Sauce

14 oz brown sugar
1 cup thick cream
9 oz butter
1 vanilla bean, split

Preheat oven to 350°F and butter a 7-inch square cake tine. Mix dates and baking soda. Pour water over dates/soda, and leave to stand. Cream butter and sugar, then add eggs, one at a time, beating well after each. Fold flour in gently, then stir in date mixture and vanilla and pour into prepared tin. Bake in center of oven for 30 to 40 minutes until cooked when tested with toothpick.

Sauce: Bring all ingredients to a boil. Reduce heat and simmer for 5 minutes. Remove vanilla bean. Pour a little sauce over warm pudding and return to oven for 2 to 3 minutes so sauce soaks in. Cut pudding into squares and pour extra sauce over.

Yield: 6 pieces
1 piece: 980 calories!!

SWEET AND SOUR STRAWBERRY DESSERT

By Judy Fulton

1 qt fresh strawberries
8 oz sour cream
1 cup firmly packed brown sugar

Wash and hull strawberries. Dry and slice. Mix brown sugar and sour cream and top strawberries.

Yield: 6 servings
1 serving: approximately 240 calories

PEANUT BUTTER BANANA SHAKE

by Tonya Boyer

1 small banana, chunked
1½ cup whole milk
¼ cup smooth peanut butter
2 tsp granulated sugar
½ tsp vanilla extract

Combine all ingredients in blender and mix until smooth and frothy.

Yield: 2 drinks
1 drink: 350 calories

SCOTCHEROOS

By Renee Exler

1 cup light corn syrup
1 cup granulated sugar
1 cup peanut butter
6 cups Rice Krispy cereal
1 cup semi-sweet chocolate chips
1 cup butterscotch morsels

Cook corn syrup and sugar over medium heat in saucepan until sugar is dissolved; stir frequently. When mixture starts to boil remove from heat, and stir in peanut butter; mix well. Add Rice Krispy cereal; stir until well coated. Press mixture into buttered 9 × 13 × 2-inch pan. Set aside.

Melt chocolate and butterscotch morsels over low heat; stirring constantly. Spread over cereal mixture. Allow to cool, then cut into 1 × 2-inch squares.

Yield: 24 squares
1 × 2 -inch square: 96 calories

CHEESECAKE SQUARES

By Amanda Ogden

1 (14 oz) can sweetened condensed milk
½ cup lemon juice or two to three lemons squeezed
1 tbsp grated lemon rind
⅔ cup shortening
1 cup brown sugar, firmly packed
1¾ cups all-purpose flour
1 tsp salt
1½ cups quick cooking oats

Blend milk, juice, and rind with electric mixer until thick; set aside. Mix together shortening and sugar. Combine flour and other dry ingredients. Blend into shortening mixture. Blend in rolled oats. Place half of the oats mixture into a 9 × 13 × 2-inch pan and press and flatten down. Spread the lemon mixture over the oats mixture. Cover with remaining oat mixture, patting lightly. Bake at 375°F for 25 to 30 minutes. Cool and cut into bars.

    Yield: 24 squares
    1 square: 203 calories

HEATH BARS

By Jane Strange

    50 to 60 soda crackers
    ¼ cup butter, melted
    1 cup (2 sticks) butter
    1 cup dark brown sugar, firmly packed
    1 (12 oz) package milk chocolate chips
    1 cup chopped nuts

Line large cookie sheet with tin foil; spread with melted butter. Place the crackers on buttered cookie sheet.

In medium saucepan cook sugar and 1 cup butter until dissolved; stirring constantly. Allow sugar and butter to boil. Pour mixture over crackers. Bake at 375°F for 7 minutes. Remove from oven and sprinkle with chocolate chips. As the chips melt, spread to smooth out. Sprinkle with nuts. Place in refrigerator to cool. Cut into bars to serve.

    Yield: 24 bars
    1 bar: 236 calories

KID PLEASIN' CHOCOLATE MOUSSE

    1 (6 oz) package chocolate instant pudding mix
    3 cups cold whole milk
    1 cup frozen whipped topping, thawed
    12 cream-filled chocolate sandwich cookies, crumbled
    8 cream-filled chocolate sandwich cookies, whole

Combine pudding mix and milk in a small mixing bowl; beat at low speed of an electric mixer until blended. Beat at low speed an additional 2 minutes. Fold in <fr1/2> cup whipped topping and cookie crumbs. Spoon mousse into eight (6 oz) dessert dishes. Cover and chill.

Garnish each serving with a drop of remaining whipped topping and a whole cookie just before serving.

    Yield: 8 (6 oz) servings
    ⅛ recipe: 276 calories

MIRACLE PUDDING

By Brenda McCullen

2 small packages chocolate instant pudding
1 (14 oz) can sweetened condensed milk
1 large container Cool Whip

Prepare pudding according to package directions. Combine remaining ingredients with pudding and mix well. Refrigerate until chilled. Any flavor pudding may be used.

Yield: 8 servings
⅛ recipe: 513 calories

PUPPY CHOW

By Brenda McCullen

1 stick (½ cup) butter
1 (12 ounce) package chocolate chips
½ cup peanut butter
8 cups Rice Chex or Crispix cereal
2 cups powdered sugar

Melt the first three ingredients in a medium saucepan. Place the cereal in a large plastic container and add the melted mixture. Shake sealed container until all the cereal is coated. Add the powdered sugar.

Yield: 12 servings
¹⁄₁₂ recipe: 500 calories

FRUIT PIZZA

By Clare Jean Haury

1 package yellow cake mix
¼ cup water
¼ cup margarine, softened
2 eggs
¼ cup packed brown sugar
½ cup pecans, chopped
2 packages Dream Whip
fresh fruit

Grease and flour two 12-inch pizza pans. Combine half the cake mix and all other ingredients except the pecans, fruit, and Dream Whip. Mix well. Add remaining cake mix and mix well. Fold in nuts. Divide evenly between the two pans and spread to the edges. Bake at 350°F for 15 to 20 minutes. Cool. Prepare Dream Whip according to directions on package. Top each cake with one package of Dream Whip and add sliced fresh fruit to decorate.

Yield: 12 servings
$\frac{1}{12}$ recipe: 350 calories

ADDITIONAL RECIPES

Additional recipes can be found in two cystic fibrosis cookbooks:

Cooking Up Calories from the Antonio J. and Janet Palumbo Cystic Fibrosis Center at Children's Hospital of Pittsburgh, **compiled by Judy Fulton, R.D.**, CF Dietitian, and **Amy Wengryn**, parent of two well-nourished grown children with CF. To order, mail $5.00 per cookbook to Judy Fulton, Cystic Fibrosis, Children's Hospital of Pittsburgh, 3705 Fifth Ave., Pittsburgh, PA 15213. Make check payable to "CF Research."

Fat And Loving It!! A Book Written for the Individual with Cystic Fibrosis, **by Gail Farmer, M.S., R.D. and Sherri Willcox,** Sponsored by Digestive Care, Jumbo Jack's Cookbooks, Audubon Media Corporation, 301 Broadway, Audubon IA 50025; tel. (800) 798-2635.

Appendix E

The History of Cystic Fibrosis

Some highlights in the history of cystic fibrosis are as follows:

1705 A book of folk philosophy states that a salty taste means that a child is bewitched.

1857 The Almanac of Children's Songs and Games from Switzerland quotes from Middle Ages: "Woe is the child who tastes salty from a kiss on the brow, for he is hexed, and soon must die."

1938 Andersen first describes cystic fibrosis (CF), calling it cystic fibrosis of the pancreas.

1946 di Sant'Agnese and Andersen report using antibiotics to treat CF lung infection.

1953 di Sant'Agnese and colleagues describe the sweat abnormality in CF.

1955 First review of use of pancreatic enzymes.

1959 Gibson and Cook describe a safe and accurate way to do sweat testing.

1964 Doershuk, Matthews, and colleagues describe a modern comprehensive treatment program.

1978 First use of enteric-coated pancreatic enzymes.

1981–1983 Description by Knowles and colleagues and Quinton and coworkers of electrolyte transport abnormalities.

1989 Tsui, Riordan, and Collins discover CF gene.

1990 Correction of chloride transport defect in CF cells in culture by adenovirus-mediated gene transfer.

1992 First trials of gene transfer in living people with CF.

1997 Establishment of Therapeutics Development Network in United States by Cystic Fibrosis Foundation.

Modified from Taussig LM. *Cystic fibrosis.* New York: Thieme-Stratton, 1984.

Appendix F

Bibliography

And Other Places to Read About Cystic Fibrosis

SUGGESTED READING

General—Textbooks

Hodson ME, Geddes DM, eds. *Cystic fibrosis.* London: Chapman & Hall Medical, 1995. A comprehensive text on cystic fibrosis; an excellent resource.

Davis PB, ed. *Cystic fibrosis.* New York: Marcel Dekker, Inc., 1993. Also an excellent text.

Orenstein DM, Stern RC, eds. *Treatment of the hospitalized cystic fibrosis patient.* New York: Marcel Dekker, Inc., 1998. In-depth medical detail, aimed at physician audience; actually covers more than just hospitalized patients.

Orenstein DM, Rosenstein BJ, Stern RC. *Cystic fibrosis medical care.* Philadelphia: Lippincott Williams & Wilkins, 2000. General overview, also aimed at professional audience.

Yankaskas JR, Knowles MR, eds. *Cystic fibrosis in adults.* Philadelphia: Lippincott–Raven Publishers, 1999. Excellent medical text, with in-depth coverage of all aspects of cystic fibrosis medical care for adults.

Doershuk CF. *Cystic fibrosis in the 20th century.* Cleveland, OH: AM Publishing, 2001. A fascinating look at the history of cystic fibrosis and cystic fibrosis science and care from the very personal viewpoints of many of the people who lived and made the history.

General—Journal Article

Davis PB, Drumm M, Konstan MW. Cystic fibrosis: state of the art. *Am J Resp Crit Care Med* 1996;154:1229–1256.

Of Historical Interest

Andersen DH. Cystic fibrosis of the pancreas and its relation to celiac disease; a clinical and pathologic study. *Am J Dis Child* 1938;356:344–395. The earliest description of cystic fibrosis as a single entity.

di Sant'Agnese PA, Darling RC, Perera GA, et al. Abnormal electrolyte composition of sweat in cystic fibrosis of the pancreas: clinical significance and relationship of the disease. *Pediatrics* 1953;12:549–563. Original description of the high salt content in cystic fibrosis sweat.

Doershuk CF, Matthews LW, Tucker AS, et al. A five-year clinical evaluation of a therapeutic program for patients with cystic fibrosis. *J Pediatr* 1964;65:677–693. The first paper to show the benefit of a comprehensive treatment program for patients with cystic fibrosis.

Gibson LE, Cooke RE. A test for concentration of electrolytes in sweat in cystic fibrosis of the pancreas utilizing pilocarpine by iontophoresis. *Pediatrics* 1959;23:545–549. Landmark report detailing a laboratory method for collection and analysis of cystic fibrosis sweat.

Knowles M, Gatzy J, Boucher R. Increased bioelectric potential difference across respiratory epithelia in cystic fibrosis. *N Engl J Med* 1981;305:1489–1495. The first of the papers to elucidate the problem with electrolyte transport across mucous membranes in CF.

Quinton PM, Bijman J. Higher bioelectric potentials due to decreased chloride absorption in the sweat glands of patients with cystic fibrosis. *N Engl J Med* 1983;308:1185–1189. Initial publication demonstrating that the problem in nose and respiratory tree also existed in sweat glands, and that it was primarily a problem with chloride not being able to pass through mucous membranes.

Rommens JM, Iannuzzi MC, Kerem B-S, et al. Identification of the cystic fibrosis gene: chromosome walking and jumping. *Science* 1989;245:1059–1065. Landmark paper announcing discovery and cloning of cystic fibrosis gene by Drs. Lap-Chee Tsui, Francis Collins, and Jack Riordan (and their colleagues), from Toronto and Michigan.

Drumm ML, Pope HA, Cliff WH, et al. Correction of the cystic fibrosis defect *in vitro* by retrovirus-mediated gene transfer. *Cell* 1990;62:1227–1233.

Rich DP, Anderson MP, Gregory RJ, et al. Expression of cystic fibrosis transmembrane conductance regulator corrects defective chloride channel regulation in cystic fibrosis airway epithelial cell. *Nature* 1990;347:358–363.

These two papers appeared almost simultaneously and showed that the CF cell defect could be cured in the laboratory with gene transfer.

For Classroom Teachers

Young A. *Cystic fibrosis in the classroom*. Distributed via Scandipharm (Birmingham, AL). Superb introduction to cystic fibrosis for teachers who have a child with cystic fibrosis in their classes.

"WEBLIOGRAPHY": SOME SELECTED SITES ON THE WORLD WIDE WEB

(To the reader, Surfer: BEWARE!! Sites may change; content of some sites you might find in a Google search may vary from superb to wacko!)

Web Site	Sponsor/Comments
http://www.cff.org	Cystic Fibrosis Foundation *Probably the best single site; up to date, reliable*
http://www.iacfa.org	International Association of Cystic Fibrosis Adults *A very good site, with international flavor; also includes topics relevant to younger patients*
http://www.cfww.org	Cystic Fibrosis Worldwide *Interchangeable with previous listing*
http://personal.nbnet.nb.ca/normap/CF.htm	Norma Kennedy Plourde, a Canadian woman with cystic fibrosis. *This site is excellent, with many useful links to other helpful sites.*

Appendix G

Cystic Fibrosis Care Centers in the United States

ALABAMA

Birmingham

UAB Cystic Fibrosis Center
The Children's Hospital
University of Alabama at Birmingham
1600 7th Avenue, South, Suite 620ACC
Birmingham, AL 35233

Appts: (205) 939-9583

Center Director:

Raymond Lyrene, M.D.
(205) 934-3574 or (205) 939-9583
Fax: (205) 975-5983
rlyrene@peds.uab.edu

Adult Program Director:

K. Randall Young, Jr., M.D.
(205) 975-0763
Fax: (205) 934-1721
ryoung@uab.edu

Mobile

USA Children's Medical Center
P. O. Drawer 40130
1504 Spring Hill Avenue
Mobile, AL 36640-0130
Appts: (334) 343-6848
Fax: (334) 340-7449

Center Director:

Lawrence J. Sindel, M.D.*
(334) 343-6848
Fax: (334) 340-7449
lsindel@zebra.net

*Preferred Mailing Address:

Pulmonary Associates of Mobile, P.A.
100 Memorial Hospital Drive, Suite 1A
Mobile, AL 36608

ALASKA

See Seattle, Washington, Children's
Hospital and Regional Medical Center.

ARIZONA

Phoenix

Cystic Fibrosis Center
Phoenix Children's Hospital
1919 East Thomas Road
Phoenix, AZ 85016

Appts: (602) 546-0354
cfcenter@phxchildrens.com

Center Director:

Peggy J. Radford, M.D.
(602) 546-0985
Fax: (602) 546-0323
peggy_radford@hotmail.com

377

Adult Program Director:

Gerald D. Gong, M.D.
(602) 546-0985
Fax: (602) 546-0323
ggong@phoenixchildrens.com

Tucson

Tucson Cystic Fibrosis Center
1501 N. Campbell Avenue,
    Room 2332
P. O. Box 245073
Tucson, AZ 85724

Appts: (520) 694-9937

Center Director:

Wayne J. Morgan, M.D.
(520) 626-7780
Fax: (520) 626-9465
wmorgan@resp-sci.arizona.edu

ARKANSAS
Little Rock

Arkansas Cystic Fibrosis Center
Arkansas Children's Hospital
800 Marshall Street
Little Rock, AR 72202-3591

Appts: (501) 320-2903

Center Director:

John Carroll, M.D.
(501) 364-1006
Fax: (501) 320-3930
carrolljohnl@uams.edu

Adult Program:

University of Arkansas for Medical
    Sciences
Pulmonary/Critical Care Medicine
4301 West Markham, Slot 555
Little Rock, AR 72205

Director:

Paula Anderson, M.D.
(501) 686-5525
Fax: (501) 686-7893
andersonpaulaj@uams.edu

CALIFORNIA
Long Beach

Cystic Fibrosis Center
Miller Children's at
Long Beach Memorial Medical Center
2801 Atlantic Avenue
P. O. Box 1428
Long Beach, CA 90801-1428

Appts: (562) 933-8567
Fax: (562) 933-8569

Center Director:

Eliezer Nussbaum, M.D.
(562) 933-8740
Fax: (562) 933-8744
enussbaum@memorialcare.net

Adult Program:

Long Beach Memorial Medical Center

Appts: (562) 933-8567

Director:

Jeffrey Riker, M.D.
jriker@memnet.org

Los Angeles

Comprehensive Cystic Fibrosis Center
Children's Hospital of Los Angeles
4650 Sunset Boulevard
Mail Stop #83
Los Angeles, CA 90027-6016

Appts: (323) 669-2287 (direct line)
        (323) 660-2450 (hospital)

Center Director:
Arnold Platzker, M.D.
(323) 669-2101

Adult Program:
University of Southern California
Ambulatory Health Care Center
1355 San Pablo Street
Los Angeles, CA 90033

Appts: (323) 442-5100

Director:
Bertrand Shapiro, M.D.
(323) 442-5100
Fax: (323) 442-5110
bshapiro@hsc.usc.edu

Affiliate Programs:
1. Kaiser-Permanente Southern
   California
   13652 Cantara Street, VC101B
   Panorama City, CA 91402

   Appts: (818) 375-2909

   (Contact: Joan Franco. Open to
   members of the Kaiser-Permanente
   Health Plan only.)

Director:
Allan S. Lieberthal, M.D.
(818) 375-2909
Fax: (818) 375-4073
allan.s.lieberthal@kp.org

2. Loma Linda University Medical
   Center
   Coleman Pavilion
   P. O. Box 2000
   Loma Linda, CA 92350

   Appts: (909) 558-2301
   Fax: (909) 824-4184

Director:
Yvonne Fanous, M.D.
(909) 796-7311

3. Pediatric Diagnostic Center
   3400 Loma Vista Road, Suite 1
   Ventura, CA 93003

   Appts: (805) 289-3333
   www.medmall.org

Director:
Chris Landon, M.D.
(805) 289-3333
Fax: (805) 289-3310
landon@rain.org

Outreach:
1. Cedars Sinai Medical Center
   8700 Beverly Boulevard
   Suite 1165, West Tower
   Department of Pediatrics
   Los Angeles, CA 90048

   Appts: (310) 423-4433

Director:
Andrew Wachtel, M.D. (adults)
wachtel@csmc.edu
2. UCLA Medical Center
   10833 Leconte Avenue
   Los Angeles, CA 90094

   Appts: (310) 267-1192
   Fax: (310) 206-3772

Director:

Oakland

1. Kaiser Permanente Medical Care
   Program
   Attn: Gail Farmer, M.S., R.D.
   Department of Pediatrics
   280 West MacArthur Boulevard
   Oakland, CA 94611

   Appts: (510) 752-6906
   (ask for Gail Farmer)
   gail.farmer@kp.org

Center Director:

Gregory F. Shay, M.D.
(510) 752-6596
Fax: (510) 752-7054
greg.shay@kp.org

(Kaiser has three locations. Call Gail Farmer for information.)

Adult Program:

Kaiser Permanente Medical Care Program
Pulmonary Medicine Division
280 West MacArthur Blvd.
Oakland, CA 94611

Director:

Bryon Quick, M.D.
(510) 752-7984
Fax: (510) 752-6882
Bryon.Quick@kp.org
2. Pediatric Pulmonary Center Children's Hospital–Oakland 747 52nd Street Oakland, CA 94609

Appts: (510) 428-3305

Center Director:

Karen A. Hardy, M.D.
(510) 428-3305
Fax: (510) 597-7154
khardy@mail.cho.org

Outreach:

Adult Program
CPMC
2351 Clay Street, Suite 501
Department of Pediatrics
San Francisco, California 94115

Director:

Christopher Brown, M.D.
(415) 923-3421
Fax: (415) 600-1414

Orange

Children's Hospital of Orange County
455 South Main Street
Orange, CA 92868

Appts: (714) 532-8622

Center Director:

David A. Hicks, M.D.
(714) 532-8622
Fax: (714) 289-4072
cfdesk@choc.com

Palo Alto

Stanford CF Center
Stanford University Medical Center
701 Welch Road, #3328
Palo Alto, CA 94304-5786

Appts: (650) 497-8841 (scheduling)
         (650) 723-5191 (message for doctor)
http://cfcenter.stanford.edu

Center Director:

Richard Moss, M.D.
(650) 723-5191
Fax: (650) 723-5201
rmoss@stanford.edu

Adult Program Director:

Noreen Henig, M.D.
(650) 498-5248
Fax: (650) 725-5489
nhenig@leland.stanford.edu

Sacramento

Cystic Fibrosis and Pediatric Respiratory Diseases Center
University of California at Davis Medical Center
Department of Pediatrics
2516 Stockton Boulevard
Sacramento, CA 95817

Appts: (916) 734-3112

Center Director:

Ruth J. McDonald, M.D.
(916) 734-3189
Fax: (916) 734-4757
peds.cfpulmo@ucdmc.ucdavis.edu

Adult Program:

University of California
Davis Medical Center
4150 V Street, Suite 3400
Sacramento, CA 95817

Director:

Carroll Cross, M.D.
(916) 734-3564
Fax: (916) 734-7924
cecross@ucdavis.edu

San Diego

San Diego Cystic Fibrosis and Pediatric
  Pulmonary Disease Center
Children's Hospital and Health Center
UCSD School of Medicine
3020 Children's Way, MC 5070
San Diego, CA 92123

Appts: (858) 966-5999

Center Director:

Mark S. Pian, M.D.
(858) 966-6790
Fax: (858) 966-8533
mpian@ucsd.edu

Adult Program:

UCSD Medical Center
200 West Arbor Drive
Mail Code 8448
San Diego, CA 92103-1990

Appts: (619) 294-6125

Director:

Douglas J. Conrad, M.D.
Fax: (619) 296-3758
dconrad@ucsd.edu

San Francisco

Cystic Fibrosis Center
University of California at
  San Francisco
505 Parnassus Avenue
Room M650
San Francisco, CA 94143-0106

Appts: San Francisco: (415) 353-2813
Walnut Creek: (925) 941-3155

Center Director:

Dennis W. Nielson, M.D., Ph.D.
(415) 641-3471
Fax: (415) 502-4186
nielsond@peds.ucsf.edu

Co-Center Director:

Nancy Lewis, M.D.

Adult Program:

University of California at San
  Francisco
505 Parnassus Avenue
Room M1093
San Francisco, CA 94143-0120

Appts: (415) 353-2244

Director:

Michael S. Stulbarg, M.D.
(415) 476-0631
Fax: (415) 476-5712
michael@itsa.ucsf.edu

Affiliate Program:

Valley Children's Hospital
Pediatric Pulmonary and Respiratory
  Care
9300 Valley Children's Place
Madera, California 93638

Appts: (559) 353-5550

Director:

Reddi Sudhakar, M.D.
Fax: (559) 353-5587
rlcsud@pol.net
slehto@valleychildrens.org

Outreach:

University of California at San Francisco
John Muir Medical Center

Appts: (925) 941-3155

Director:

Nancy C. Lewis, M.D.

COLORADO

Denver

The Children's Hospital
1056 East 19th Avenue
Box B395
Denver, CO 80218-1088

Appts: (303) 861-6182, option 1

Center Director:

Frank J. Accurso, M.D.
(303) 837-2522
Fax: (303) 837-2924
accurso.frank@tchden.org

Adult Program:

University of Colorado Health Sciences
   Center
4200 East 9th Avenue
Box B-133
Denver, CO 80262

Appts: (303) 315-6026
Fax: (303) 270-2206

Director:

David Rodman, M.D.
(303) 315-4473
david.rodman@.uchsc.edu

Outpatient Program:

(303) 315-6026

Outreach Program:

Billings Clinic
2825 8th Avenue, North
Billings, MT 59101

Appts: (406) 237-4280

CONNECTICUT

Hartford

Cystic Fibrosis Center
Pediatric Pulmonology Division
Connecticut Children's Medical Center
282 Washington Street
Hartford, CT 06107

Appts: (860) 545-9440

Center Director:

Craig D. Lapin, M.D.
(860) 545-9436
Fax: (860) 545-9445
clapin@ccmckids.org

Adult Program Director:

Rick Knauft, M.D.
(860) 547-1876
Fax: (860) 520-1379
rknauft@harthosp.org

New Haven

Cystic Fibrosis Center
Yale University School of Medicine
333 Cedar Street, Fitkin 511
New Haven, CT 06520-8064

Appts: (203) 785-4081

Center Director:

Regina M. Palazzo, M.D.
(203) 785-2480
Fax: (203) 785-6337
regina.palazzo@yale.edu

Associate Director:

Marie E. Egan, M.D.
(203) 785-2480
Fax: (203) 785-6337
marie.egan@yale.edu

Adult Program Director:

Caroline S. Kim, M.D., M.P.H.

DELAWARE

Wilmington

Alfred I. duPont Hospital for Children
1600 Rockland Road
P. O. Box 269
Wilmington, DE 19899

Appts: (302) 651-4200

Center Director:

Raj Padman, M.D.
(302) 651-6400
Fax: (302) 651-6408
aszymans@nemours.org
dmjohnso@nemours.org

Center Codirector:

Aaron Chidekel, M.D.
achidek@nemours.org

DISTRICT OF COLUMBIA

Metropolitan D.C. Cystic Fibrosis Center
for Care, Training and Research
Children's National Medical Center
111 Michigan Avenue, N.W.
Washington, D.C. 20010-2970

Appts: (202) 884-2610

Interim Center Director:

Holly Chaney, M.D.
(202) 884-2128
Fax: (202) 884-5864
hchaney@cnmc.org

FLORIDA

Gainesville

Cystic Fibrosis and Pediatric Pulmonary
Disease Center
University of Florida
1600 SW Archer Road
P. O. Box 100296
Gainesville, FL 32610-0296

Appts: (352) 392-4458
harvelr@peds.ufl.edu

Center Director:

Mary H. Wagner, M.D.
Fax: (352) 392-4450
wagneam@peds.ufl.edu

Adult Program Director:

Arundhati Foster, M.D.
(352) 392-2666
Fax: (352) 392-0821
fostera@medicine.ufl.edu

Affiliate Program:

Joe DiMaggio Children's Hospital
Cystic Fibrosis Clinic
3435 Hayes Street
Hollywood, FL 33321

Appts: (954) 986-6333

Director:

Morton N. Schwartzman, M.D.
(954) 986-6333
Fax: (954) 961-7027
jdcf@mhs-net.com

Jacksonville

Nemours Children's Clinic
807 Children's Way
Jacksonville, FL 32207

Appts: (904) 390-3788
cfc@nemours.org

Center Director:

Bonnie B. Hudak, M.D.
(904) 390-3676
Fax: (904) 390-3422
bhudak@nemours.org

Affiliate Program:

Nemours-Pensacola
Pensacola, FL

Appts: (850) 505-4700

Director:

Kevin D. Maupin, M.D.
kmaupin@nemours.org

Miami

Batchelor Children's Research Institute
  University of Miami School of Medicine
1580 N.W. 10th Avenue
Miami, FL 33136

Appts: (305) 243-6641

Center Director:

Giovanni Piedimonte, M.D.
(305) 243-3176
Fax: (305) 243-1262
gpiedimo@med.miami.edu

Associate Director:

Michael Light, M.D.
(305) 243-6641
mlight@med.miami.edu

Adults Program:

University of Miami School of Medicine

Appts: (305) 243-6641

Adult Program Director:

Debra Fertel, M.D.
(305) 585-7340
dfertel@exchange.med.miami.edu

Orlando

Cystic Fibrosis Center
The Nemours Children's Clinic
83 West Columbia Street
Orlando, FL 32806

Appts: (407) 650-7366

Center Director:

David Geller, M.D.
(407) 650-7270
Fax: (407) 650-7277
dgeller@nemours.org

Adult Program:

Central Florida Pulmonary Group

Appts: (407) 841-1100, ext. 112

Adult Program Director:

Martin A. Kubiet, M.D.
teresam_cfpg@hotmail.com

St. Petersburg

Cystic Fibrosis Center
All Children's Hospital
880 Sixth Street South, Suite 390
St. Petersburg, FL 33701

Appts: (727) 892-4146

Center Director:

Juan Martinez, M.D.
(727) 892-4146
Fax: (727) 892-4218
martinez@allkids.org

Adult Program:

University of South Florida
Adult Cystic Fibrosis Center
880 6th Street, S, Suite 390
St. Petersburg, FL 33701

Appts: (727) 892-4146

Director:

Mark Rolfe, M.D.
(813) 974-7551
Fax: (813) 907-1060
mwrolfe@aol.com

Affiliate Programs:

1. St. Mary's Medical Center
   P. O. Box 24620
   901 45th Street
   West Palm Beach, FL 33407

   Appts: (561) 840-6065

Director:

Sue S. Goldfinger, M.D.
(561) 881-2911
Fax: (561) 882-1078
ljmidd@ihswpb.com

2. Division of Pulmonology
   Miami Children's Hospital
   MOB #203, 3200 S.W. 60th Court
   Miami, FL 33155

   Appts: (305) 662-8380

Director:

Carlos E. Diaz, M.D.
(305) 662-8380
Fax: (305) 663-8417
carlos.diaz@mch.com

3. University of South Florida
   Department of Pediatrics
   17 Davis Boulevard, Suite 200
   Tampa, FL 33606

   Appts: (813) 259-8767
   ksulliva@comq.ed.usf.edu

Director:

Bruce M. Schnapf, D.O.
(813) 276-5520
Fax: (813) 272-2995
bschnapf@com1.med.usf.edu

Outreach Clinics:

1. New Port Richey Specialty Care
   Clinic
   5640 Main Street
   New Port Richey, FL 34652
2. Sarasota Clinic
   5881 Rand Boulevard
   Sarasota, FL 34238
3. Tampa Clinic
   12220 Bruce B. Downs Boulevard
   Tampa, FL 33612
4. Lakeland Clinic
   3310 Lakeland Hills Boulevard
   Lakeland, FL 33805

   Appts: (727) 892-4146

GEORGIA

Atlanta

Emory University CF Center
Emory University School of Medicine
Department of Pediatrics
2040 Ridgewood Drive, NE
Atlanta, GA 30322

Appts: (404) 727-5728
Fax: (404) 727-4828
joy_dangerfield@oz.ped.emory.edu

Center Director:

Gerald Teague, M.D.
rhonda_thompson@oz.ped.emory.edu

Augusta

Medical College of Georgia
Pediatric Pulmonology Section
1120 15th Street
Augusta, GA 30912-3755

Appts: (706) 721-2635
krhodes@mail.mcg.edu

Center Director:

Margaret F. Guill, M.D.
(706) 721-2635
Fax: (706) 721-8512
mguill@mail.mcg.edu

Adult Program Director:

Amy R. Blanchard, M.D.

Appts: (706) 721-1450
Fax: (706) 721-3069
ablancha@mail.mcg.edu

Affiliate Program:

Children's Healthcare of Atlanta
1001 Johnson Ferry Road, N.
Atlanta, GA 30342

Appts: (404) 250-2038
Fax: (404) 257-3291
barbara.crews@choa.org

Director:

Peter H. Scott, M.D.
(404) 252-7339
Fax: (404) 257-0337
pscott@jppa.net

Outreach Clinics:

1. Ware County Health Department
   Daisy Clinic
   Waycross, GA 31501

   Appts: (706) 721-2635
2. John Archbold Memorial Hospital
   Thomasville, GA 31799

   Appts: (706) 721-2635
3. Children's Medical Services
   Albany, GA 31701

   Appts: (706) 721-2635

HAWAII

See San Antonio, Texas
Tripler Army Medical Center

IDAHO

See Salt Lake City, Utah
(Meridian, Pocatello, and Idaho Falls)

ILLINOIS
Chicago

1. Cystic Fibrosis Center
   Children's Memorial Hospital
   Northwestern University
   2300 Children's Plaza, Box 43
   Chicago, IL 60614

   Appts: (773) 880-4382
   www.childrenscf.org

Center Director:

Susanna A. McColley, M.D.
(773) 880-4382
Fax: (773) 880-6300
smccolley@northwestern.edu

Adult Program:

Northwestern Memorial Hospital
303 E. Superior Street, Suite 774
Chicago, IL 60611

Appts: (312) 695-2003

Director:

Manu Jain, M.D.
(312) 908-4233
m-jain@northwestern.edu
2. University of Chicago Cystic
   Fibrosis Center
   University of Chicago Children's
   Hospital
   5841 South Maryland Avenue
   Mail Code 4064, Room L444
   Chicago, IL 60637-1470

   Appts: (773) 702-6178

Center Director:

Young-Jee Kim, M.D.

Adult Program:

University of Chicago Hospitals
5841 South Maryland Avenue
MC6076, Room W659
Chicago, IL 60637-1470

Appts: (773) 702-3815

Adult Program Director:

Eugene Geppert, M.D.
egeppert@medicine.bsd.uchicago.edu
3. Rush Cystic Fibrosis Center
   1653 W. Congress Parkway, #451-PAV
   Chicago, IL 60612

   Appts: (312) 563-2270
   Fax: (312) 563-2299

Center Codirector:

Lucille A. Lester, M.D.
Lucille_A_Lester@rush.edu

Center Codirector:

John D. Lloyd-Still, M.D.
John_D_Lloyd-Still@rush.edu

Adult Program:

Rush Medical Center

Appts: (312) 563-2270

Adult Program Director:

Peter Szidon, M.D.
jan.szidon@worldnet.att.net

Maywood

Cystic Fibrosis Center
Loyola University Medical Center
2160 S. First Avenue
Maywood, IL 60153

Appts: (708) 327-9134

Pediatric Program Director:

Youngran Chung, M.D.
(708) 327-9073
Fax: (708) 327-9160
ychung@lumc.edu

Center Director

Adult Program Director:

Edward R. Garrity, Jr., M.D.
egarrit@lumc.edu

Park Ridge

Cystic Fibrosis Center
Lutheran General Children's Hospital
Victor Yacktman Children's Pavilion
1775 W. Dempster Street
Park Ridge, IL 60068

Appts: (847) 318-9330

Center Director:

Gabriel Aljadeff, M.D.
(847) 723-5578
Fax: (847) 723-2325
gabriel.aljadeff-md@advocatehealth.com

Adult Program:

Lutheran General Hospital
Adult Cystic Fibrosis Center
8780 WW Golf Road, Suite 204
Niles, IL 60714

Appts: (847) 759-4770

Director:

Arvey Stone, M.D.
(847) 759-4770
Fax: (847) 759-8824
alja4@aol.com

Peoria

Cystic Fibrosis Center
Saint Francis Medical Center
320 E. Armstrong, 2nd Floor
Peoria, IL 61603

Appts: (309) 624-9680

Center Director:
Umesh C. Chatrath, M.D.*
(309) 624-9680
Fax: (309) 624-9757
marie.green@osfhealthcare.org
uchatra@uic.edu

*Preferred Mailing Address:
320 E. Armstrong, 2nd FloorAQ3
Peoria, IL 61603

Adult Program:
St. Francis Medical Center
320 E. Armstrong, 2nd Floor
Peoria, IL 61603

Appts: (309) 624-9680

Adult Program Director:
W. Anthony Sauder, M.D.
wasauder@insightbb.com

Springfield

See Washington University School of
Medicine, St. Louis, Missouri.

Urbana

See Washington University School of
Medicine, St. Louis, Missouri.

INDIANA

Indianapolis

Cystic Fibrosis Center
Riley Hospital for Children
Indiana University Medical Center
702 Barnhill Drive, Room 2750
Indianapolis, IN 46202-5225

Appts: (317) 274-7208
Fax: (317) 274-5791

Center Director:
Michelle Howenstine, M.D.
(317) 274-7208
mhowenst@iupui.edu

Clinic Coordinator:
Judy Hollingsworth, M.S.N., R.N.
jlhollin@iupui.edu

Adult Program:
Indiana University
1481 West 10th Street
VA111 P
Indianapolis, IN 46202-2884

Director:
Veena Antony, M.D.
(317) 554-000, ext. 2513
vantony@indyunix.iupui.edu

Affiliate Program:
Lutheran Hospital
c/o Cystic Fibrosis and Pediatric
Pulmonary Clinic
7950 West Jefferson Boulevard
Ft. Wayne, IN 46804-4160

Appts: (219) 435-7123
Fax: (219) 435-6947

Director:
Pushpom James, M.D.

Cystic Fibrosis Program Coordinator:
Eva Fish, R.R.T.
efish@lutheran-hosp.com

Adult Care Provider:
Fred Rasp, M.D.

Adult Clinic Coordinator:
Paul Kuras, R.R.T.

Appts: (219) 435-7711

Outreach:

Deaconess Hospital
600 Mary Street
Evansville, IN 47747

Appts: (812) 450-2176

South Bend

Cystic Fibrosis and Chronic Pulmonary
Disease Clinic of St. Joseph's
Regional Medical Center
720 E. Cedar Street, Suite 440
South Bend, IN 46617-1935

Appts: (574) 239-6126
figgl@sjmrc.com

Center Director:

James Harris, M.D.*
(574) 237-9216
Fax: (574) 239-1451
jbharrismd@aol.com

Preferred Mailing Address:

Cystic Fibrosis and Chronic Pulmonary
Disease Clinic of St. Joseph's Regional
Medical Center
720 E. Cedar Street, Suite 440
South Bend, IN 46617-1935

Attn: Lynn Figg, R.N.

Adult Care Provider:

Matthew Koscielsk

IOWA

Des Moines

Cystic Fibrosis Center
Blank Children's Health Center
1212 Pleasant Street, Suite 300
Des Moines, IA 50309

Appts: (515) 241-8925
Fax: (515) 241-8728

Center Director:

Veljko Zivkovich, M.D.
(515) 244-7229
Fax: (515) 244-7233
wellenjm@ihs.org

Iowa City

Cystic Fibrosis Center
Pediatric Allergy and Pulmonary Division
Department of Pediatrics
200 Hawkins Drive
University of Iowa Hospitals and Clinics
Iowa City, IA 52242-1083

Appts: (319) 356-2229
Fax: (319) 356-7171
elizabeth-dowd@uiowa.edu

Center Director:

Miles M. Weinberger, M.D.
(319) 356-3485
Fax: (319) 356-7171
miles-weinberger@uiowa.edu

Center Codirector:

Richard C. Ahrens, M.D.
(319) 356-4050
Fax: (319) 356-7171
richard-ahrens@uiowa.edu

Adult Program Director:

Douglas Hornick, M.D.
(319) 356-8266
Fax: (319) 353-6406
douglas-hornick@uiowa.edu

Affiliate Program:

McFarland Clinic
Mary Greeley Hospital
1215 Duff
Ames, IA 50010

Appts: (515) 239-4482

Director:

Edward G. Nassif, M.D.
mcfarlandclinic.com

KANSAS

Kansas City

Cystic Fibrosis Center
Kansas University Children's Center
3901 Rainbow Boulevard
Kansas City, KS 66160-7330

Appts: (913) 588-6377

Center Director:

Joseph Kanarek, M.D.
(913) 588-6377
Fax: (913) 588-6280
alieberg@kumc.edu

Center Codirector:

Gayln Perry, M.D.
(913) 588-6377
Fax: (913) 588-6320
gperry@kumc.edu

Adult Program:

University of Kansas Medical Center
3901 Rainbow Blvd.
Kansas City, Kansas 66160-7381

Appts: (913) 588-6044

Adult Program Director:

Steven Stites, M.D.
Fax: (913) 588-4098
sstites@kumc.edu

Adult Program Assistant Director:

Gayln Perry, M.D.
gperry@kumc.edu

Wichita

Cystic Fibrosis Care and Teaching Center
Via Christi, St. Francis Campus
929 North St. Francis
Outpatient Clinic/CF Clinic
Wichita, KS 67218

Appts: (800) 362-0070 x5040

Center Director:

Maria Riva, M.D*
(316) 689-9264
Fax: (316) 689-9140
mariariva@pol.net

*Preferred Mailing Address:

Wichita Clinic
3311 East Murdock
Wichita, KS 67208

Adult Program Director:

Daniel Doornbos, M.D.
1120 N. Rutland Street
Wichita, KS 67206
(316) 689-9355
Fax: (316) 689-9363
drdand@kscable.com

KENTUCKY

Lexington

Cystic Fibrosis Center
University of Kentucky
Division of Pediatric Pulmonology
740 South Limestone
J410 Kentucky Clinic
Lexington, KY 40536-0284

Appts: (859) 323-6211, ext. 1

Center Director:

Jamshed F. Kanga, M.D.
(859) 257-5536
Fax: (859) 257-7706
jfkk@pop.uky.edu

Adult Program Director:

Michael I. Anstead, M.D.
mianstq@pop.uky.edu

Louisville

Kosair Children's Cystic Fibrosis Center
University of Louisville
234 East Gray Street, Suite 270
Louisville, KY 40202

Appts: (502) 629-8830

Center Director:

Nemr S. Eid, M.D.*
(502) 852-3772
Fax: (502) 852-4051
nseid@louisville.edu

*Preferred Mailing Address:
571 S. Floyd Street, Suite 414
Louisville, KY 40202

LOUISIANA

New Orleans

Tulane University Cystic Fibrosis Center
Tulane University Hospital and Clinic
1415 Tulane Avenue
New Orleans, LA 70112

Patient Appts:
Pediatric: (504) 587-7625
Adults: (504) 588-5800

Center Director:

Scott H. Davis, M.D.
Department of Pediatrics SL-37
Tulane University School of Medicine
1430 Tulane Avenue
New Orleans, LA 70112
(504) 588-5601
Fax: (504) 588-5490
shdavis@tulane.edu

Adult Program Director:

Blesilda C. Quiniones, M.D.
Department of Medicine SL-9
Tulane University School of Medicine
1430 Tulane Avenue
New Orleans, LA 70112
(504) 588-2250
Fax: (504) 587-2144
bquinio@tulane.edu

Shreveport

Cystic Fibrosis and Pediatric Pulmonary
  Center
Louisiana State University Health
  Sciences Center
1501 Kings Highway
P. O. Box 33932
Shreveport, LA 71130-3932

Appts: (318) 675-6094
Fax: (318) 675-7668

Center Director:

Kimberly Jones, M.D.
(318) 675-6094
kjone1@lsuhsc.edu

MAINE

Portland

MMC Cystic Fibrosis Center
Maine Pediatric Specialty Group
887 Congress Street, Suite 320
Portland, ME 04102

Appts: (207) 828-8226
lefebj@mmc.org

Center Director:

Anne Marie Cairns, D.O.*
(207) 828-8226
Fax: (207) 775-6024
cairna@mmc.org

*Preferred Mailing Address:

Maine Pediatric Specialty Group
295 Forest Avenue
Portland, ME 04101

Adult Program Director:

Jonathan Zuckerman, M.D.
(207) 871-2770
Fax: (207) 871-4691
zuckej@mail.mmc.org

Affiliate Programs:

1. Cystic Fibrosis Clinical Center
   Eastern Maine Medical Center
   417 State Street, Suite 305
   Bangor, ME 04401

   Appts: (207) 973-7559
   Fax: (207) 973-7674

Director:

Thomas Lever, M.D.
(207) 947-0147
Fax: (207) 990-3365
tflever@pol.net

2. Central Maine Cystic Fibrosis Center
   Central Maine Medical Center
   300 Main Street
   Lewiston, ME 04240

   Appts: (207) 795-2630
   Fax: (207) 795-5679

Director:

Ralph V. Harder, M.D.
(207) 784-5489
Fax: (207) 777-7241
rharder@cochs.com

Associate Director:

David Baker, M.D.
(207) 795-5730
Fax (207) 795-5679
dbaker@cmhc.org

Center Coordinator:

Shelly Jo Stone, R.N.C.
(207) 795-2630

MARYLAND

Baltimore

The Johns Hopkins Hospital
600 N. Wolfe Street, Park 315
Baltimore, MD 21287-2533

Appts: (410) 955-2795

Center Director:

Peter Mogayzel, M.D.
(410) 955-2795
Fax: (410) 955-1030

Center Codirector:

Pamela L. Zeitlin, M.D., Ph.D
(410) 955-2795
Fax: (410) 955-1030
pzeitli@jhmi.edu

Adult Program:

Johns Hopkins Adult CF Program
Jefferson B1-170
600 N. Wolfe Street
Baltimore, MD 21287-8922

Appts: (410) 502-7044

Director:

Michael P. Boyle, M.D.
(410) 502-7043
Fax: (410) 502-7048
mboyle@mail.jhmi.edu

Bethesda

Cystic Fibrosis Center
National Institute of Diabetes and Digestive and Kidney Diseases
National Institutes of Health
Building 10, Room 8C438
Bethesda, MD 20892

Appts: (301) 496-3434

Center Director:

Milica S. Chernick, M.D.
(301) 496-3434
Fax: (301) 496-9943
milica_chernick@nih.gov

MASSACHUSETTS

Boston

1. Cystic Fibrosis Center Pulmonary
   Division
   Children's Hospital
   300 Longwood Avenue
   Boston, MA 02115

Appts: (617) 355-7881

Center Director:

Mary Ellen Wohl, M.D.
(617) 355-6105
Fax: (617) 566-7810
maryellen.wohl@hub.tch.harvard.edu

Adult Care Program Director:

Craig Gerard, M.D., Ph.D.
(617) 355-6953
craig.gerard@tch.harvard.edu

2. Cystic Fibrosis Center
   Massachusetts General Hospital
   ACC 707
   15 Parkman Street
   Boston, MA 02114

Appts: (617) 726-8707

Center Director:

Henry L. Dorkin, M.D.
(617) 726-8707
Fax: (617) 724-0581
hdorkin@partners.org

Adult Program Director:

Marcy Ruddy, M.D.
(617) 726-8707
Fax: (617) 726-6878
mruddy@partners.org

3. Cystic Fibrosis Center
   New England Medical Center
   750 Washington Street, Box 343
   Boston, MA 02111
   Appts: (617) 636-7917

Center Director:

Thomas Martin, M.D.
(617) 636-7917
Fax: (617) 636-7760

Adult Program Director:

Leonard Sicilian, M.D.
(617) 636-7917
lsicilian@lifespan.org

Springfield

Baystate Medical Center
3300 Main Street, Suite 4A
Springfield, MA 01199

Appts: (413) 794-7040

Center Director:

Robert S. Gerstle, M.D.
(413) 794-7341
Fax: (413) 794-7140
robert.gerstle@bhs.org

Worcester

UMass Memorial Health Care
Pediatric Pulmonary, Asthma, and Cystic
   Fibrosis Center
Room S5-860
55 Lake Avenue, North
Worcester, MA 01655

Appts: (508) 856-4155

Center Director:

Brian P. O'Sullivan, M.D.
(508) 856-4155
Fax: (508) 856-2609
osullivb@ummhc.org

Associate Director:

Robert G. Zwerdling, M.D.

MICHIGAN

Ann Arbor

University of Michigan Health System
Department of Pediatric Pulmonology
1500 East Medical Center Drive
Room L2221-0212
Ann Arbor, MI 48109-0212

Appts: (734) 764-4123 (Pediatrics)
(734) 936-5580 (Adult)

Center Director:

Samya Nasr, M.D.
Fax: (734) 764-4123
snasr@umich.edu

Adult Program Director:

Richard H. Simon, M.D.*
(734) 764-4554
Fax: (734) 764-4556
richsimo@umich.edu

Preferred Mailing Address:

University of Michigan Medical Center
Division of Pulmonary and Critical Care
6301 MSRB-3, Box 0642
1150 West Medical Center Drive
Ann Arbor, MI 48109-0642

Detroit

Children's Hospital of Michigan
Cystic Fibrosis Care, Teaching and
Resource Center
3901 Beaubien Boulevard
Detroit, MI 48201

Appts: (313) 745-5541

Center Director:

Debbie Toder, M.D.
(313) 745-5541
Fax: (313) 993-2948
dtoder@med.wayne.edu

Adult Programs:

1. Wayne State University
   Harper University Hospital
   3990 John R. Street, 3 Brush Center
   Detroit, MI 48201

   Appts: (313) 745-9151
   Fax: (313) 966-7178

Center Coordinator:

Yvette LeFlore, R.N.
(313) 745-9151
Fax: (313) 966-7178
yleflore@int.med.wayne.edu

Director:

Dana Kissner, M.D.
(313) 745-0895
Fax: (313) 993-0562
dkissner@intmed.wayne.edu
2. Providence Hospital
   16001 Nine Mile Road
   DePaul Center, 3 West
   Southfield, MI 48075

Director:

Bohdan M. Pichurko, M.D.
Appts: (248) 424-5718
Fax: (248) 424-5726
bopich@aol.com

Center Coordinator:

Rajesh Joseph
(248) 424-5718
Fax: (248) 424-5726

Affiliate Program:

Hurley Children's Clinic at Mott
   Children's Health Center
806 Tuuri Place
Flint, MI 48503

Appts: (810) 257-9344
Fax: (810) 762-7308

Director:

Cem Demerci, M.D.

Appts: (810) 257-9278
Fax: (810) 762-7030
CDemerci1@hurleymc.edu

Grand Rapids

Cystic Fibrosis Care Center of Grand
Rapids
Helen DeVos Women and Children's
Center
330 Barclay, N.E., Suite 200
Grand Rapids, MI 49503

Appts: (616) 391-2125
Fax: (616) 391-2131

(Contact Person: Marion Schaefer)

Center Codirector:

Adrian O'Hagan, M.D.
(616) 391-2125
Fax: (616) 391-2131
john.schuen@spectrum-health.org

Center Codirector:

Susan L. Millard, M.D.
(616) 391-2125
Fax: (616) 391-2131
susan.millard@spectrum-health.org

Adult Program Director:

Adrian R. O'Hagan, M.D.
(616) 391-2125
Fax: (616) 391-2131
adrian.o'hagan@spectrum-health.org

Kalamazoo

Michigan State University
Kalamazoo Center for Medical Studies
1000 Oakland Drive
Kalamazoo, MI 49008

Appts: (616) 337-6430

Center Director:

Douglas N. Homnick, M.D.
(616) 337-6430
Fax: (616) 337-6474
homnick@kcms.msu.edu

Contact Person:

Marlene Pryson

Lansing

Michigan State University Cystic Fibrosis
Center
1200 East Michigan Avenue, Suite 145
Lansing, MI 48912-1811

Appts: (517) 364-5440
Fax: (517) 364-5413
Information E-Mail:
kathleen.king@ht.msu.edu

Center Director:

Richard E. Honicky, M.D.
(517) 353-5042
Fax: (517) 364-5413
honicky@msu.edu

MINNESOTA

Minneapolis

University of Minnesota
CF Center
420 Delaware Street, S.E., MMC 742
Minneapolis, MN 55455-0392

Appts: (612) 624-0962

Director:

Carlos E. Milla, M.D., M.P.H.
(612) 626-2963
Fax: (612) 626-0696
milla005@tc.umn.edu

Adult Program Director:

Jordan Dunitz, M.D.
(612) 626-1112
Fax: (612) 624-0696
dunit001@umn.edu

Affiliate Program:

Children's Hospitals and Clinics,
    Minneapolis
2545 Chicago Avenue, South
Suite 617
Minneapolis, MN 55404

Appts: (612) 863-3226
Fax: (612) 863-3153

Director:

John J. McNamara, M.D.
doctors@crccs.com

MISSISSIPPI

Jackson

University of Mississippi Medical
    Center
Department of Pediatrics
Pediatric Pulmonary Division
2500 North State Street
Jackson, MS 39216-4505

Appts: (601) 984-5205

Center Director:

Lynn Walker, M.D.
Fax: (601) 815-1050
lwalker@ped.umsmed.edu

Adult Program Director:

Glenda Patterson, M.D.
(601) 984-5650
Fax: (601) 984-5658
gpatterson@medicine.umsmed.edu

MISSOURI

Columbia

Children's Hospital
University of Missouri Health Sciences
    Center
Department of Child Health
Division of Pulmonary Medicine and
    Allergy
Room M668
One Hospital Drive
Columbia, MO 65212

Appts: (573) 882-6921

Center Director:

Peter König, M.D., Ph.D.
(573) 882-6978
Fax: (573) 882-2742
konigp@missouri.edu

Outreach Clinics:

1. St. John's Specialty Clinic
   Fremont Medical Building
   1961 South Fremont Avenue
   Springfield, MO 65804

   Appts: (573) 882-6978
   Contact: Connie Fenton, R.N., B.S.N.
2. Southeast Missouri Hospital
   1701 Lacey Street
   Cape Girardeau, MO 63701

   Appts: (573) 882-6978
   Contact: Connie Fenton, R.N., B.S.N.

Kansas City

The Children's Mercy Hospital
University of Missouri at Kansas City
Pediatric Pulmonology Section
2401 Gillham Road
Kansas City, MO 64108

Appts: (816) 234-3066
Sweat Test Only: (816) 234-1530

Center Director:
Michael McCubbin, M.D.
(816) 234-3033
Fax: (816) 234-3590
mmccubbin@cmh.edu

St. Louis

1. Cystic Fibrosis and Pediatric
   Pulmonary Center
   Cardinal Glennon Children's Hospital
   St. Louis University School of Medicine
   1465 South Grand Boulevard
   St. Louis, MO 63104

   Appts: (314) 268-6439
   Judy_Consolino@SSHMC.com

Center Director:
Anthony J. Rejent , M.D.
(314) 268-6439
Fax: (314) 268-2798
rejentaj@slu.edu

Adult Program:
St. Louis University Health Sciences
   Center
3635 Vista Avenue at Grand Boulevard
P. O. Box 15250
St. Louis, MO 63110-0250

Director:
Mary Ellen Kleinhenz, M.D.
(314) 577-8856
Fax: (314) 577-8859
kleinhme@slu.edu
2. Washington University School of
   Medicine
   St. Louis Children's Hospital
   Cystic Fibrosis Center
   One Children's Place
   St. Louis, MO 63110

   Appts: (314) 454-2694
           (314) 454-8764 (adults)
           (314) 454-6248 (sweat test
           only)
   Fax: (314) 454-2515

Center Director:
Thomas Ferkol, M.D.
(314) 454-2694
Fax: (314) 454-2515
ferkol_t@kids.wustl.edu

Pediatric Coordinator:
Jane A. Quante, R.N., B.S.
(314) 454-2694
quante_j@kids.wustl.edu

Adult Program:
Washington University School of
   Medicine
Division of Pulmonary/Critical Care
   Medicine
660 South Euclid Avenue, Box 8052
St. Louis, MO 63110

Director:
Daniel Rosenbluth, M.D.
(314) 454-8764
Fax: (314) 454-8768
rosenbluth@msnotes.wustl.edu

Adult Coordinator:
Joan Zukosky, R.N., B.S.N.
(314) 454-8640

Affiliate Programs:
1. Southern Illinois University School
     of Medicine
   Division of Pulmonary Medicine
   P. O. Box 19636
   701 North First Street
   Springfield, IL 62794

   Appts: (217) 524-3880;
           (217) 782-0182;
           (800) 246-3458

Director:
Lanie E. Eagleton, M.D.
(217) 782-0187
Fax: (217) 788-5543
bmorris@siumed.edu

Coordinator:

Joni Colle, R.N., R.R.T.
(217) 788-3383
jcolle@siumed.edu

2. Carle Clinic Association
   Department of Pediatrics
   602 W. University Avenue
   Urbana, IL 61801

   Appts: (217) 383-3100

Director:

Donald F. Davison, M.D.
(217) 383-3100
Fax: (217) 383-4468
donald.davison@carle.com

MONTANA

See Denver, Colorado.

NEBRASKA

Omaha

University of Nebraska Medical Center
985190 Nebraska Medical Center
Omaha, NE 68198-5190

Appts: (402) 559-4389
necfcntr@unmc.edu

Center Director:

John L. Colombo, M.D.
(402) 559-6275
Fax: (402) 559-7062
jcolombo@unmc.edu

Adult Program:

University of Nebraska Medical Center
Department of Pulmonary and Critical
Care Medicine
985300 Nebraska Medical Center
Omaha, NE 68198-5300

Appts: (402) 559-4015

Adult Program Director:

Peter J. Murphy, M.D.
(402) 559-4087
Fax: (402) 559-8210
pjmurphy@unmc.edu

Adult Coordinator:

Jill Fliege, M.S., A.P.R.N.
(402) 559-4087
Fax: (402) 559-8210
jfliege@unmc.edu

NEVADA

Las Vegas

University of Nevada School of Medicine
Childrens Lung Specialists, Ltd.
3838 Meadows Lane
Las Vegas, NV 89107

Appts: (702) 598-4411

Center Director:

Ruben P. Diaz, M.D.
(702) 598-4411
Fax: (702) 598-1988
docdiaz@aol.com

Adult Program Director:

Angelica E. Honsberg, M.D.
(702) 598-4411
Fax: (702) 598-1488
docdiaz@aol.com

NEW HAMPSHIRE

Lebanon

New Hampshire CF Program
Dartmouth Hitchcock Medical Center
1 Medical Center Drive
Lebanon, NH 03756

Appts: (603) 650-6244 (Lebanon) or
           (603) 695-2560 (Manchester)
linda.jackman@hitchcock.org

Center Director:

H. Worth Parker, M.D.
(603) 650-5541
Fax: (603) 650-8601
lynn.m.feenan@hitchcock.org

Adult Program Director:

H. Worth Parker, M.D.
(603) 650-5533
Fax: (603) 650-4437
h.worth.parker@hitchcock.org
priscilla.robichaud@hitchcock.org

NEW JERSEY

Long Branch

Cystic Fibrosis and Pediatric Pulmonary
  Center
Monmouth Medical Center
279 Third Avenue, Suite 604
Long Branch, NJ 07740

Appts: (732) 222-4474

Center Director:

Robert L. Zanni, M.D.
(732) 222-4474
Fax: (732) 222-4472
rzanni@monmouth.net

Adult Program Director:

Chandler D. Patton, M.D.
(732) 571-5151
Fax: (732) 571-6367
DL-Patton@comcast.net

New Brunswick

Pediatric Pulmonary and Cystic Fibrosis
  Center
Bristol-Myers Squibb Children's Hospital
  at Robert Wood Johnson University
  Hospital
P. O. Box 19, 1 Robert Wood Johnson Place
MEB, Room 339
  New Brunswick, New Jersey 09803-0019

Appts: (732) 235-7899

Center Director:

Lourdes Laraya-Cuasay, M.D.
(732) 235-7899
Fax: (732) 235-7077
cuasaylr@umdnj.edu

NEW MEXICO

Albuquerque

University of New Mexico School of
  Medicine
Department of Pediatrics
Ambulatory Care Center
2211 Lomas Boulevard, N.E., ACC 3rd
  Floor
Albuquerque, NM 87131-5311

Appts: (505) 272-6633 or
  (888) UNM-PULM (866-7856)

Center Director:

Elizabeth Perkett, M.D
(505) 272-0330
eperkett@salud.unm.edu

Adult Program Director:

David S. James, M.D.
(505) 272-4751
Fax: (505) 272-8700
dsjames@medusa.unm.edu

NEW YORK

Albany

Pediatric Pulmonary and Cystic Fibrosis
  Center
Albany Medical College
Department of Pediatrics, Mail Code 112
47 New Scotland Avenue
Albany, NY 12208

Appts: (518) 262-6880
Fax: (518) 262-688

Center Director:

Robert A. Kaslovsky, M.D.

(518) 262-6880

Fax: (518) 262-6884

kaslovr@mail.amc.edu

Adult Program Director:

Jonathan M. Rosen, M.D.

(518) 262-5196

Fax: (518) 262-5555

rosenj@mail.amc.edu

Brooklyn

Long Island College Hospital
340 Henry Street
Brooklyn, NY 11201

Appts: (718) 780-1025 or
(718) 780-1026
Fax: (718) 780-2989

Center Director:

Robert Giusti, M.D.

(718) 780-1025

Fax: (718) 780-2989

giucfdoc@pol.net

Adult Program Director:

Peter Smith, M.D.

(718) 780-2905

Fax: (718) 780-1256

CF Coordinator:

Christine Mavara, R.N.

(718) 780-1025

Fax: (718) 780-2989

Buffalo

Children's Lung and Cystic Fibrosis Center
Children's Hospital of Buffalo
219 Bryant Street
Buffalo, NY 14222

Appts: (716) 878-7524 (pediatrics and
adults)
After hours: (716) 878-7000

Center Director:

Drucy Borowitz, M.D.

(716) 878-7561

Fax: (716) 888-3945

dborowitz@upa.chob.edu

Adult Program Director:

James Cronin, M.D.

(716) 878-7655

Fax: (716) 888-3945

jpcronin@acsu.buffalo.edu

New Hyde Park

Cystic Fibrosis Care and Teaching
Center
Schneider Children's Hospital
North Shore Long Island Jewish Health
System
269-01 76th Avenue
New Hyde Park, NY 11040

Pediatric Appts: (718) 470-3305
cystic.fibrosis@lij.edu
Adult Appts: (718 or 516) 470-4245

Center Director:

Joan K. DeCelie-Germana, M.D.

(718) 470-3305

Fax: (718) 962-9057

germana@lij.edu

Adult Program Director:

Rubin Cohen, M.D.

(718) 470-7231

Fax: (718) 470-1035

rcohen@lij.edu

New York City

1. Cystic Fibrosis and Pediatric
   Pulmonary Center
   Mount Sinai School of Medicine
   One Gustave L. Levy Place, Box 1202B
   New York, NY 10029-6574

   Appts: (212) 241-7788

Center Directors:

Richard J. Bonforte, M.D.
Meyer Kattan, M.D.

Adult Program Director:

Maria Padilla, M.D.
(212) 241-5656
Fax: (212) 987-7259
maria/padilla@mssm.edu

Affiliate Program:

St. Joseph's Children's Hospital
703 Main Street
Paterson, NJ 07503

Appts: (973) 754-2550

Director:

Roberto Nachajon, M.D.
(973) 754-2550
Fax: (973) 754-2548
2. Children's Lung and CF Center
    Children's Hospital of New York
    Columbia University
    630 West 168th Street, BH-7S
    New York, NY 10032

Appts: (212) 305-5122

Center Director:

Lynne M. Quittell, M.D.
(212) 305-6551
Fax: (212) 305-6103
lmq1@columbia.edu

Adult Program Director:

Emily DiMango, M.D.
(212) 305-0290
Fax: (212) 305-7063
ead3@columbia.edu
3. The Cystic Fibrosis Center
    Saint Vincent Catholic Medical
    Centers
    St. Vincent's Manhattan
    36 Seventh Avenue, Suite 509
    New York, NY 10011

Appts: (212) 604-8895
Fax: (212) 604-3899
SVHCF@aol.com

Center Codirector:

Maria Berdella, M.D.
(212) 604-8895

Adult Program Director:

Patricia Walker, M.D.
PAWCF@aol.com

Rochester

University of Rochester Medical Center
Strong Memorial Hospital
Department of Pediatrics
601 Elmwood Avenue, Box 667
Rochester, NY 14642-8667

Appts: (716) 275-2464

Center Codirectors:

Karen Z. Voter, M.D.
karen_voter@urmc.rochester.edu
Clement L. Ren, M.D.
clement_ren@urmc.rochester.edu
Fax: (716) 275-8706

Affiliate Program:

Samaritan Medical Center
Child and Adolescent Health
    Associates
513 Washington Street
Watertown, NY 13601

Appts: (315) 788-2211

Director:

Ronald Perciaccante, M.D.
(315) 788-2211
Fax: (315) 788-0956
pereocon@pol.net

Stony Brook

University Medical Center at Stony Brook
Department of Pediatrics
Health Sciences Center T11, Room 080
Stony Brook, NY 11794-8111

Appts: (631) 444-KIDS

Center Director:

Catherine Tayag-Kier, M.D.
(631) 444-8340
Fax: (631) 444-6045

Syracuse

Robert C. Schwartz Cystic Fibrosis Center
SUNY Upstate Medical University
750 East Adams Street
Syracuse, NY 13210

Appts: (315) 464-6323 (pediatrics)
(315) 464-4189 (adults)

Center Director:

Ran D. Anbar, M.D.
(315) 464-6323
Fax: (315) 464-6322
anbarr@upstate.edu

Adult Program Director:

James Sexton, M.D.
sextonj@upstate.edu

Valhalla

The Armond V. Mascia Cystic Fibrosis
Center
The Children's Hospital at Westchester
Medical Center
New York Medical College
Munger Pavilion, Room 106
Valhalla, NY 10595

Appts: (914) 493-7585

Center Director:

Allen Dozor, M.D.
(914) 493-7585
Fax: (914) 594-4336
pedpulm@nymc.edu

NORTH CAROLINA

Chapel Hill

University of North Carolina at Chapel Hill
Department of Pediatrics, CB #7220
635 Burnett-Womack Building
Chapel Hill, NC 27599-7220

Appts: (919) 966-1401 (pediatrics)
(919) 966-7933 [adults (18 years
and older)]

Center Director:

Margaret W. Leigh, M.D.
(919) 966-1055
Fax: (919) 966-6179
mleigh@med.unc.edu

Center Codirector:

George Retsch-Bogart, M.D.
gzrb@med.unc.edu

Adult Program:

Cystic Fibrosis/Pulmonary Research
and Treatment Center
University of North Carolina at Chapel
Hill
7019 Thurston Bowles Building,
CB# 7248
Chapel Hill, NC 27599-7248

Codirectors:

Michael Knowles, M.D.
James R. Yankaskas, M.D.
(919) 966-1077
Fax: (919) 966-7524
knowles@med.unc.edu
pwsjry@med.unc.edu

Affiliate Program:

Western Carolinas Cystic Fibrosis Center
411 Billingsley Road
Suite 104
Charlotte, NC 28211

Appts: (704) 338-9818
Fax: (704) 338-9023

Codirectors:

William S. Ashe, M.D.
Hugh R. Black, M.D.
(704) 338-9818
Fax: (704) 338-9023
r.macfetrich@worldnet.att.net

Outreach Program:

The Ruth and Billy Graham
Children's Health Clinic
50 Doctors Drive
Suite 105
Asheville, NC 28801

Appts: (828) 213-1740

Director:

Kristi Gott, P.N.P.
(828) 213-1759
msjchckkg@memo.msj.org

Durham

Cystic Fibrosis and Pediatric Pulmonary
Center
Duke University Medical Center
Bell Building, Room 302
P. O. Box 2994
Durham, NC 27710

Appts: (919) 684-3364 or
        (919) 681-3364 or
        (919) 668-4000

Center Director:

Maria D. Martinez, M.D.
Fax: (919) 684-2292

Center Codirector:

Thomas Murphy, M.D.
(919) 684-2292
murph016@mc.duke.edu

Adult Program:

Duke University Medical Center
Box 31166
Durham, NC 27710

Director:

Peter S. Kussin, M.D.
(919) 684-3202 or (919) 684-8049
Fax: (919) 681-7837
kussi001@mc.duke.edu

Affiliate Program:

Children's Respiratory Center
58 Bear Drive
Greenville, SC 29605

Appts: (864) 220-8000

Director:

Jane V. Gwinn, M.D.
Fax: (864) 220-8009
jgwinn_crc@msn.com

Winston-Salem

Wake Forest University Baptist Medical
Center
Department of Pediatrics
Medical Center Boulevard
Winston -Salem, NC 27157

Appts: (336) 716-4126

Center Director:

Michael S. Schechter, M.D., M.P.H.
(336) 716-0512
Fax: (336) 716-9229
mschech@wfubmc.edu

Center Codirector:

Bruce K. Rubin, M.D.
brubin@wfubmc.edu

Adult Center Director:

Michael Larj, M.D.
mlarj@wfubmc.edu

NORTH DAKOTA

Bismarck

Heart and Lung Clinic
P. O. Box 2698
Bismarck, ND 58502-2698

Appts: (800) 932-8848 or
        (701) 530-7502

Center Director:

James A. Hughes, M.D.
(701) 530-7500
Fax: (701) 530-7560
jhughea@aol.com

OHIO

Akron

Lewis H. Walker Cystic Fibrosis Center
Children's Hospital Medical Center
  of Akron
One Perkins Square
Akron, OH 44308

Appts: (330) 543-3249
Fax: (330) 543-8890

Center Director:

Gregory J. Omlor, M.D.
(330) 543-8885
gomler@chmca.org

Adult Program Director:

Thomas G. Olbrych, M.D.
(330) 543-3249
Fax: (330) 543-8890
olbrycht@summa-health.org

Cincinnati

Cincinnati Children's Hospital Medical
  Center
Pulmonary Medicine, OSB 5
3333 Burnet Avenue
Cincinnati, OH 45229-3039

Appts: (513) 636-7987
Appts: (513) 475-8520 (adults)

Center Director:

James D. Acton, M.D.
(513) 636-6771
Fax: (513) 636-4615
james.acton@chmcc.org

Adult Program Director:

Patricia M. Joseph, M.D.
University of Cincinnati
(513) 558-4831
Fax: (513) 558-0835
patricia.joseph@uc.edu

Cleveland

Rainbow Babies and Children's Hospital
Case Western Reserve University,
  Room 3001
Pediatric Pulmonary Division
Mail Code: RBC 6006
11100 Euclid Avenue
Cleveland, OH 44106

Appts: (216) 844-3267

Center Director:

Michael W. Konstan, M.D.
(216) 844-3267
Fax: (216) 844-5916
mwk3@po.cwru.edu

Adult Program Director:

Michael D. Infeld, M.D.
(216) 844-3267
Fax: (216) 368-4223
mdi@po.cwru.edu

Columbus

Cystic Fibrosis Center
Columbus Children's Hospital
Section of Pulmonary Medicine
700 Children's Drive
Columbus, OH 43205-2696

Appts: (614) 722-4766

Center Director:

Karen S. McCoy, M.D.
(614) 722-4766
Fax: (614) 722-4755
mccoyk@pediatrics.ohio-state.edu

Adult Program Director:

John S. Heintz, M.D.
(614) 722-4766
Fax: (614) 722-4755
jheintzl@columbus.rr.com

Dayton

Cystic Fibrosis Center
The Children's Medical Center
One Children's Plaza
Dayton, OH 45404-1815

Appts: (937) 641-3376

Center Director:

Fred Royce, M.D.
(937) 641-3440
Fax (937) 641-5390
roycef@cmc-dayton.org

Adult Program:

Wright State University School of
Medicine

Adult Program Director:

Gary M. Onady, M.D., Ph.D.
(937) 775-3875
Fax: (937) 775-2261
gmonady@pol.net

Toledo

Toledo Children's Hospital
2142 North Cove Boulevard
Toledo, OH 43606

Appts: (419) 291-2207 or
        (800) 227-2959

Center Director:

Pierre A. Vauthy, M.D.
(419) 471-4549
Fax: (419) 479-6092
suisse3@aol.com

Adult Program Director:

Jeffrey Lewis, M.D.
(419) 471-2367
Fax: (419) 749-6952
jeff.lewis.md@promedica.org

OKLAHOMA

Oklahoma City

Children's Hospital of Oklahoma
University of Oklahoma Health Science
    Center
Cystic Fibrosis Center
940 N.E. 13th Street, Room 3B3314
Oklahoma City, OK 73104

Appts: (405) 271-6390

Center Director:

James Royall, M.D.
(405) 271-6390
Fax: (405) 271-2873
james-royall@ouhsc.edu

Affiliate Program:

Tulsa Cystic Fibrosis Center
University of OK Health Science
    Center/Pediatric Clinic
2815 S. Sheridan Road
Tulsa, OK 74129

Appts: (918) 838-4820
Fax: (918) 838-4822

Director:

John C. Kramer, M.D.
(918) 481-8100
Fax: (918) 481-8128
JCKramer@pol.net

Codirector:

T. L. Carey, M.D.
(918) 481-8100
Fax: (918) 481-8128

OREGON

Portland

Oregon Health Sciences University UHN 56
Cystic Fibrosis Center
3181 S.W. Sam Jackson Park Road
Portland, OR 97201-3098

Appts: (503) 418-5747

Center Director:

Michael Wall, M.D.
(503) 494-8023
Fax: (503) 494-8898
wallm@ohsu.edu

Coordinator:

Lana Sheinkman, R.N.

Outreach Clinics:

1. Medford CF Clinic
    Rogue Valley Hospital
    Medford, OR 97501
2. Eugene CF Clinic
    Sacret Heart Hospital
    Eugene, OR 97401

Adult Program Director:

Mark Chesnutt, M.D.
(503) 494-7680
Fax: (503) 494-6670
chesnutm@ohsu.edu

Affiliate Program:

Kaiser Permanente–Northwest Region
3550 N. Interstate Avenue
Portland, OR 97227
(503) 285-9321
Fax: (503) 331-5286

Director:

Richard C. Cohen, M.D.
richard.cohen@kp.org

PENNSYLVANIA

Harrisburg

Pediatric and Adult Cystic Fibrosis Center
Harrisburg Hospital
Brady Medical Arts Building, 4th Floor
205 South Front Street
Harrisburg, PA 17101

Appts: (717) 231-8670

Center Director:

Muttiah Ganeshananthan, M.D.
(717) 231-8670
Fax: (717) 231-8676
kbynum@pinnaclehealth.org

Adult Program Director:

William M. Anderson, M.D.
(717) 782-4105
Fax: (717) 782-2798
wander1@netscape.net

Hershey

Hershey Medical Center
Department of Pediatrics
Pennsylvania State University
500 University Drive
P. O. Box 850
Hershey, PA 17033

Appts: (717) 531-5338

Center Director:

Bettina Hilman, M.D.
(717) 531-5338
Fax: (717) 531-0761

Adult Program Director:

Robert Vender, M.D.

Affiliate Program:

Geisinger Medical Center
Pediatric Allergy, Immunology
  & Pulmonary Medicine
100 N. Academy Avenue
Danville, PA 17822-1339

Appts: (570) 271-7910

Director:

Carlos Perez, M.D.
(570) 271-6266
Fax: (570) 271-7833
cperez@geisinger.edu

Philadelphia

1. Children's Hospital of Philadelphia
   University of Pennsylvania
   Abramson Research Center,
    Room 402G
   34th Street and Civic Center Boulevard
   Philadelphia, PA 19104-4318

Appts: (215) 590-3749/3510
     (Monday–Friday: 8:30–4:30;
     evenings and weekends: ask for
     physician on call)

Center Director:

Thomas F. Scanlin, M.D.
(215) 590-3608
Fax: (215) 590-4298
scanlin@email.chop.edu

Adult Program:

Hospital of the University of
  Pennsylvania
Pulmonary Medicine/Critical Care
  Medicine
835 West Gates Building
3600 Spruce Street
Philadelphia, PA 19104-4283

Appts: (215) 662-8766

Director:

David A. Lipson, M.D.
(215) 349-5478
Fax: (215) 614-0869

2. St. Christopher's Hospital for Children
   Erie Avenue at Front Street
   Philadelphia, PA 19134-1095

Appts: (215) 427-5183

Center Director:

Laurie Varlotta, M.D.
(215) 427-5183
Fax: (215) 427-4621
Laurie.Varlotta@Drexel.edu

Associate Director:

Suzanne Beck, M.D.
suzannebeck@tenethealth.com

Adult Program:

Pulmonary/Critical Care Division
Medical College of Pennsylvania
  Hospital
3300 Henry Avenue
Philadelphia, PA 19129

Appts: (215) 842-7748

Director:

Stanley Fiel, M.D.
(215) 842-7748
Fax: (215) 843-1705
Stanley.Fiel@Drexel.edu

Outreach Clinic:

St. Luke's Hospital
Health Network
Pediatric Specialists
153 Broadhead Road
Bethlehem, PA 18017

Pittsburgh

Cystic Fibrosis Center
Children's Hospital of Pittsburgh
University of Pittsburgh School of
  Medicine
3705 Fifth Avenue at DeSoto Street
Pittsburgh, PA 15213

Appts: (412) 692-5661

Center Director:

David M. Orenstein, M.D.
(412) 692-5184
Fax: (412) 692-6645
davido+@pitt.edu

Adult Program Director:

Joel Weinberg, M.D.
(412) 621-1200
Fax: (412) 621-9958

PUERTO RICO

San Juan

Cystic Fibrosis Center
Pediatric Pulmonary Program of
San Juan
Cardiovascular Center of Puerto Rico
  and Caribbean
P. O. Box 366528
Fax: (787) 754-8500, ext. 1261, 1229, or
  1215
San Juan, PR 00936-6528

Appts: (787) 754-8500, ext. 1229 or 3010

Center Director:

Jose R. Rodriguez-Santana, M.D.
Fax: (787) 743-1917 or (787) 758-2780
jr@pedasthma.com

RHODE ISLAND

Providence

Brown University Medical School
Cystic Fibrosis Center
Rhode Island Hospital Child
  Development Center
593 Eddy Street, 6th Floor APC
  Building
Providence, RI 02903

Appts: (401) 444-5685

Center Director:

Mary Ann Passero, M.D.
(401) 444-5685
Fax: (401) 444-6115
mary_passero@brown.edu

Adult Program Director:

Walter Donat, M.D.

SOUTH CAROLINA

Charleston

Cystic Fibrosis Center
Medical University of South Carolina
Division of Pediatric Pulmonology,
  Allergy & Immunology
135 Rutledge Avenue
P. O. Box 250561
Charleston, SC 29425

Appts: (843) 876-0444

Center Director:

C. Michael Bowman, M.D., Ph.D.
(843) 876-1555
Fax: (843) 876-1583
bowmanm@musc.edu

Adult Program:

Adult CF Center
Medical University of South Carolina
Division of Pulmonary and Critical
  Care
96 Jonathan Lucas Street, Suite 812-CSB
P. O. Box 250623
Charleston, SC 29425

Appts: (843) 792-0729

Director:

Patrick Flume, M.D.
(843) 792-0729
Fax: (843) 792-0732
flumepa@musc.edu

Columbia

Pediatric Pulmonary Associates
3 Medical Park, Suite 270
Columbia, SC 29203

Appts: (803) 748-7555

Center Director:

Daniel C. Brown, M.D.
(803) 748-7555
Fax: (803) 748-9555
danielbrown@pol.net

Greenville

See Durham, North Carolina, Duke
University Medical Center.

SOUTH DAKOTA

Sioux Falls

Cystic Fibrosis Center
Sioux Valley Hospital
1100 South Euclid Avenue
P. O. Box 5039
Sioux Falls, SD 57117-5039

Appts: (605) 333-7188
Fax: (605) 333-1585
husmank@siouxvalley.org

Center Director:

James Wallace, M.D.
(605) 333-7199
Wallace_James@msn.com

Adult Program Director:

Rodney R. Parry, M.D.*
rparryL@usd.edu

Preferred Mailing Address:

University of South Dakota School
  of Medicine
1400 West 22nd Street
Sioux Falls, SD 57105-1570

TENNESSEE

Memphis

Memphis Cystic Fibrosis Center
University of Tennessee College of
  Medicine
Le Bonheur Children's Medical Center
50 North Dunlap
Memphis, TN 38103-2893

Appts: (901) 572-5222

Center Director:

Robert A. Schoumacher, M.D.
(901) 572-5222
Fax: (901) 572-3337
rschoumacher@utmem.edu

Adult Program Director:

Richard Boswell, M.D.
121 Union Avenue, Suite 120
Memphis, TN 38104

Appts: (901) 725-5533
Fax: (901) 278-7053
bpajrhrlb@bellsouth.net

Nashville

Cystic Fibrosis Center
Vanderbilt Children's Hospital
Vanderbilt University Medical Center
1161 21st Street
S-0119 MCN
Nashville, TN 37232-2586

Appts: (615) 343-7617
Fax: (615) 343-7727

Center Director:

Thomas A. Hazinski, M.D.
(615) 343-7617
Fax: (615) 343-7727
tom.hazinski@mcmail.vanderbilt.edu

Adult Program:

Vanderbilt University Medical Center
Cystic Fibrosis Center
T-1217 MCN
Nashville, TN 37232-2650

Appts: (615) 322-2386

Director:

Bonnie S. Slovis, M.D.
(615) 322-2386
Fax: (615) 343-3749
bonnie.slovis@mcmail.vanderbilt.edu

Affiliate Programs:

1. East Tennessee Children's Hospital
   Cystic Fibrosis Clinic
   2018 Clinch Avenue
   Knoxville, TN 37916

Appts: (865) 525-2640

Director:

John S. Rogers, M.D.
(865) 541-8583
Fax: (865) 525-9536
pedpulmonology@etch.com
2. T.C. Thompson Children's Hospital
   910 Blackford Street
   Chattanooga, TN 37403

Appts: (423) 778-6511

Director:

Joel C. Ledbetter, M.D.
(423) 778-6501
Fax: (423) 778-6215
ledbetjc@erlanger.org

TEXAS

Dallas

Children's Medical Center of Dallas
Cystic Fibrosis Center
1935 Motor Street, Room D304
Dallas, TX 75235

Appts: (214) 456-2361 or
        (214) 456-2362

Center Director:

Claude B. Prestidge, M.D.
(214) 456-2361
Fax: (214) 456-2563
npratt@childmed.dallas.tx.us

Adult Program:

St. Paul Medical Center
5939 Harry Hines Boulevard, Suite 711
Dallas, TX 75235

Director:

Randall Rosenblatt, M.D.
(214) 879-6555
Fax: (214) 879-6312
rosie@pol.net

Affiliate Programs:

1. Allergy Alliance of the Permian Basin
   606B North Kent Street
   Midland, TX 79701

Appts: (915) 561-8183

Director:

John D. Bray, M.D.
(915) 561-8183
Fax: (915) 684-7003
jdavidbrayl@aol.com

2. Scott & White Clinic
   2401 South 31st Street
   Temple, TX 76508

Appts: (254) 724-2144

Director:

John Pohl, M.D.
(254) 724-5504
Fax: (254) 724-0721

3. The University of Texas Health
   Center at Tyler
   11937 US Hwy 271
   Tyler, TX 75708

   Appts: (903) 877-7220
           (current patients) or
           (903) 877-7170
           (new patients)

Director:

Rodolfo Amaro, M.D.
(903) 988-7219
Fax: (903) 877-7218

Fort Worth

Cystic Fibrosis Center
Cook Children's Medical Center
901 Seventh Avenue
Fort Worth, TX 76104

Appts: (817) 885-4207
Shirleyd@cookchildrens.org

Center Codirectors:

James C. Cunningham, M.D.
Nancy N. Dambro, M.D.
(817) 810-1621
Fax: (817) 885-1090
jccunningham@cookchildrens.org
ndambro@cookchildrens.org

Outreach Clinic:

Texas Tech University Health Sciences
  Center
1400 Coulter, Building E, Suite 703
Amarillo, TX 79106

Appts: (806) 354-5437
Fax: (806) 354-5689

Codirectors:

James C. Cunningham, M.D.
Maynard Dyson, M.D.

Houston

Baylor College of Medicine
One Baylor Plaza
Houston, TX 77030

Appts: (832) 824-3330

Center Director:

Peter W. Hiatt, M.D.*
(832) 822-3300
Fax: (832) 825-3308
pwhiatt@texaschildrenshospital.org

*Preferred Mailing Address:

Baylor Cystic Fibrosis Care Center
6621 Fannin, CC1040.00
Houston, TX 77030

Center Codirector:

Dan Seilheimer, M.D.
dkseilhe@texaschildrenshospital.org

Adult Program:

The Methodist Hospital
Department of Medicine–Pulmonary
6550 Fannin, Suite 1236
Houston, TX 77030

Appts: (713) 394-3800

Director:

Kathryn A. Hale, M.D.
(713) 790-2076
Fax: (713) 790-3648
khale@bcm.tmc.edu

Affiliate Program:

Children's Hospital of Austin
Specialty Care Center
1400 N IH 35
Austin, TX 78701

Appts: (512) 324-8835

Director:
Allan L. Frank, M.D.*
(512) 454-3387
ajfrank@flash.net

Preferred Mailing Address:
Capital Pediatric Group Associates
1100 West 39 1/2 Street
Austin, TX 78756

San Antonio

1. Cystic Fibrosis–Chronic Lung Disease
   Center
   Christus Santa Rosa Children's Hospital
   333 N. Santa Rosa Street
   San Antonio, TX 78207

   Appts: (210) 704-2335 or
   (210) 704-2596

Center Director:
Donna Beth Willey-Courand, M.D.*
(210) 271-0321
Fax: (210) 271-0880
courandd@uthscsa.edu

Preferred Mailing Address:
343 W. Houston Street, Suite #906
San Antonio, TX 78205

Affiliate Program:
Cystic Fibrosis Program
Methodist Children's Hospital
Methodist Plaza
7700 Floyd Curl
San Antonio, TX 78229

Appts: (210) 575-7371 or
(800) 297-1021
Fax: (210) 575-7374

Director:
Amanda Dove, M.D.

Assistant Director:
Martha Morse, M.D.
2. Tri-Services Military CF Center
   Department of Pediatrics
   Wilford Hall USAF Medical Center
   2200 Bergquist Drive, Suite 1
   59MDW / MMNP|
   Lackland AFB, TX 78236-5200

   Appts: (210) 292-7585

Center Director:
Dr. Kenneth M. Olivier, LTC, USAF, MC
(210) 292-3170
Fax: (210) 292-6180
olivier@whmc-lafb.af.mil

Affiliate Programs:
1. Naval Medical Center–San Diego
   Department of Pediatrics
   34800 Bob Wilson Drive
   San Diego, CA 92134-5000

   Appts: (619) 532-6896

Director:
Henry Wojtczak, M.D.
(619) 532-6883
Fax: (619) 532-9582
hwojtcza@snd10.med.navy.mil
2. Tripler Army Medical Center
   Department of Pediatrics
   1 Jarrett White Road
   Tripler AMC, HI 96859-5000

   Appts: (808) 433-9226 or
   (808) 433-6697

Director:
Dr. Charles Callahan, COL, MC
(808) 433-6407
Fax: (808) 433-4837
charles_w.callahan@tamc.chcs.amedd.
army.mil

3. National Naval Medical Center
Pediatric Clinic, Building 9,
Room 123
8901 Wisconsin Avenue
Bethesda, MD 20889-5000

Appts: (301) 295-4919

Director:

Dr. Donna R. Perry, CAPT, MC, USN
(301) 295-4915
Fax: (301) 295-6173
DRPerry@bth20.med.navy.mil
4. USAF (Keesler) Medical Center
81st MDOS/SGOCC
301 Fisher Street
Keesler AFB, MS 39534-2519

Appts: (800) 700-8603

Director:

Major Keith Graham, M.D.
(228) 377-1249
Fax: (228) 377-6535
keith.graham@keesler.af.mil
5. Naval Medical Center, Portsmouth
Charette Health Care Center
Pediatric Pulmonary Clinic
27 Effingham Street
Portsmouth, VA 23708-2197

Appts: (757) 953-2955

Director:

Capt. John A. McQueston, M.D.
(757) 953-0220-0201
Fax: (757) 953-0858
JAMcQueston@mar.med.navy.mil
6. Madigan Army Medical Center
Department of Pediatrics
Pediatric Pulmonary Medicine
Tacoma, WA 98431

Appts: (800) 404-4506

Director:

Dr. Donald Moffitt, COL, MC, USA
Direct: (253) 968-1881
(253) 968-1980 (receptionist)
Fax: (253) 968-0384
*donald_r.moffitt@mamc.chcs.amedd.ar
my.mil*

UTAH

Salt Lake City

Intermountain Cystic Fibrosis Center
Department of Pediatrics
University of Utah Health Sciences Center
100 North Medical Drive, 2C 454 SOM
Salt Lake City, UT 84132-0001

Appts: (801) 588-2621
permatin@ihc.com

Center Director:

Barbara A. Chatfield, M.D.

Pediatric Coordinator:

Raheleh Matinkhah, R.N., B.S.N.
(801) 588-2716
Fax: (801) 588-2640

Appts: (801) 585-2804
      (801) 581-2410
Fax: (801) 581-4920
barbara.chatfield@hsc.utah.edu

Adult Program:

Intermountain Cystic Fibrosis Center
University of Utah Health Sciences
Center
50 North Medical Drive, 711 Wintrobe
Building
Salt Lake City, UT 84132-0001

Director:

Ted Liou, M.D.
(801) 581-7806
Fax: (801) 585-3355

Adult Coordinator:

Kristin Bleyl, R.N., B.S.N.
(801) 585-3187
Fax: (801) 585-2661
Kristin.Bleyl@hsc.utah.edu

Affiliate Programs:

1. Children's Special Health Program
   St. Luke's CF Clinic
   100 East Idaho, Suite 200
   Boise, ID 83712

   Appts: (208) 381-7092

Director:

Henry Thompson, M.D.
(208) 381-7092
Fax: (208) 381-7002
thompshe@slrmc.org

Nurse Coordinator:

Mary E. Nelson, R.N., B.S.N., J.D.
(208) 381-7092

2. Pocatello Children's & Adolescent
   Clinic
   500 S. 11th Avenue
   P. O. Box 4730
   Pocatello, ID 83205

   Appts: (208) 232-1443

Director:

Don McInturff, M.D.
(208) 232-1443
Fax: (208) 239-3434
mcdon@isu.edu

3. Medical Center for Children
   890 Oxford Avenue
   Idaho Falls, ID 83401-4280

   Appts: (208) 523-3060

Director:

George H. Groberg, M.D.
(208) 523-3060
Fax: (208) 523-0028

VERMONT

Burlington

Cystic Fibrosis and Pediatric Pulmonary
  Center
The Children's Specialty Center, FAHC
111 Colchester Avenue
Burlington, VT 05401

Appts: (802) 847-8600
Fax: (802) 847-5805

Center Director:

Thomas Lahiri, M.D.
(802) 847-8600
thomas.lahiri@vtmednet.org

Adult Program Director:

Laurie Whittaker, M.D.

VIRGINIA

Charlottesville

Division of Respiratory Medicine
Department of Pediatrics, Box 800386
University of Virginia Health System
Charlottesville, VA 22908

Appts: (434) 924-2613

Center Director:

Deborah K. Froh, M.D.
Barringer Building, Room 5411
(434) 924-2250
Fax: (434) 243-6618
dkf2x@virginia.edu

Adult Center Director:

Mark K. Robbins, M.D.
Private Clinic Building Room 6569B
(434) 924-9687
Fax: (434) 924-9682
mkr3j@virginia.edu

Appts: (434) 924-9687

Affiliate Program:

Pediatric Lung Center
Fairfax, VA 22031

Appts: (703) 289-1410

Affiliate Program Director:

John P. Osborn, M.D.
(703) 289-1410
Fax: (703) 289-1420
mcosborn@erols.com

Norfolk

Eastern Virginia Medical School
Children's Hospital of the King's Daughters
601 Children's Lane
Norfolk, VA 23507

Appts: (757) 668-7137

Center Director:

Karl Karlson, M.D.
(757) 668-7426
Fax: (757) 668-9644
kkarlson@chkd.com

Adult Program Director:

Ignacio Ripoll, M.D.
(757) 668-7137
Fax: (757) 668-9644
iripoll@aol.com

Clinic Coordinator:

Connie Sigley
(757) 668-7137
cssigley@chkd.com

Richmond

Cystic Fibrosis Center
VCU Health System–Medical College of
 Virginia
401 N. 12th Street
P. O. Box 980315
Richmond, VA 23298

Appts: (804) 828-2980

Center Director:

Greg Elliott, M.D.
(804) 828-2980
Fax: (804) 828-2980
grelliott@hsc.vcu.edu

WASHINGTON

Seattle

Cystic Fibrosis Center
Division of Pediatric Pulmonary Medicine
Children's Hospital and Regional Medical
 Center
P. O. Box 5371, CH-18
4800 Sand Point Way, N.E.
Seattle, WA 98105

Appts: (206) 987-2101

Center Director:

Ronald Gibson, M.D., Ph.D.
(206) 987-2024
Fax: (206) 987-2639
rgibso@chmc.org

Associate Director:

Bonnie Ramsey, M.D.
bramsey@u.washington.edu

Clinic Coordinator:

Melinda Garbenich
(206) 526-2024
mgarb1@chmc.org

Clinical Nurse Specialist:

Janine Cassidy, R.N., M.S.N.
(206) 526-2024
jcassi@chmc.org

Adult Program:

Cystic Fibrosis Clinic
Division of Pulmonary and Critical
 Care Medicine
University of Washington Medical Center
Box 356522, Health Sciences Center,
 BB1253
Seattle, WA 98195

Appts: (206) 598-4615

Director:

Moira Aitken, M.D.
(206) 543-3166
Fax: (206) 685-8673
moira@u.washington.edu

Clinic Coordinator:

Gwen McDonald, R.N., M.S.
(206) 598-8446
Fax: (206) 598-2105
gwen@u.washington.edu

Affiliate Programs:

1. Anchorage Cystic Fibrosis Clinic
   Providence Medical Center
   3200 Providence Drive
   P. O. Box 196604
   Anchorage, AK 99519-6604

   Appts: (907) 561-5440

Director:

Dion Roberts, M.D.*
Fax: (907) 562-0412
dmrobert@alaska.net

*Preferred Mailing Address:
4001 Dale Street, Suite 210
Anchorage, AK 99508
2. Mary Bridge Children's Health Center
   311 South L Street
   Mailstop B1-OC
   Tacoma, WA 98405

   Appts: (253) 403-1469 or 1415
   Fax: (253) 403-4979
   mbontemps@multicare.org

Codirectors:

Lawrence A. Larson, D.O.
rickerdh@aol.com
David Ricker, M.D.
dricker@mbcha.net
3. Deaconess Medical Center
   West 800 Fifth Avenue
   P. O. Box 248
   Spokane, WA 99210-0248

Appts: (509) 473-7300
Fax: (509) 473-2512

Director:

Michael M. McCarthy, M.D.
mccartm@empirehealth.org

WEST VIRGINIA
Morgantown

Mountain State Cystic Fibrosis Center
West Virginia University
P. O. Box 9214
Morgantown, WV 26506

Appts: (304) 293-1217

Nurse Coordinator:

Linda Baer, R.N.
(304) 293-1227
lbaer@hsc.wvu.edu

Center Director:

Kathryn S. Moffett, M.D.
(304) 293-1217
Fax: (304) 293-1216
kmoffett@hsc.wvu.edu

Adult Program:

Section of Pulmonary and Critical Care
    Medicine
Box 9166
West Virginia University and School of
    Medicine
Morgantown, WV 26506-9166

Appts: (304) 293-4661

WISCONSIN
Madison

University of Wisconsin
Cystic Fibrosis/Pediatric Pulmonary Center
Clinical Sciences Center, KU/938
600 Highland Avenue
Madison, WI 53792-9988

Appts: (608) 263-8555
Info./Appts: camoodie@facstaff.wisc.edu

Center Director:

Michael J. Rock, M.D.
Fax: (608) 263-0510
mjrock@wisc.edu
Madison, WI 53792-9988

Adult Program:

University of Wisconsin
Adult Cystic Fibrosis Program
Clinical Sciences Center, H6/380
600 Highland Avenue
Madison, WI 53792

Appts: (608) 263-7203
Fax: (608) 263-9103
lrwill@facstaff.wisc.edu

Director:

Guillermo A. doPico, M.D.
(608) 263-3612
Fax: (608) 263-3104
gad@medicine.wisc.edu

Adult Nurse Coordinator:

Lorna Will, R.N., M.A.
(608) 263-9740
lrwill@facstaff.wisc.edu

Affiliate Programs:

1. St. Vincent's Hosopital
835 South Van Buren
Green Bay, WI 54301

Appts: (920) 496-4700

Director:

Peter Holzwarth, M.D.
Fax: (920) 433-8355
peterh@prevea.com
2. Marshfield Clinic
1000 North Oak Street
Marshfield, WI 54449

Appts: (800) 782-8581, ext. 75251

Director:

Bradley J. Sullivan, M.D.
sullivab@mfldclin.edu

Milwaukee

Children's Hospital of Wisconsin
Medical College of Wisconsin
Cystic Fibrosis Clinic
9000 West Wisconsin Avenue, Box 1997
MS #211
Milwaukee, WI 53201

Appts: (414) 266-6730

Center Director:

Mark Splaingard, M.D.
(414) 266-6730
Fax: (414) 266-6742
splain@mcw.edu

Adult Program Director:

Julie A. Biller, M.D.
(414) 266-6730
Fax: (414) 266-6742
jbiller@post.itsmcw.edu

The information in this appendix was kindly provided by the Cystic Fibrosis Foundation and is intended to serve as a resource for patients with cystic fibrosis and their families.

Appendix H

Cystic Fibrosis Care Centers Worldwide

ARGENTINA

Centro Nacional De Genetica Medica
Dpto. Genética Experimental
Av. Las Heras 2670–4° Piso
1425 Ciudad de Buenos Aires
Tel: 54.11.48012326/54.11.48092000
    (int. 2163)
Fax: 54.11.48014428
pivetta@genes.gov.ar

Hospital De Neuquén
Buenos Aires 353
8400 Neuquén

Hospital De Niños "Ricardo Gutierrez"
Centro Respiratorio
Sánchez de Bustamante 1399
1425 Ciudad de Buenos Aires
Tel: 54.11.49629212/54.11.49629229/
    54.11.49629232

Hospital De Niños/Sor Maria Ludovica
Calle 14 entre 65 y 66
1900 La Plata (Pcia. Buenos Aires)
Tel: 54.0221.4210448

Hospital De Pediatria/Dr. Pedro De Elizalde
Av. Montes de Oca 40
1270 Ciudad de Buenos Aires
Tel: 54.11.43074788/54.11.43075553/
    54.11.43075842

Hospital De Pediatria/Prof. Dr. Juan
    Garrahan
Combate de los Pozos 1881
1245 Ciudad de Buenos Aires
Tel: 54.11.49431455

Hospital Maria Ferrer
Dr. Enrique Finochietto 849
1272 Ciudad de Buenos Aires
Tel: 54.11.43071445

Hospital De Niños de Córdoba
Corrientes 643
5000 Córdoba

Hospital De Niños/Dr. O. Alassia
Mendoza 4551
3000 Santa Fe

Hospital/J.B. Iturraspe
Boulevard Pellegrini 3551
3000 Santa Fe

Hospital De Niños/Víctor J. Vilela
Virasoro 1855
2000 Rosario (Pcia. Santa Fe)
Tel: 54.0341.4808125

Hospital Provincial/Del Centenario
Urquiza 3101
2000 Rosario (Pcia. Santa Fe)
Tel: 54.0341.4307320

Hospital Escuela/Eva Perón
Ruta 11 s/No
2152 Granadero Baigorria (Pcia. Santa Fe)
Tel: 54.0341.4710940

Hospital/Emilio Civit
Parque Gral. San Martìn
5300 Mendoza

AUSTRALIA

Cystic Fibrosis Adult Clinic, Page Chest
  Pavilion
Prof. Peter Bye
Royal Prince Alfred Hospital
Missenden Road
Camperdown NSW 2050
Tel: 61.2.95157427
Fax: 61.2.95158196

Dept. of Respiratory Medicine, New
  Children's Hospital
Dr. Peter Cooper
Hawkesbury Road
Westmead NSW 2145
Tel: 61.2.98453395
Fax: 61.2.98453396

Cystic Fibrosis Adult Clinic, Westmead
  Hospital
Dr. Peter Middleton
Hawkesbury Road
Westmead NSW 2145
Tel: 61.2.98456797
Fax: 61.2.98457286

The Sydney Children's Hospital Cystic
  Fibrosis Clinic
Dr. John Morton
High Street
Randwick NSW 2131
Tel: 61.2.93821477
Fax: 61.2.93821580

Prince of Wales Hospital (adults)
Dr. Frank Maccioni
High Street
Randwick NSW 2131
Tel: 61.2.93824631
Fax: 61.2.93824627

John Hunter Children's Hospital
Dr. D. Cooper/Dr. Peter Gibson
Lookout Road
New Lambton Heights NSW 2305
Tel: 61.2.49213676
Fax: 61.2.49213599

Gosford District Hospital Cystic Fibrosis
  Clinic
Dr. J. Pendergast
Holden Street
Gosford NSW 2250
Tel: 61.2.43245077
Fax: 61.2.43250629

The Alfred Hospital CF Adult Clinic
Professor John Wilson
Commercial Road
Prahran VIC 3181
Tel: 61.3.92763476
Fax: 61.3.92763434

Royal Children's Hospital
Dr. Phil Robinson
Flemington Road
Parkville VIC 3052
Tel: 61.3.93455844
Fax: 61.3.93491289

Dept. of Paediatric Respiratory Medicine
Dr. David Armstrong/Dr. Peter Solin
Monash Medical Centre
Locked Bag 29
Clayton VIC 3168
Tel: 61.3.95942045
Fax: 61.3.95945415

Sir Charles Gairdner Hospital Adult CF
  Clinic
Dr. Gerard Ryan
Verdun Street
Nedlands WA 6009
Tel: 61.8.93463251
Fax: 61.8.93463606

Princess Margaret Hospital for Children
Dr. Barry Clements
GPO Box D184
Perth WA 6001
Tel: 61.8.93408830
Fax: 61.8.93408983

The Royal Adelaide Hospital CF Adult
  Clinic
Dr. Hugh Greville
275 North Terrace
Adelaide SA 5000
Tel: 61.8.82225132
Fax: 61.8.82225957

Women's & Children's Hospital
Dr. James Martin
King William Road
North Adelaide SA 5006
Tel: 61.8.82047234
Fax: 61.8.82047050

Royal Hobart Hospital
Dr. Ian Stewart and Dr. Colin Sherrington
48 Liverpool Street
Hobart TAS 7000
Tel: 61.3.62228475
Fax: 61.3.62228951

Launceston General Hospital
Dr. J. Markos
Charles Street
Launceston TAS 7250
Tel: 61.3.63327111
Fax: 61.3.63327577

Royal Children's Hospital
Dr. Paul Francis
Herston Road
Herston QLD 4006
Tel: 61.7.36365270
Fax: 61.7.36361958

Mater Children's Hospital
Dr. Ian Robertson/Dr. Simon Bowler
Raymond Terrace
South Brisbane QLD 4101
Tel: 61.7.38394870/61.7.38401178
Fax: 61.7.38328201/61.7.32172312

The Prince Charles Hospital (adults)
Dr. Scott Bell
Rode Road
Chermside QLD 4032
Tel: 61.7.33508406
Fax: 61.7.33508510

Royal Brisbane Hospital
Dr. I Brown
Herston QLD 4006
Tel: 61.7.32538111
Fax: 61.7.32571765

Allamanda Medical Centre (children)
Dr. Darrell Price
Suite 5
25 Spendelove Avenue
Southport QLD 4215
Tel: 61.7.55327755
Fax: 61.7.55329413

Gold Coast Hospital (adults)
Dr. Iain Feather
Nerang Street
Southport QLD 4215
Tel: 61.7.55718649
Fax: 61.7.55718996

Bundaberg Base Hospital
Dr. J Williams and Dr. C Ryan
Bundaberg QLD 4760

Tel: 61.7.41520699

Rockhampton Base Hospital
Dr. L. Gray
Rockhampton QLD 4700
Tel: 61.7.49206211

Mackay Base Hospital
Dr. M. Williams
Mackay QLD 4740
Tel: 61.7.49686000

Townsville Base Hospital
Dr. W. Frischmann and Dr. P. Ryan
Townsville QLD 4810
Tel: 61.7.47819211

Flecker House
Dr. R. Messer
5 Upward Street
Cairns QLD 4870
Tel: 61.7.40515430
Fax: 61.7.40310686

Dr. G. Simpson
130 Abbott Street
Cairns QLD 4870
Tel: 61.7.40314095
Fax: 61.7.40518411

BELGIUM

A.Z. V.U.B. Children's Hospital
Prof. Dr. I. Dab and Prof. Dr. A. Malfroot
   (children and adults)
Laarbeeklaan 101
1090 Bruxelles
Tel: 32 2 477 41 11
Fax: 32 2 477 58 00

U.C.L. Saint-Luc
Dr. Lebecque (children)
avenue Hippocrate 10
1200 Bruxelles

Tel: 32.2.7641385
Fax: 32.2.7648911

Hôpital Erasme
Dr. Cnoop (adults)
route de Lennik 808
1070 Bruxelles
Tel: +32 2 526 39 85
Fax: +32 2 555 44 14

Zeepreventorium
Dr. H. Franckx
Koninklijke Baan 5
8420 De Haan
Tel: 32 59 23 39 11
Fax: 32 59 23 40 57

U.Z. Gent
Prof. D. R. Robberecht and Prof. F.
   De Baets (children and adults)
De Pintelaan 185
9000 Gent
Tel: 32.9.2402111
Fax: 32.9.2403875

U.Z. Gasthuisberg
Prof. Dr. C. de Boeck (children and adults)
Herestraat 49
3000 Leuven
Tel: 32.16.332211
Fax: 32.16.343842

U.Z.A.
Prof. Kristine Desager (children)
Wilrijkstraat 10
2650 Edegem
Tel: 32.3.8213537
Fax: 32.3.8291194

St. Vincentiusziekenhuis
Dr. L. Van Schil (adults)
St. Vincentiusstraat 20
2018 Antwerpen
Tel: 32 3 285 20 00
Fax: 32 3 285 28 85

Hôpital Universitaire Des Enfants Reine
  Fabiola
Dr. Casimir (children)
Place Van Gehuchten
1020 Bruxelles
Tel: +32 2 477 21 11
Fax: +32 2 477 32 78

Centre Hospitalier Régional de la Citadelle
Dr. Leclercq
bld. du 12è de Ligne 1
4000 Liege
Tel. : 32 41 25 61 11
Fax : 32 41 26 47 47

Revalidatiecentrum Voor Kinderen
  En Jongeren
Dr. Schuddinck
Reebergenlaan 4
2240 Pulderbos
Tel: 32.3.4843600
Fax: 32.3.4845770

CANADA

Alberta

Alberta Children
Lisa Semple
1820 Richmond Road S.W.
Calgary AB T2T 5C7
Tel: 1.403.2097319
Fax: 1.403. 2297647

Southern Alberta Adult CF Clinic
University of Calgary Medical
Clinic–Area 6
Foothills Hospital
1403-29 Street N.W.
Calgary AB T2N 2T9
Tel: 1.403.6704365
Fax: 1.403.2702772

University of Alberta Hospitals
Joan Tabak
112 Street and 84th Avenue
7-109 Clinical Sciences Building
Edmonton AB T6G 2B7
Tel: 1.780.4076745
Fax: 1.780.4073112

British Columbia

St. Paul's Hospital
Janet Hopkins
1081 Burrard Street
Vancouver BC V6Z 1Y6
Tel: 1.604.8068522
Fax: 1.604.8068122

B.C. Children
Anna Gravelle
4480 Oak Street
Vancouver BC V6H 3V4
Tel: 1.604.8752146
Fax: 1.604.8752349

Victoria General Hospital
Eleanor Shambrook/Sharon Wiltse
35 Helmcken Road
Victoria BC V8Z 6R5
Tel: 1.250.7274187/1.250.7274223
Fax: 1.250.7274221

Manitoba

Children's Hospital of Winnipeg
Marilyn Lowe
840 Sherbrook Street
Winnipeg MB R3A 1S1
Tel: 1.204.7872401
Fax: 1.204.7871944

Health Science Centre
Tamara Wells
810 Sherbrook Street
Winnipeg MB R3A 1R8
Tel: 1.204.7871521
Fax: 1.204.7872420

New Brunswick

Saint John Regional Hospital
Diana Peacock
P. O. Box 2100
Saint John NB E2L 4L2
Tel: 1.506.6486793
Fax: 1.506.6486060

The Janeway Child Health Centre
Elizabeth Sheppard
710 Newfoundland Drive
St. John
S NB A1A 1R8
Tel: 1.709.7784389
Fax: 1.709.7784333

Nova Scotia

IWK Grace Health Centre
Paula Barrett
5850 University Avenue
Halifax NS B3J 3G9
Tel: 1.902.4288219
Fax: 1.902.4283223

Queen Elizabeth II Health Sciences Centre
Fran Gosse
1796 Robie Street
Halifax NS B3H 3A7
Tel: 1.902.4734147
Fax: 1.902.4736202

Hamilton Health Sciences Corporation
Rosamund Hennessey
McMaster Campus
Department of Pediatrics
1200 Main Street West Room 3f18
Hamilton ON L8N 3Z5
Tel: 1.905.5212100/1.905.5273086
Fax: 1.905.5212654

Ontario

Children's Hospital of Eastern Ontario
Anne Smith
401 Smyth Road
Ottawa ON K1H 8L1
Tel: 1.613.7372214
Fax: 1.613.7384832

Children's Hospital of Western Ontario
Elizabeth Hunter
London Health Sciences Centre
800 Commissioners Road East
London ON N6A 4G5
Tel: 1.519.6858500, ext. 52692
Fax: 1.519.6858130

Hotel Dieu Hospital
Darlene McCulloch
166 Brock Street
Kingston ON K7L 5G2
Tel: 1.613.5443400
Fax: 1.613.5448320

Hotel Dieu Grace Hospital
Dagmar Ray
1030 Ouellette Avenue
Windsor ON N9A 1E1
Tel: 1.519.9734431
Fax: 1.519.2589918

Kitchener-Waterloo Health Centre of
    Grand River Hospital
Joy Geiger
835 King Street West
Kitchener ON N2G 1G3
Tel: 1.519.7494300/1.519.7492622
Fax: 1.519. 7494317

Laurentian Hospital
Charlene Piche
41 Chemin Du Lac Ramsey
Sudbury ON P3E 5J1
Tel: 1.705.5222200/1.705.5223263
Fax: 1.705.5237089

The Hospital for Sick Children
Louise Taylor
555 University Avenue
Toronto ON M5G 1X8
Tel: 1.416.8135826
Fax: 1.416.8136246

St. Michael's Hospital
Anna Tsang
30 Bond Street
Toronto ON M5B 1W8
Tel: 1.416.8645409
Fax: 1.416. 8645651

Ottawa General Hospital
Kathleen Devecseri
501 Smyth Road
Ottawa ON K1H 8L6
Tel: 1.613.7378198
Fax: 1.613.7396266

Québec

Centre Hospitalier De Gatineau
Thérèse Faucher
909 Boul. De La Vérendrye Ouest
C.P. 2000
Gatineau (Québec) J8P 7H2
Tel: 1.819.5618195
Fax: 1.819.5618390

Centre Hospitalier Régional De
L'outaouais
Denise Lévesque
116 Boul. Lionel Émond
Hull (Québec) J8Y 1W7
Tel: 1.819.5956053
Fax: 1.819.5951582

Centre Hospitalier Régional De Rimouski
Francine Raymond
150 Av. Rouleau
Rimouski (Québec) G5L 5T1
Tel: 1.418.7248561
Fax: 1.418.7248615

Centre Hospitalier De L'Universite Laval
Manon Roussin
2705 Boul. Sir Wilfrid-Laurier
Ste-Foy (Québec) G1V 4G2
Tel: 1.418.6564141/1.418.6567730
Fax: 1.418.6542137

Centre Universitaire De Santé De L
Marguerite Plante
3001 12e Av. Nord
Fleurimont (Québec) J1H 5N4
Tel: 1.819.3461110/1.819.3412820
Fax: 1.819.8206454

Hôpital De Chicoutimi
Suzanne Mignault
C.P. 5006
Chicoutimi (Québec) G7H 5H6
Tel: 1.418.5411037
Fax: 1.418. 5411134

Hôpital Sainte-Justine
Diane Dupont
3175 Chemin De La Côte-Ste-Catherine
Montréal (Québec) H3T 1C5
Tel: 1.514.3454724
Fax: 1.514.3454804

Hôtel-Dieu De Montréal
Jocelyne Lavallée
Service De Pneumologie
3840 Rue Saint-Urbain
Montréal (Québec) H2W 1T8
Tel: 1.514.8432670
Fax: 1.514.8432769

Centre Hospitalier Thoracique De Montréal
France Paquet
3650 Rue Saint-Urbain
Montréal (Québec) H2X 2P4
Tel: 1.514.8495201/1.514.8495280
Fax: 1.514. 8432076

Hôpital De Montréal Pour Enfants
Jackie Townshend
2300 Rue Tupper
Montréal (Québec) H3H 1P3
Tel: 1.514.9344400/1.514.9342643
Fax: 1.514.9344364

Centre Hospitalier Rouyn-Noranda
Louise Boucher
4 9e Rue
Rouyn-Noranda (Québec) J9X 2B2
Tel: 1.819.7620995
Fax: 1.819.7976837

Saskatchewan

Regina General Hospital
Marlene Hall
1440-14th Avenue
Regina SK S4P 0W5
Tel: 1.306.7664289
Fax: 1.306.7664946

University Hospital
Cathy Turtle
Saskatoon SK S7N 0X0
Tel: 1.306.9668120
Fax: 1.306.9753767

CUBA

Comision Cubana De Fibrosis Quistica
Hospital Pediatrico J. M. Marquez
Ave. 31 esq. 76 Marianao CP 11400
Ciudad de La Habana
Tel./Fax: 53-7-330-145

CZECH REPUBLIK

Pediatric Department University Hospital
Dr. Antonin Kolek
I.P. Pavlova 6
775 20 Olomouc
Tel: 420.68.5853560/420.68.5852929/
420.68.5853559

Pediatric Department
Dr. Alena Holcikova
Cernopolni 9
662 63 Brno
Tel: 420.5.4512562/420.5.4512245

Pediatric Department Bata Hospital
Dr. Lenka Toukalkova
Havlickovo n. 600
760 01 Zlin
Tel: 420.67.7552019/420.67.7552913

Pediatric Department University Hospital
Dr. Hubert Vanicek
500 36 Hradec Kralove
Tel: 420.49.583.3433

Pediatric Department University Hospital
Dr. Helena Honomichlova
Dr. E. Benese 13
305 99 Pzen
Tel: 420.19.7402916

Department TRN ILF Masaryk Hospital
Dr. Ivana Tumova
401 13 USTI nad Labem Bukov
Tel: 420.47.5682325

Pediatric Department ILF
Dr. Ivana Sekyrova
B. Nemcove 54
370 87 Ceske Budejovice
Tel: 420.38.7878737

Pediatric Department ILF
Dr. Jaroslava Hubova
Syllabove 19
703 86 Ostrava
Tel: 420.69.6924378

2nd Pediatric Department University Hospital Motol
Dr. Vera Vavrova Dr. Jana Bartosova
V Uvalu 84
150 18 Praha 5 - Motol
Tel: 420.2.24432269/420.2.24432253
Fax: 420.2.24432220

Pediatric Department
Dr. Jiri Biolek
Tylova 2067
436 01 Litvinov
Tel: 420.35.6173486

Nutarch Podunajske Biskupice
Krajinska 101
825 56 Bratislava
Pediatric Executive: Mudr. Jaroslava
Orosova; Tel.: 421.2.40 251 155
Pediatric Executive: Mudr. Hana Kay-
serova; Tel.: 421.2.40 251 566
Adult Executive: Mudr. Branislav
Drugda; Tel.: 421.2.40 251 458
Adult Executive: Mudr. Branislav Remis;
Tel.: 421.2.40 251 677

DENMARK

Cystic Fibrosis Center Copenhagen
Dr. Christian Koch
Dept. of Pediatrics GGK-5003
Rigshospitalet
Blegdamsvej 9
DK-2100 Copenhagen
Tel: 45.3545.4832/45.3545.5006
Fax: 45.3545.6717

Cystic Fibrosis Center Aarhus
Prof. P. O. Schiotz
Dept. of Pediatrics A
Skejby Sygehus
Brendstrupgaardsvej 100
DK-8200 AARHUS
Tel: 45.8949.6740
Fax: 45.8949.6023

FINLAND

Helsinki University Hospital/Hospital for
Children and Adolescents
Dr. Erkki Savilahti and Dr. Merja
Kajosaari
Stenbäckinkatu 11
FIN-00290 Helsinki
Tel: +358 9 4711
www.hus.fi
erkki.savilahti@hus.fi/merja.kajosaari@
hus.fi

International Physiotherapy Group for
Cystic Fibrosis (IPG/CF)/Pulmonary
Association Heli
Leena Jokinen Coordinator S.R.PT
Hoikka Resource Centre
Hoikantie 15
FIN 38100 Karkku
Tel: +358 3 5121273
Fax: +358 3 5121220
leena.jokinen@hoikkacentre.fi
www.hengitysliitto.fi/www.hoikkacentre.fi
leena.jokinen@hoikkacentre.fi

FRANCE

Hôpital de Hautepierre
Dr. Lionel Donato
Service de Pédiatrie 2
avenue Molière
67098 Strasbourg Cedex
Tel: 33.3.88.127785
Fax: 33.3.88.127132
leonard-donato@chru-strasbourg.fr

Hôpital de Hautepierre–Centre de Soins
Adultes
Dr. Romain Kessler
Service de Pneumologie
avenue Molière
67098 Strasbourg Cedex
Tel: 33.3.88.116768
Fax: 33.3.88.127827
romain.kessler@chru-strasbourg.fr

Centre Muco Adulte Aquitaine
Dr. Philippe Domblides
17 rue de Rivière
33000 Bordeaux
Tel: 33.5.56.443451
Fax: 33.5.56.793226
domblide@infonie.fr

CHU–Groupe Pellegrin
Dr. Michaël Fayon
Hùpital des Enfants
Place Amélie Raba Léon
33076 Bordeaux Cedex
Tel: 33.5.57.970505
Fax: 33.5.57.970500
bordeaux1@eunet.mail.fr

Hôpital du Haut-lévêque–Adult.
Dr. Claire Dromer
Service de Chirurgie Thoracique
Maison du Haut-Lévêque–avenue de Magellan
33604 Pessac Cedex
Tel: 33.5.56.555051
Fax: 33.5.56.555021
claire.dromer@chu-aquitaine.fr

CHG de Dax
Dr. Richard Barbier
Service de Pédiatrie
Boulevard Yves du Manoir–BP 323
40107 Dax Cedex
Tel: 33.5.58914976
Fax: 33.5.58913996

Hôtel Dieu–Pavillon Hacquart
Prof. André Labbé
Pédiatrie A
avenue Vercingétorix–BP 69
63003 Clermont Ferrand Cedex 1
Tel: 33.4.73750027
Fax: 33.4.73354172
alabbé@chu-clermontferrand.fr

Hôpital d'Enfants du Bocage
Prof. Frédéric Huet
Service de Pédiatrie 1
10 Bd du Mal de Lattre de Tassigny
21034 Dijon Cedex
Tel: 33.3.80293415
Fax: 33.3.80293803
frederichuet@chu-dijon.fr

CHU–Hôpital Augustin Morvan Péd.
Dr. Jean-Marie Lefur
Service de Pédiatrie Marfan
5 avenue Foch–BP 824
29609 Brest Cedex
Tel: 33.2.98223659
Fax: 33.2.98223494

Centre Hé Marin–Clinique Mucoviscidose
Dr. Gilles Rault
Presqu'île de Perharidy
29684 Roscoff Cedex
Tel: 33.2.98293916
Fax: 33.2.98293424
admissions@chm-roscoff.fr

CHRU–Hôpital Sud–Péd.
Prof. Michel Roussey
Annexe Pédiatrique–Centre de Soins de Muco.
16 Boulevard de Bulgarie–BP 56129
35056 Rennes Cedex 2
Tel: 33.2.99266756
Fax: 33.2.23302764
hop-ren@mail.eunet.fr

CHRU–Hôpital Sud–Adult.
Prof. Benoît Desrues
Pneumologie Adultes–Centre de Soin Muco.
16 Boulevard de Bulgarie–BP 56129
35056 Rennes Cedex 2
Tel: 33.2.23302764
Fax: 33.2.23302766
benoit.desrues@chu-rennes.fr

Centre Hospitalier Prosper Chubert
Dr. Valérie Moisan-Petit
Service de Pédiatrie
Boulevard du Général Guillaudot
56017 Vannes Cedex
Tel: 33.2.97014160
Fax: 33.2.2.97014369

CHU Clocheville
Prof. Jean-Claude Rolland
Service de Pédiatrie R
49 Boulevard Béranger
37044 Tours Cedex
Tel: 33.2.47474747
Fax: 33.2.47664370

CHU Bretonneau
Dr. Françoise Varaigne
Service de Pneumologie Adultes
Unité Muco. Fonction.–2 Bd Tonnellé
37044 Tours Cedex 1
Tel: 33.2.47476936
Fax: 33.2.2.47473882
eb@med.univ-tours.fr

CHU–American Memorial Hospital
Dr. Michel Abely
Service de Pédiatrie A
47 rue Cognacq-Jay
51092 Reims Cedex
Tel: 33.3.26787007
Fax: 33.3.26788262
mabely@chu-reims.fr

Hôpital Saint Jacques
Dr. Marie-Laure Dalphin
Service de Pédiatrie
2 place Saint-Jacques
25030 Besançon Cedex
Tel: 33.3.81218143
Fax: 33.3.81218830

Hôpital de Saint Pierre
Dr. Michel Renouil
Service de Pédiatrie
Le Tampon 350
97448 Saint Pierre Cedex
Tel: 33.0.262359143
Fax: 33.0.262359234
michel.renouil@wanadoo.fr

Hôpital d'Enfants
Dr. Jean-François Lesure
Service de Pédiatrie
60 rue Bertin–BP 840
97476 Saint Denis Cedex
Tel: 33.0.262908700
Fax: 33.0.262908710
hop.enfants@guetali.fr

Hôpital Arnaud de Villeneuve
Prof. Daniel Rieu
Service de Pédiatrie II
371 avenue du Doyen Gaston Giraud
34090 Montpellier Cedex 5
Tel: 33.4.67336571
Fax: 33.4.67547148
d-rieu@chu-montpellier.fr

Institut Saint Pierre
Dr. Bernard Rolin
Service de Pédiatrie
rue Giniez Mares
34250 Palavas Les Flots
Tel: 33.4.67077558
Fax: 33.4.67680990

Centre Hospitalier Général de Brive
Dr. Philippe Gautry
Service de Pé
Boulevard du Dr. Verlhac–BP 432
19100 Brive Cedex
Tel: 33.5.55926043
Fax: 33.5.55926189

CHU Dupuytren
Prof. Lionel de Lumley
Service de Pédiatrie 1
2 avenue Martin Luther-King
87042 Limoges Cedex
Tel: 33.5.55056801
Fax: 33.5.55056795
delumley@unilim.fr

Hôpitaux de Brabois Pneumo.
Dr. Philippe Scheid
Service de Pneumologie A
rue du Morvan
54511 Vandoeuvre Les Nancy Cedex
Tel: 33.3.83153400
Fax: 33.3.83153564
p.scheid@chu-nancy.fr

Hôpitaux de Brabois Pédiat.
Dr. Jocelyne Derelle
Srvce Pédiatrie 3 & Génétique Clinique
Höpital d'Enfants–rue du Morvan
54511 Vandoeuvre les Nancy Cedex
Tel: 33.3.83154747
Fax: 33.3.83154647
m.vidailhet@chu-nancy.fr

Mucozenne
Dr. Bernard Sablayrolles
Pneumologie et Allergologie de l'Enfant
2 rue Ozenne
31000 Toulouse
Tel: 33.5.61526436
Fax: 33.5.61331174
michelpiot@yahoo.fr

CHU Purpan–Hôpital des Enfants
Dr. François Brémont
Maladies respirat. et allerg. de l'Enfant
330 avenue de Grande Bretagne–BP 3119
31026 Toulouse Cedex 3
Tel: 33.5.34558586
Fax: 33.5.34558589
bremont.f@chu-toulouse.fr

CHU de Rangueil–Pneumo
Dr. Marlène Murris-Espin
Service de Pneumologie-Allergologie
avenue du Pr Jean Poulhès
31403 Toulouse Cedex 4
Tel: 33.5.61322771
Fax: 33.5.61322957
MURRIS.M@chu-toulouse.fr

Hôpital Saint Antoine
Dr. Manuëla Scalbert
Service de Pédiatrie
329 Boulevard Victor Hugo–BP 255
59019 Lille Cedex
Tel: 33.3.20783114
Fax: 33.3.20783195
hsa.pediatrie@nordnet.fr

H. Calmette–Clinique Maladies Respirat.
Prof. Benoît Wallaert
Service de Pneumo. Immuno-Allergologie
Unité EFR
59037 Lille Cedex
Tel: 33.3.20445036
Fax: 33.3.20446693
bwallaert@nordnet.fr

Hôpital Jeanne de Flandres
Prof. Dominique Turck
Clinique de Pédiatrie
Gastroenté–Mucoviscidose
59037 Lille Cedex
Tel: 33.3.20446885
Fax: 33.3.20446134
dturck@chru-lille.fr

Centre Hospitalier de Valenciennes
Dr. Elisabeth Tassin
Service de Pédiatrie
Avenue Desandrouins
59322 Valenciennes Cedex
Tel: 33.3.27143026
Fax: 33.3.27143462

CHG de Dunkerque
Dr. Guy-André Loeuille
Srvce de Pé et Médecine de l'ados
130 avenue Louis Herbeaux–BP 6-367
59385 Dunkerque Cedex 01
Tel: 33.3.28285693
Fax: 33.3.28285936

Centre Hospitalier de Lens
Dr. Anne Sardet
Service de Pédiatrie
99 route de la Bassée
62307 Lens
Tel: 33.3.21691105
Fax: 33.3.21691534
ismedical1@ch-lens.fr

CHU Clémenceau
Prof. Jean-François Duhamel
Service de Pédiatrie A
avenue Georges Clémenceau
14033 Caen Cedex
Tel: 33.2.31272594
Fax: 33.2.31272655

CHG Robert Bisson
Dr. Marcel Guillot
Service de Pédiatrie
4 rue Roger Aini
14100 Lisieux
Tel: 33.2.31613213
Fax: 33.2.31613318
eckart14@aol.com

CHG des Feugrais
Dr. Kamel Lashinat
Service de Pédiatrie
rue du Dr. Villers–BP 346
76503 Elbeuf Cedex
Tel: 33.2.32963540
Fax: 33.2.35873687

CHU–Hôpital Charles Nicolle Adult.
Dr. Stéphane Dominique
Clinique Pneumologique
1 rue de Germont
76031 Rouen Cedex
Tel: 33.2.32888247
Fax: 33.2.32888240
dominique@chu-rouen.fr

CHU–Hôpital Charles Nicolle Péd.
Dr. Olivier Mouterde
Service de Pédiatrie
1 rue de Germont
76031 Rouen Cedex
Tel: 33.2.32888216
Fax: 33.2.32888188
Olivier.Mouterde@chu-rouen.fr

C.H. du Havre–Hôpital de Jour
Dr. Bernard Le Luyer
Service de Pédiatrie
55 bis rue Gustave Flaubert–BP 24
76600 Le Havre
Tel: 33.2.32733630
Fax: 33.2.32733636
bleluyer@hps.tm.fr

Hôpital l'Archet
Prof. Marc Albertini
Service de Pédiatrie
151 rte St Antoine Ginestière–BP 117
06003 Nice Cedex
Tel: 33.4.92036073
Fax: 33.4.93447178

Hôpital Sainte Marguerite–Adult.
Dr. Martine Reynaud-Gaubert
Service de Chirurgie Thoracique
270 Boulevard Sainte-Marguerite
13274 Marseille Cedex 9
Tel: 33.4.91744619
Fax: 33.4.91744590

Hôpital d'Enfants de la Timone–Ped.
Prof. Jacques Sarles
Service de Pédiatrie
264 rue Saint Pierre
13385 Marseille Cedex 5
Tel: 33.4.91386743
Fax: 33.4.91386736
jsarles@ap-hm.fr

CHG d'Aix en Provence
Dr. Dominique Théveniau
Service de Pédiatrie
avenue des Tamaris
13616 Aix en Provence Cedex 1
Tel: 33.4.42335031
Fax: 33.4.42335185
d.theveniau@ch-aix.fr

Hôpital Renée Sabran
Dr. Jean-Pierre Chazalette
Unité de soins pour mucoviscidose
Boulevard Edouard Herriot
83406 Giens Cedex
Tel: 33.4.94381740
Fax: 33.4.94381887

Hôpital Cochin
Dr. Dominique Hubert
Service de Pneumologie
27 rue du Faubourg Saint-Jacques
75014 Paris
Tel: 33.1.58412372
Fax: 33.1.46338253
dominique.hubert@cch.ap-hop-paris.fr

Hôpital Robert Debré
Prof. Jean Navarro
Gastroentérologie pédiatrique
48 Boulevard Sérurier
75019 Paris
Tel: 33.1.40034788
Fax: 33.1.40032353
jean.navarro@rdb.ap-hop-paris.fr

Hôpital Trousseau
Prof. Annick Clément
Service Pédiatrique/Pneumo. de l'Enfant
26 avenue du Dr. Arnold Netter
75571 Paris Cedex 12
Tel: 33.1.44736668
Fax: 33.1.44736718
annick.clement@trs.ap-hop-paris.fr

H. Necker Enfants Malades Pneumo.
Prof. Pierre Scheinmann
Service Pneumo. Allergo. Pédiatrique
149 rue de Sèvres
75730 Paris Cedex 15
Tel: 33.1.44484942
Fax: 33.1.44381740
pneumo.allergo@nck.ap-hop-paris.fr

H. Necker Enfants Malades Péd.
Prof. Gérard Lenoir
Unité de Pédiatrie Générale
149 rue de Sèvres
75743 Paris Cedex 15
Tel: 33.1.44494882
Fax: 33.1.47833226

Hôpital André Mignot
Dr. Pierre Foucaud
Service de Pé
177 rue de Versailles
78157 Le Chesnay Cedex
Tel: 33.1.39638944
Fax: 33.1.39639396
pediatrie@ch-versailles.fr

Centre de Pneumologie de l'Enfant
Dr. Bertrand Delaisi
104 avenue Victor Hugo
92100 Boulogne
Tel: 33.1.46999898
Fax: 33.1.46999897
resppanif@yahoo.com

Hôpital Foch–Pneumo.
Prof. Isabelle Caubarrére
Service de Pneumologie
40 rue worth–BP 36
92151 Suresnes Cedex
Tel: 33.1.46252635
Fax: 33.1.42043281
i.caubarrere@hopital-foch.org

Centre Intercommunal de Créteil
Prof. Philippe Reinert
Service de Pédiatrie
40 avenue de Verdun
94010 Créteil Cedex
Tel: 33.1.45175420
Fax: 33.1.45175426

Hôpital Mère-Enfant
Dr. Valérie David
Service de Pédiatrie médicale
Quai Moncousu
44093 Nantes Cedex 01
Tel: 33.2.40083172
Fax: 33.2.40083483
vdavid@chu-nantes.fr

Hôpital G. et R. Laënnec–Adult.
Dr. Alain Haloun
Unité de Transplantation Thoracique
BP 1005
44093 Nantes Cedex 01
Tel: 33.2.40165092
Fax: 33.2.40165092
haloun.alain@chu-nantes.fr

CHR de Saint Nazaire
Dr. Georges Picherot
Service de Pé
Boulevard Laënnec–BP 414
44606 Saint Nazaire Cedex
Tel: 33.2.40906100
Fax: 33.2.40905201

CHU–Centre Robert Debré
Prof. Jean-Louis Giniès
4 rue Larrey
49033 Angers Cedex 01
Tel: 33.2.41354987
Fax: 33.2.41354173
jlginies@pediatrie.net

CHD Les Oudairies
Dr. Pierre Blanchard
Service de Pédiatrie
85025 La Roche sur Yon
Tel: 33.2.51446201
Fax: 33.2.51446298

CHU Nord
Dr. Jean-Claude Pautard
Srvce Pédiatrie I–Unité Pneumo. Infantile
Place Victor Pauchet
80054 Amiens Cedex
Tel: 33.3.22668260
Fax: 33.3.22668483

Centre Hospitalier de Saintes
Dr. Marc Besson-Léaud
Service de Pédiatrie
9 place du 11 novembre–BP 326
17108 Saintes Cedex
Tel: 33.5.46927676
Fax: 33.5.46927791

CHU–La Milètrie
Dr. Catherine Gambert
Service de Pédiatrie
350 avenue Jacques Coeur–BP 577
86021 Poitiers Cedex
Tel: 33.5.49.444390
Fax: 33.5.49443820
d.oriot@chu.univ-poitiers.fr

CHU de Grenoble–Péd.
Dr. Isabelle Pin
Département de Pédiatrie–Centre Muco
BP 217
38043 Grenoble Cedex 9
Tel: 33.4.76765469
Fax: 33.4.76765830
isabelle.pin@ujf-grenoble.fr

CHU de Grenoble–Adult
Dr. Isabelle Pin
Service de Pneumologie–Centre Muco
BP 217x
38043 Grenoble Cedex 9
Tel: 33.4.76768732
Fax: 33.4.76765617
isabelle.pin@ujf-grenoble.fr

CH de Voiron
Dr. Jean-Pierre Gout
Service de Pédiatrie
38500 Voiron
Tel: 33.4.76671416
Fax: 33.4.76671597

CH Lyon Sud–Péd.
Prof. Gabriel Bellon
Service de Pédiatrie–Unité Pneumologie
165 chemin du Grand Revoyet
69495 Pierre Bénite Cedex
Tel: 33.4.78861557
Fax: 33.4.78865724

C.H. Lyon Sud–Adult
Dr. Isabelle Durieu
Srvce Médecine Interne–Bât 1K Giraud
165 Chemin du Grand Revoyet
69495 Pierre Bénite Cedex
Tel: 33.4.78861354
Fax: 33.4.78863264
isabelle.durieu@chu-lyon.fr

ITALY

C.R.R. Divisione di Pediatria
Dr. Paolo Moretti
Ospedale di Teramo
Abruzzo-Molise
Tel: 39.861.4291

S.R.R.–Attivita' di Supporto presso
    Divisione Pediatrica
Dr. Rosaria Abate
Dr. Donatello Salvatore
Ospedale di Villa
85100 Potenza
Basilicata
Tel: 39.975.352845/39.975.312111
    (int. 236)

C.R.R. Attivita' di Supporto presso
    Divisione Pediatrica
Ospedale di Soverato
88100 Catanzaro
Calabria
Tel: 39.967.539111

C.R.R. Clinica Pediatrica della II Facolta'
    di Medicina
Prof. Giorgio De Ritis
Via Pansini 5
80100 Napoli
Campania
Tel: 39.81.7463273/39.81.7463500

C.R.R. Centro di Fisiopatologia
    Respiratoria Infantile
Prof. Augusta Battistini
Universita' di Parma
Via Gramsci 14
43100 Parma
Emilia
Tel: 39.521.991198/39.521.290461
Fax: 39.521.290458

C.R.R. Divisione Pediatria
Dott.ssa Brevella Giglio
Instituto per l'Infanzia Burlo Garofolo
Via dell'Istria 65
34100 Trieste
Friuli Venezia Giulia
Tel: 39.40.3785111
Fax: 39.40.3785210

C.R.R. Servizio fibrosi Cistica e
    Fisioterapia
Instituto Clinica Pediatrica
Prof. Mariano Antonelli
Policlinico Umberto I Viale Regina
    Elena 312
00100 Roma
Lazio
Tel: 39.6.497891 (int. 289)/39.6.4454898

Centro di diagnosi e Terapia della Fibrosi
    Cistica
Dr. Massimo Castro
Dr. Lucidi
Divisione Pediatrica di Gastroenterologia
    Ospedale Bambino Gesu'
Piazza S. Onofrio 4 00100
Roma
Lazio
Tel: 39.6.66859.2330/39.6.66859.2296

C.R.R. Centro Regionale per le Malattie
    Endocrine e Metaboliche dell'Eta'
    Evolutive
Prof. Cesare Romano
Sez. Fibrosi Cistica
Clinica Pediatrica 1a Instituto G. Gaslini
Via Largo Gerolamo Gaslini 5
16100 Genova
Liguria
Tel: 39.10.387496/39.10.5636366/
    39.10.3776590

C.R.R. IIa Clinica Pediatrica De Marchi
    Instituti clinici di Perfezionamento di
    Milano
Prof. Annamaria Giunta
Via della Commenda 9
20100 Milano
Lombardia
Tel: 39.2.55111043/39.2.57992456
Fax: 39.2.55195341

C.R.R. Centro Fibrosi Cistica
Prof. Guiseppe Caramia
Dr. Rolando Gagliardini
Divisione di Pediatria e Neonatologia
    Ospedale dei Bambini
g. Salesi ULSS n. 12
Marche
Tel: 39.71.5962351/39.71.5962354

C.R.R. Settore minori: Centro
    Dipartimentale Clinico-Ospedaliero per
    la Fibrosi
Cistica
Prof. Nicoletta Ansaldi
Prof. Domenico Castello
Ospedale Infantile Regina Margherita
Piazza Polonia 94
10100 Torino
Piemonte–Valle d'Aosta
Tel: 39.11.69227247/39.11.69227267/
    39.11.69227765

C.R.R. Servizio di Prevenzione e Cura
    della Mucoviscidosi
Prof. Nicola Rigillo
Clinica Pediatrica Iia–Policlinico
Piazza Giulio Cesare
70100 Bari
Puglia
Tel: 39.80.5527527
Fax: 39.80.278911

C.R.R. Centro per la Fibrosi Cistica
    Divisione di Pediatria e Patologia
    Neonatale
Prof. Giancarlo Biasini Dr. Angelo Miano
Ospedale M. Bufalini
ULSS n. 39
47023 Cesena (FO)
Romagna
Tel: 39.547.352837.302322

C.R.R Divisione di Pediatria
Prof. Mario Silvetti
Ospedale G. Brotzu
ULSS n. 21 Regione Sardegna
Via Peretti 09100 Cagliari
Sardegna
Tel: 39.70.539551
Fax: 39.70.539682

C.R.R. Servizio per la Diagnosi e Cura
    della Fibrosi Cistica
Prof. Vincenzo Balsamo Ospedale dei
    Bambini
G. De Cristina Piazza Porta Montalto
90100 Palermo
Sicilia
Tel: 39.91.6666074/39.91.6666226

C.R.R. Instituto Clinica Pediatrica
Prof. Giuseppe Magazzu'
Policlinico Universitario
98100 Messina
Sicilia
Tel: 39.90.2935007
Fax: 39.90.2935007

Centro Regionale Toscano per la
    Fibrosi Cistica
Prof. Lore Marianelli
Dipartimento di Pediatria Ospedale Meyer
    Via L. Giodano 13
50100 Firenze
Toscana
Tel: 39.55.56621
Fax: 39.55.570380

C.R.R. Servizio Supporto Fibrosi
  Cistica e Fisioterapia
Dr. Angelo Cosimi
Ospedale Calai–Divisione di Pediatria
06023 Gualdo Tadino (PG)
Umbria
Tel: 39.75.9109301

C.R.R. Centro Regionale Veneto di Ricerca
Prof. B.H. Assael
Prevenzione Riabilitazione ed
  Insegnamento per la Fibrosi Cistica
Ospedale Civile Maggiore
Piazzale Stefani 1
37100 Verona
Veneto
Tel: 39.45.8072370
Fax: 39.45.8072042

Attivita di Supporto presso
Dr. Luigi Ratclif
Divisione Pediatrica Ospedale di
  Cerignola (FG)
Puglia
Tel: 39.885.419111

Attivita di Supporto presso Divisione
  Pediatrica
Ospedale di Acquaviva Delle Fonti, Bari
Dr. Nicola D'Andrea
Puglia
Tel: 39.80.760374

Attivita di Supporto presso Divisione
  Pediatrica
Dr. Germano Pio Ercolino
Ospedale di San Giovanni Rotondo (FG)
Puglia
Tel: 39.882.853721/39.882.853621

Attivita di Supporto presso Divisione
  Pediatrica
Dr. Maria Vittoria Perez
Ospedale di Livorno
Toscana
Tel: 39.586.418111

Attivita di Supporto presso Divisione
  Pediatrica
Dr. Adalberto Campagna
Ospedale di Grosseto
Toscana
Tel: 39.564.485329

Attivita di Supporto presso Divisione
  Pediatrica
Dr. Lydia Pescolderung
Ospedale di Bolzano
Trentino Alto Adige
Tel: 39.471.908111

C.R.R. Settore adulti: Centro Fibrosi Cistica
Reparto Pneumologia Clinica
  Universitaria Tisiologica
Reg. Gonzole Ospedale S. Luigi
10043 Orbassano (TO)
Piemonte–Valle D'Aosta
Tel: 39.11.9026432/39.11.9038674/
  39.11.9038639

JORDAN

The Medical School
Dr. M Rawashdeh
University of Science & Technology
PO Box 3030
Irbid

Ibn Al-Haytham Hospital
Dr. M Rawashdeh
Amman
Tel: 962.6.5516823

THE NETHERLANDS

Academisch Ziekenhuis VU
  Adults–Children
De Boelelaan 1117
P.O. Box 7057
1007 MB Amsterdam
Tel: 31.20.4444444
Fax: 31.20.4444645

Ziekenhuis Leijenburg–Adults
Leyweg 275
Postbus 40551
2504 LN Den Haag
Tel: 31.70.3592000
Fax: 31.70.3595040

Ac. Medisch Centrum (AMC) Adults
Meibergdreef 9
1105 AZ Amsterdam
Tel: 31.20.5669111
Fax: 31.20.5664440

Ac. Ziekenhuis Rotterdam (AZR)–Adults
Dr. Molewaterplein 40
Postbus 2040
3000 CA Rotterdam
Tel: 31.10.4639222
Fax: 31.10.4635305

Universitair Medisch Centrum
   (UMC)–Adults
Heidelberglaan 100
Postbus 85500
3508 GA Utrecht
Tel: 31.30.2509111

Ac. Ziekenhuis Maastricht
   (AZM)–Children
P. Debyelaan 25
Postbus 5800
6202 AZ Maastricht
Tel: 31.43.3876543
Fax: 31.43.3878787

Ac. Ziekenhuis Groningen
(AZG)–Adults/Children
Hanzeplein 1
Postbus 30001
9700 RB Groningen
Tel: 31.50.3619111
Fax: 31.50.3614351

AMC/Emma Kinderziekenhuis–Children
Meibergdreef 9
1105 AZ Amsterdam
Tel: 31.20.5669111
Fax: 31.20.5664440

Medisch Centrum Alkmaar–
   Adults/Children
Wilhelminalaan 12
Postbus 501
1800 AM Alkmaar
Tel: 31.72.5484444
Fax: 31.72.5482179

Juliana Kinderziekenhuis–Children
Sportlaan 600
Postbus 60605
2566 MJ Den Haag
Tel: 31.70.3127200
Fax: 31.70.3126161

AZR/Sophia Kinderziekenhuis–Children
Dr. Molewaterplein 60
Postbus 2060
3000 CB Rotterdam
Tel: 31.10.4636363
Fax: 31.10.4636800

UMC/Wilhelmina
Kinderziekenhuis–Children
Lundlaan 6
Postbus 85090
3508 AB Utrecht
Tel: 31.30.2504000

NEW ZEALAND

Starship Children's Hospital
Dr. Alison W Wesley
Private Bag 92024
Auckland
Tel: 64.9.3074949/64.9.3076480
Fax: 64.9.3074913

Green Lane Hospital
Dr. John Kolbe
Private Bag
Auckland 3
Tel: 64.9.6389919/64.9.6383896
Department of Paediatrics
Dr. Philip Pattemore
Christchurch Hospital
Private Bag 4710
Christchurch
Tel: 64.3.3640734
Fax: 64.3.3640919

Respiratory Physician
Dr. Peter Thornley
Christchurch Hospital
Private Bag 4710
Christchurch
Tel: 64.3.3640919

Dunedin Hospital
Dr. Christopher Hewitt
Private Bag 1921
Dunedin
Tel: 64.3.4740999
Fax: 64.3.4747623

Waikato Hospital
Dr. David Graham
Private Bag 3200
Hamilton
Tel: 64.7.8398899

Waikato Hospital
Dr. Graeme Mills
Private Bag 3200
Hamilton
Tel: 64.7.8398899

Capital Coast Healthcare
Dr. Alan Farrell
Private Bag 7902
Wellington South
Tel: 64.4.3855999
Fax: 64.4.43855856

Capital Coast Healthcare
Dr. David Jones
Private Bag 7902
Wellington South
Tel: 64.4.3855999
Fax: 64.4.3855856

NORWAY

Dept. of Pediatrics
Olav Trond Storrosten, M.D.
Ulleval Hospital
0407 Oslo
Norway
Tel: 47.23.01.5591

ROMANIA

Clinic II Paediatrics University of
    Medicine and Pharmacy
Prof. Dr. Ioan Popa
Paltinis Street 1-3
1900 Timisoara
Tel: 40.56.194529
Fax: 40.56.194529

County Hospital Pediatric Departament
Dr. Laura Dracea
Nicopole Street 45
2200 Brasov
Tel: 40.68.415130

Children's Hospital
Dr. Rodica Mihalceanu
Ostasilor Street 12
3700 Oradea
Tel: 40.59.441844
Fax: 40.59.442687

Clinic I Paediatrics University of
    Medicine and Pharmacy Cluj–Napoca
Prof. dr. Paula Grigorescu–Sido
Motilor Street 68
3400 Cluj–Napoca
Tel: 40.64.197706
Fax: 40.64.192446

County Hospital Clinic II Paediatrics
    Faculty of Medicine Craiova
Senior lecturer Dr. Eva Nemes
Maresal Antonescu Street 60
1100 Craiova
Tel: 40.51.132498

Children's Hospital Clinic III Pediatrics
Prof. Dr. Dan Moraru
Vasile Lupu Street 62
6600 Iasi
Tel: 40.32.175740
Fax: 40.32.177309

County Hospital Pediatric Departament
Dr. Nelia Munteanu
Cosbuc Street 31
4800 Baia–Mare
Tel: 40.62.426031
Fax: 40.62.426859

County Hospital New Born Departament
Dr. Camelia Balas
22 Decembrie Street
2700 Deva
Tel: 40.54.215050

County Hospital Pediatric Departament
Dr. Mihaela Mînascurta
Revolutiei Avenue 23
2500 Alba–Iulia

SLOVAK REPUBLIK

FNsP Kosice
Executive: Dr. Anna Feketeova
  (Tel: 421.55.640 4151)
Trieda SNP 1
040 11 Kosice
Tel: 421.55.640 4137

Nemocnica F.D.Roosevelta
Pediatric. Dept
Executive: Dr. Adriana Zigova (Tel:
421.48.441.3375)
974 00 Banska Bystrica
Tel: 421.88.4413375

SOUTH AFRICA

Johannesburg Hospital–Paediatric CF Clinic
Dr. Susan Klugman
Tel: 27.11.4883983

Johannesburg Hospital–Adult Respiratory
  Clinic
Dr. Mervyn Mer
Tel: 27.11.4884911/27.11.4883496
  (page no. 1025)

Sandton Clinic
Dr. Dave Richard
Tel: 27.11.706 6060

Pretoria Academic Hospital–CF Clinic
Dr. Fanie Naude
Tel: 27.12.354 6244/27.12.3541564

Addington Hospital (Durban)–CF Clinic
Dr. Graham Ducasse
Tel: 27.31.3322111

St. Augustine
Dr. Jonathan Egner
Tel: 27.31.2010215

Red Cross Childrens Hospital (Cape Town)
S Hospital (Durban)
Prof. John Ireland/Dr. Tony Westwood
Tel: 27.21.6585111

Groote Schuur (Cape Town) Adult CF
  Clinic
Prof. Paul Willcox
Tel: 27.21.4044369

Port Elizabeth Greenacres Hospital
Dr. Paul Gebers
Tel: 27.41.3633900

SPAIN

Hospital San Juan de la Cruz
Dr. Antonio Torres Torres
Ctra. de Linares Km. 1
23400 Ubeda
Jaén
Tel: 953797100

Hospital Santa Ana
Dr. Eduardo Ortega Paez
Ctra. Antigua de Granada s/n
18600 Motril
Granada
Tel: 958603506

Hospital Valle de Pedroches
Dr. Juan Amor Truejos
Av. De la Constitución s/n
14400 Pozoblanco
Córdoba
Tel: 957771511

Hospital La Linea de la Concepción
Pediatria
C/menendez Pelayo 103
11300 La Linea de la Concepción
Cádiz
Tel: 956175550

Hospital Punta de Europa
Dr. Julio Guerrero Vázquez
Ctra. de Getafe s/n
11207 Algeciras
Cádiz
Tel: 956580420

Hospital Severo Ochoa
Dra. Gonzalez Alvarez
Av. De Orellana s/n
28911 Leganes
Madrid
Tel: 916944811

Hospital de Ponferrada
Pediatria
C/ de la Dehesa s/n
24411 Fuentesnuevas
Ponferrada (León)
Tel: 987455200

Hospital de Terrasa
Dra. Socorro Uriz Urzainqui
Ctra. Torrebonica
08221 Terrasa
Barcelona
Tel: 937310007

Hospital Naval San Carlos
Dr. Juan M. Garc¡a-Cubillana
Capitan Conforto s/n
11100 San Fernando
Cádiz
Tel: 956599000

Hospital Principes D Espanyo
Dr. Federico Manresa Presas
Feria Llarga s/n
08950 Esplugues de Llobregat
Barcelona
Tel: 933357011

Hospital Torrecardenas
Dr. Morales Ferrer
Pasaje Torrecardenas s/n
04009 Almeria
Almeria
Tel: 951212100

Hospital General de Elche
Dr. Jesus Garde Garde
Partida Huertos y Molinos s/n
03071 Elche
Alicante
Tel: 966606000
Fax: 966606108

Hospital General de Elda
Dra. Isabel Ortin Septien
Ctra. Elda-Sax s/n
03600 Elda
Alicante
Tel: 966989000

Hospital Comarcal La Vilajolosa
Dra. Amparo Gomez Granell
Partida Galandu 5
03570 Villajoyosa
Alicante
Tel: 966859200
Fax: 966859300

Hospital Virgen de los Lirios
Dr. Fernando Clemente
Poligono de Caramanxel s/n
03800 Alcoy
Alicante
Tel: 966527400
Fax: 966527448

Hospital General de Alicante
Dr. Juan Gonzalez Perabá
Maestro Alonso 109
03010 Alicante
Alicante
Tel: 965908300
Fax: 965245971

Hospital Clinico San Juan
Dra. Mercedes Juste
Ctra. Alicante-Valencia s/n
03550 San Juan de Alicante
Alicante
Tel: 965938700
Fax: 965908652

Hospital de Francesc de Borja
Dr. Manuel Oltra Benavent
Passeig de les Germanies 71
46700 Gandia
Valencia
Tel: 963875936
Fax: 962959200

Hospital General
Dr. Miguel Calabuig
Av. Tres Cruces s/n
46014 Valencia
Valencia
Tel: 963862900

Hospital Cantabria
Dr. Pedro Fernandez
Cazona s/n
39008 Santander
Santander
Tel: 942202520

Hospital Provincial Universitario
Dr. Fernando Sanchez Gascon
Av. Intendente Jorge Palacios
20003 Murcia
Murcia
Tel: 968256900

Hospital Materno Infantil
Dr. Luis Pe§a
Av. Maritima del Sur s/n
35016 Las Palmas de Gran Canaria
Las Palmas de Gran Canaria
Tel: 928444500

Hospital Ciudad de Ja,n
Dra. Antonia Pizarro
Av. Ejercito Español 10
23007 Jaén
Jaén
Tel: 953299000

Hospital Juan Ramon Jimenez
Dr. Garcia Martin
Ronda Exterior Zona Norte
21005 Huelva
Huelva
Tel: 959201000

Hospital de Vinaroz
Dra. Rabasco
Av. Gil de Atrocillo s/n
12005 Vinaroz
Castellón
Tel: 964400032
Fax: 964400736

Hospital General de Castellón
Dr. Eduardo Bues
Av. Benicasim s/n
12004 Castellón
Castellón
Tel: 964200100
Fax: 964252345

Hospital Virgen del Rocio
Dr. Dapena
Av. Manuel Siurot s/n
41013 Sevilla
Sevilla
Tel: 954247642

Hospital Marques Valdecilla
Dr. Zubano
Av. Valdesilla 25
39008 Santander
Santander
Tel: 942202520

Hospital Virgen del Camino
Dr. Jose Emilia Olivera
Irunlarrea 4
31008 Pamplona
Pamplona
Tel: 948429400

Hospital Puerta del Mar
Dr. Mena/Dr. Antonio Alienza
Av. Ana de Villa 21
11009 Cádiz
Cádiz
Tel: 956242100

Hospital Infanta Cristina
Dr. Antonio Serrano
Ctra. Madrid-Lisboa s/n
06080 Badajoz
Badajoz
Tel: 924218100

Hospital Cristal Piñor
Dr. Tabares
Ramon Puga 54
32005 Orense
Orense
Tel: 988385500

Hospital San Pedro Alcantara
Dra. Lopez
Av. de Millan Astray s/n
10003 Cáceres
Cáceres
Tel: 927256200
Fax: 927256202

Hospital de Jerez
Dr. Garcia Chesa
Ctra. de Circunvalación s/n
11407 Jerez de la Frontera
Cádiz
Tel: 956358000

Hospital La Macarena
Dr. Navarro
Av. Dr. Fedriani 3
41071 Sevilla
Sevilla
Tel: 954557400

Clinico Universitario
Dra. Lázaro
Av. Gomez Laguna s/n
50009 Zaragoza
Zaragoza
Tel: 976556400

Infantil Miguel Servet
Dra. Heredia
Paseo Isabel la catolica s/n
50009 Zaragoza
Zaragoza
Tel: 976355700

Clinico Universitario
Dra. Calvo
Av. Ramon y cajal 7
47005 Valladolid
Valladolid
Fax: 983420000

Clinico Universitario
Dra. Escribano
Av. Blasco Ibañez 17
46010 Valencia
Valencia
Tel: 963862600
Fax: 963862600

La F
Dr. Ferrer
Av. Campanar 21
46009 Valencia
Valencia
Tel: 963862700

Hospital Ntra. Sra. Candelaria
Dr. Ortigosa
Ctra. Gral. del Rosario s/n
38010 Sta. Cruz de Tenerife
Sta. Cruz de Tenerife
Tel: 922602000

Univer. Canarias
Dr. Honorio de Armas
Ofra–La Laguna
38320 Sta.Cruz de Tenerife
Sta. Cruz de Tenerife
Tel: 922678000

Hospital Son Dureta
Dr. Juan Figuerola Mulet
Andrea Doria 55
07014 Palma de Mallorca
Palma de Mallorca
Tel: 971750000

Hospital Ntra. Sra. Covadonga
Dr. Carlos Bousoño
Celestino Villamil s/n
33006 Oviedo
Oviedo
Tel: 985108019

Hospital Virgen de la Arreixaca
Dr. Manuel López Sanchez Solís
Ctra. Madrid-Cartagena
30120 El Palmar
Murcia
Tel: 968369582

Hospital Carlos Haya
Dr. Javier Perez Frias
Av. Arroyo de los Angeles s/n
29010 Málaga
Málaga
Tel: 952390400

Hospital Gregorio Marañon
Dra. Hubert
Dr. Esquerdo 46
28007 Madrid
Madrid
Tel: 915868000

Hospital La Princesa
Dra. Girón
Diego de León 62
28006 Madrid
Madrid
Tel: 915202277

Hospital Doce de Octubre
Dr. Manzanares
Ctra. de Andalucia km 5400
28041 Madrid
Madrid
Tel: 913908323

Hospital Ramon y Cajal
Dr. Maiz
Ctra. de Colmenar km. 9100
28034 Madrid
Madrid
Tel: 913368092
Fax: 913580614

Hospital La Paz
Dra. Antelo
Paseo de la Castellana 261
28046 Madrid
Madrid
Tel: 913580851

Hospital Niño Jesus
Dr. Salcedo
Menendez y Pelayo 65
28009 Madrid
Madrid
Tel: 915735200, ext. 276

Hospital Teresa Herrera
Dr. Leopoldo Garcia Alonso
Ctra. de las Xubias
15006 La Coruña
La Coruña
Tel: 981178000

Hospital Virgen de las Nieves
Dr. Valenzuela
Av. Constitución 100
18012 Granada
Granada
Tel: 958241100

Hospital Reina Sofia
Dr. Vaquero
Av. Menendez Pidal s/n
14004 Córdoba
Córdoba
Tel: 957217000

Infantil de Cruces
Dr. Carlos Vazquez
Pl. Barrio de Cruces
48903 Bilbao
Bilbao
Tel: 944850086

Hospital Nen Jesus
Dr. Oscar Asensio de la Cruz
Bonaigua 31
08208 Sabadell
Barcelona
Tel: 937237358

Hospital Sant Joan de Deu
Dr. Jose Luis Seculi
Paseo Sant Joan de Deu 2
08950 Esplugues de Llobregat
Barcelona
Tel: 932804000

Hospital Vall dHebron
Dr. Nicolas Cobos
Passeig Vall dHebron s/n
08023 Barcelona
Barcelona
Tel: 934893170

Hospital Universitario de Getafe
Dra. Madruga
Ctra. de Toledo km. 12500
28021 Getafe
Madrid
Tel: 916839360

Hospital Virgen de la Vega
Dr. Grande
Paseo de San Vicente 58-182
37007 Salamanca
Salamanca
Tel: 923291200

Hospital Clinico
Dra. Martinez
Paseo de San Vicente 58-182
37007 Salamanca
Salamanca
Tel: 923291100

SWEDEN

Pediatric Clinic University Hospital
Lena Hjelte
Stockholms CF Center B 59
141 86 Huddinge
Tel: 46.8.58587359
Fax: 46.8.58581410

CF Center Medical/Lung Clinic
Leif Eriksson
University Hospital
221 85 Lund
Tel: 46.46.171490
Fax: 46.46.146793

CF Center Pediatric Clinic
Anders Lindblad
University Hospital
SU/Östra
416 85 Göteborg
Tel: 46.31.3435624
Fax: 46.31.3435184

CF Center Pediatric Clinic
Marie Johannesson
University Hospital
751 85 Uppsala
Tel: 46.18.665929
Fax: 46.18.665853

SWITZERLAND

Kinderklinik Kantonsspital
PD Dr. Hanspeter Gnehm/Dr. P. Eng
5001 AARAU
Tel: 41.62.8384004

Universitäts-Kinderspital
PD Dr. med. Jürg Hammer
Römergasse 8
4005 Basel
Tel: 41.61.6912626

Universitäts-Kinderklinik Inselspital
Prof. Dr. Richard Kraemer/Prof. Dr.
  M.-H. Schöni
3010 Bern
Tel: 41.31.6329493
Fax: 41.31.6329468

Alpine Kinderklinik
Dr. med. Bruno Knöpfli
Scalettastrasse 5
7270 Davos-Platz
Tel: 41.81.4157070

Hôpital Cantonal Universitaire
Prof. Dr. Dominique Belli/Prof. Dr.
  Thierry Rochat/Prof. Dr. Susanne Suter
30 Bd. de la Cluse
1211 Geneve 4
Tel: 41.22.3729902

Centre Hospitalier Universitaire Vaudois
  CHUV
PD Dr. Michel Roulet
Service de Pédiatrie
1011 Lausanne
Tel: 41.21.3145631

Pädiatrische Klinik
Dr. J. Spalinger
Kinderspital/Kantonsspital
6000 Luzern 16
Tel: 41.41.2053151

Ostschweiz. Kinderspital
Dr. med. P. Eng
Claudiusstrasse 6
9000 ST.Gallen
Tel: 41.71.3244111

Universitäts-Kinderspital
PD Dr. Christian Braegger/Prof. Dr. F.
  Sennhauser
Steinwiesstrasse 75
8032 Zurich
Tel: 41.1.2661111

UNITED KINGDOM

The Children's Hospital
Dr. P Weller (Children)
Ladywood Middleway
Birmingham B16 8ET
Tel: 0121 333 9999
Fax: 0121 333 8201

The Cardiothoracic
CentreLiverpool–NHS Trust
Dr. M. Walshaw (adults)
Thomas Drive
Liverpool L14 3PE
Tel: 0151 293 2390
Fax: 0151 228 5539

Addenbrooke's Hospital Hills Road
Dr. R. Ross-Russell (children)
Cambridge CB2 2QQ
Tel: 01223 216020/012232 216878
Fax: 01223 216020/01223 216878, Dr. R
Iles (children)

Seacroft Hospital
Dr. D. Peckham (adults)/Dr. S. Conway
  (adults)
York Road
Leeds LS14 6UH.
Tel: 0113 206 2088/Tel: 0113 206 3513
Fax: 0113 206 3738/Fax: 0113 206 3738

Birmingham Heartlands Hospital
Dr. D. Honeybourne/Dr. D. Stableforth
  (adults)
Bordesley Green East
Birmingham B9 5SS
Tel: 0121 776 6611, ext. 4475/0121 766
6611, ext. 4478
Fax: 0121 772 0292/0121 772 0292

St. James's and Seacroft University
  Hospital NHS
Dr. K. Brownlee (Children)/Dr. S.
  Conway (Children)
Trust Beckett Street
Leeds LS9 7TF
 Fax: 0113 206 5405/0113 206 3540

Royal Hospital for Sick Children
Dr. S. Langton-Hewer (children)
St. Michael's Hill
Bristol BS2 8BJ
Fax: 0117 928 5693

Royal Devon and Exeter Hospital
Dr. C. Sheldon (adults)/Dr. P. Oades
  (children)/Dr. J. Tripp (children)
Barrack Road
Exeter EX2 5DW
Tel: 01392 402132/01392 402665/
  01392 403147
Fax: 01392 402152/01392 402668/
  01392 403158

Leicester Royal Infirmary
Dr. C. O'Callaghan (children)
Infirmary Square
Leicester LE1 5WW
Fax: 0116 258 7657

Papworth Hospital
Dr. D. Bilton (adults)
Papworth Everard
Cambridge CB3 8RE
Tel: 01480 830541
Fax: 01480 460969

Frimley Park Hospital
Dr. R. Knight (adults)
Portsmouth Road
Frimley
Surrey GU16 5UJ
Tel: 01276 604122
Fax: 01276 604148

Royal Liverpool Children's
Hospital–Alder Hey
Prof. R. Smyth (children)/Dr. D. Heaf
  (children)
Eaton Road
Liverpool L12 2AP
Fax: 0151 252 5929/Fax: 0151 252 5929

Dr. C. Wallis (children)/Dr. R. Dinwiddie
  (children)
Great Ormond Street
London WC1N 3JII
Tel: 020 7405 9200, ext. 5453/020 7405
9200, ext. 5453
Fax: 020 7829 8634/020 7829 8634

The Hospital for Sick Children
Dr. C. Wallis (children)/Dr. R. Dinwiddie
  (children)
Great Ormond Street
London WC1N 3JH
Tel: 020 7405 9200, ext. 5453/020 7405
9200, ext. 5453
Fax: 020 7829 8634/020 7829 8634

Royal Manchester Children's Hospital
Dr. M. Super (children)/Dr. G. Hambleton
  (children)
Pendlebury
Manchester M27 4HA
Tel: 0161 727 2335
Fax: 0161 727 2333/0161 727 2191

The Royal Brompton Hospital
Prof. M. Hodson (adults)/Prof. D. Geddes
  (adults)/Dr. A. Bush (children)
Sydney Street
London SW3 6NP
Tel: 020 7352 8121 bleep 1006/
  020 7351 8182/020 7351 8232
Fax: 020 7352 8052/020 7351 8999/
  020 7351 8763

University Hospital Lewisham
Dr. C. Daman-Willems and Dr. J.
  Stroobant (children)
High Street
Lewisham
London SE13 6LH
Tel: 020 8333 3136
Fax: 020 8690 1963

Royal Victoria Infirmary
Dr. C. O'Brien (children)/Dr. D. Spencer
  (children)
Queen Victoria Road
Newcastle Upon Tyne NE1 4LP
Tel: 0191 232 5131,
  ext. 25089/0191 284 3111
Fax: 0191 201 0155/0191 213 2167

Barts and the Royal London Hospital–
 CF Unit
Dr. D. Empey (adults)/Dr. S. Carr (children)
Fielden House
Whitechapel
London E1 1BB
Tel: 020 7377 7605/020 7377 7462
Fax: 020 7377 7033/020 7377 7433

Wythenshawe Hospital
Dr. A. K. Webb (adults)
Southmoor Road
Manchester M23 9LT
Tel: 0161 291 2154
Fax: 0161 291 2080

Norfolk and Norwich Hospital
Dr. C. Upton (children)
Brunswick Road
Norwich
Norfolk NR1 3SR
Tel: 01603 287544
Fax: 01603 287584

King's Healthcare
King's College Hospital
Dr. G. Ruiz (children)/Prof. J. Price
 (children)
Denmark Hill
London SE5 9RS
Tel: 020 7346 3562,
 ext. 3431/020 7346 3215
Fax: 020 7346 4217/020 7346 3657

Manchester Children's Hospital NHS Trust
Dr. L. Patel (children)/Prof. T. David
 (children)
Booth Hall
Charlestown Road
Manchester M9 7AA
Tel: 0161 220 5093/0161 220 5093
Fax: 0161 795 7542/0161 795 7542

Nottingham City Hospital
Prof. A. Knox (adults)/Dr. A Smyth
 (children)
Hucknall Road
Nottingham NG5 1PB
Tel: 0115 840 4775/0115 969 1169,
 ext. 46475
Fax: 0115 840 4771/0115 962 0564

Oxford Radcliffe NHS Trust.
Dr. A Thomson (children)
John Radcliffe Hospital
Headington
Oxford OX3 9DU
Tel: 01865 221496
Fax: 01865 220479

Southampton University Hospital NHS
 Trust
Dr. M. Carroll (adults)/Dr. G. Connett
 (children)
Tremona Road
Southampton S016 6YD
Tel: 023 80796801/023 80794862
Fax: 023 80794762/023 80794750

Northern General Hospital
Dr. F Edenborough (adults)
Herries Road
Sheffield S5 7AU
Tel: 0114 271 4770
Fax: 0114 226 6280

Sheffield Children's Hospital Western Bank
Prof. C. Taylor (children)
Sheffield S10 2TH
Fax: 0114 275 5364

North Staffs City General Hospital
Dr. W. Lenney (children)/Dr. C. Campbell
 (children)
Newcastle Road
Stoke On Trent ST4 6QC
Tel: 01782 552572/01782 718392
Fax: 01782 713946/01782 710791

Royal Belfast Hospital for Sick Children
Dr. A. Redmond (children)
Falls Road
Belfast BT12 6BE
Fax: 028 90235340

Belfast City Hospital–Adult CF Unit
Dr. S. Elborn (adults)
Belfast BT9 7AB
Tel: 028 90 329241
Fax: 028 90263546 (326614)

Royal Aberdeen Children's Hospital
Dr. R. Brooker (children)
Cornhill Road
Aberdeen AB9 2ZG
 Fax: 01224 840727

Ninewells Hospital and Medical School
Dr. A. Mehta (children)/Prof. R. Olver
  (children)
Dundee DD1 9SY
Tel: 01382 632179/01382 632179
Fax: 01382 632597/01382 632597

Western General Hospital
Dr. A. Innes (adults)/Dr. A. Greening
  (adults)
Crewe Road
Edinburgh EH4 2XU
Tel: 0131 537 1783
Fax: 0131 343 3989

Royal Hospital for Sick Children
Dr. T. Marshall (children)
Sciennes Road
Edinburgh EH9 1LF
Tel: 0131 536 0000
Fax: 0131 536 0171

Royal Hospital for Sick Children
Dr. N. Gibson (children)/Dr. J. Paton
  (children)/Dr. J. Evans (children)
Yorkhill
Glasgow G3 8SJ.
Tel: 0141 201 0035/0141 201 0035/
  0141 201 0314
Fax: 0141 201 0671 (for all)

Gartnavel General Hospital
Dr. B. Stack (adults)
Great Western Road 1053
Glasgow G12 0YN
Tel: 0141 211 3247
Fax: 0141 211 3464

University Hospital of Wales
Dr. I. Doull (children)
Heath Park
Cardiff CF14 4XW
Tel: 02920 743530
Fax: 02920 743587

Llandough Hospital Penarth
Prof. D. Shale (adults)/Dr. I. Campbell
  (adults)
Cardiff CF6 1XX
Tel: 02920 716947/02920 715417
Fax: 02920 712284/02920 350056

Royal Gwent Hospital Newport
Dr. I. Bowler (children)/Dr. S. Maguire
  (children)
Gwent NP9 2UB
Tel: 01633 234613X/01633 238965
Fax: 01633 234788 (243788)/01633
234920

Subject Index

Note: Page numbers followed by f indicate figures; those followed by t indicate tables.